MW00837726

BIOSECURITY IN ANIMAL PRODUCTION AND VETERINARY MEDICINE

Biosecurity

in animal production and veterinary medicine

From principles to practice

Edited by **Jeroen Dewulf** and **Filip Van Immerseel**

Acco Leuven / Den Haag

First print: 2018

Published by
Uitgeverij Acco, Blijde Inkomststraat 22, 3000 Leuven, België
E-mail: uitgeverij@acco.be – Website: www.acco.be

For The Netherlands:
Acco Nederland, Westvlietweg 67 F, 2495 AA Den Haag, Nederland
E-mail: info@uitgeverijacco.nl

Cover design: Frisco-ontwerpbureau
Book layout: Karakters

© 2018 by Acco (Academische Coöperatieve Vennootschap cvba),
Leuven (België)

No part of this book may be reproduced in any form, by mimeograph,
film or any other means without permission in writing from the publisher.

D/2017/0543/407   NUR 840   ISBN 978-94-6344-378-4

Contributors

Preface

CONTRIBUTORS

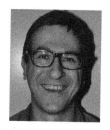

Prof. Dr. Filip Van Immerseel is professor at the Department of Pathology, Bacteriology and Avian Diseases at the Faculty of Veterinary Medicine of Ghent University in Belgium. Being a scientist with a research group on host-bacterium interactions in animals, he has specific interest in prophylaxis of infectious diseases. His group focusses on intestinal health and diseases in production animals and is involved in a variety of research projects on alternatives to antibiotics. He is lecturer of Biosecurity and Hygiene for veterinary students.

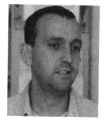

Prof. Dr. Jeroen Dewulf is professor in Veterinary Epidemiology at the Faculty of Veterinary Medicine of Ghent University in Belgium. His main research interests are quantitative epidemiology and control of zoonoses with a specific emphasis on antimicrobial use and resistance animals, as well as the prevention of epidemic and endemic diseases with a focus on the application of biosecurity measures. He is the main developer of the Biocheck.ugent risk based biosecurity scoring system which has been used in over 5000 farms in more than 30 countries around the world.

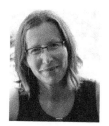

Associate Professor Magdalena Dunowska (DVM, PhD) is an Infectious Disease Group leader at the Institute of Veterinary, Animal and Biomedical Sciences at Massey University (IVABS), New Zealand. Her research interests include viral diseases of veterinary and public health importance. In addition to teaching virology and biosecurity to veterinary students, Dr. Dunowska also chairs IVABS Infection Control committee, and has extensive practical experience in implementation of infection control measures and biosecurity related research gained during 4 years of employment as an Infection Control officer at the Veterinary Teaching Hospital at Colorado State University, USA.

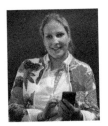

Dr. Merel Postma is postdoctoral researcher at the Veterinary Epidemiology Unit of the Faculty of Veterinary Medicine of Ghent University in Belgium and innovation manager at Livar BV in the Netherlands. Her main research interests are the application of biosecurity and herd health optimization measures in pig production in relation to a reduction of antimicrobial usage. She is furthermore interested in veterinary epidemiology and is a diplomate of the European College of Veterinary Public Health.

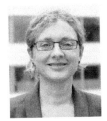

Prof. Dr. Katharina Stärk is professor in Veterinary Public Health Policy at the Royal Veterinary College, London. She also is Director Science & Quality at SAFOSO AG, a private consultancy company based in Bern, Switzerland. Katharina's work focuses on public health risks linked to animal-derived foods using risk analysis frameworks. In this context, she has worked and published on antibiotic resistance for more than a decade.

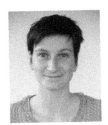

Dr. Lucie Collineau is a junior consultant at SAFOSO AG in Bern, Switzerland. Her main background is in veterinary epidemiology and food safety. She completed a PhD on the reduction of antimicrobial usage in pig production, with a focus on the socio-economic aspects of implementing alternative measures to antimicrobials. Her main research interests relate to the risk analysis and risk management of antimicrobial resistance along the food chain.

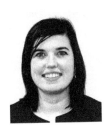

Bo Vanbeselaere is working as veterinarian at CID LINES NV in Ieper, Belgium. She gives technical support for the pig and poultry industry with a special focus on biosecurity and antimicrobial resistance. In collaboration with the Veterinary Epidemiology unit of the Faculty of Veterinary Medicine of Ghent University, she is also working on the Biocheck.UGent, a risk-based scoring system to evaluate the quality of the on-farm biosecurity.

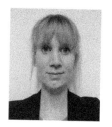

Dr. Kaat Luyckx completed her PhD degree at the Faculty of Veterinary Medicine of Ghent University in Belgium. Her work focused on the evaluation and impliciation of internal biosecurity, more specifically on cleaning and disinfection on broiler and pig farms as it is of high importance for the prevention of diseases.

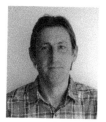

Dr. Koen De Reu is senior researcher and food microbiologist at the Institute for Agricultural, Fisheries and Food Research (ILVO) in Melle, Belgium. His research group works in the broad field of microbiological quality and safety in the entire agro-food chain. Special attention is given to microbiology in the poultry chain, shigatoxin producing E. coli, cleaning, disinfection and biofilms in the agro-food chain, biocide and antibiotic resistance.

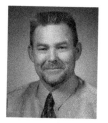

Steven J. Hoff, PhD, PE is a professor of agricultural and Biosystems engineering at Iowa State University. Dr. Hoff's expertise is in the areas of animal housing ventilation design, sensor development, and control system logic development. Dr. Hoff has focused his career on developing methods to better characterize the housed thermal environment for efficient animal production systems. Dr. Hoff has been at Iowa State University since 1990, with a balance of duties between undergraduate and graduate education and research. Dr. Hoff has five patents and numerous patent disclosures, all related to animal housing ventilation systems.

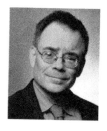

Dr. Steven C. Ricke is the Donald Wray Endowed Chair in Food Safety and Director-Center for Food Safety at the University of Arkansas. He is also a faculty member of the Dept. of Food Science, and the Cellular and Molecular Graduate program. Dr. Ricke's research program is primarily focused on virulence and pathogenic characteristics of foodborne pathogens. Dr. Ricke's research projects have emphasized studies on the growth, survival and pathogenesis of foodborne pathogens under conditions encountered during food animal production and processing.

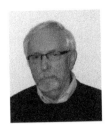

Dr. Olkowski is a research scientist with a wide-ranging interest in biomedical sciences. His research interest is centered on the patho-physiology of health problems in farm animals. He has been the lead investigator on several projects of major economic significance related to health problems in ruminants and poultry. His research interests also include drinking water physiology and metabolism, water hygiene, and metabolic and health effects of drinking water contaminants.

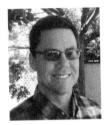

Dr. Alec Gerry is a Professor of Veterinary Entomology in the Department of Entomology at the University of California at Riverside. His research interests focus on the biology and management of arthropod pests of animals, with particular emphasis on control of filth flies and the role of biting flies in the transmission of animal pathogens. He teaches courses in Medical and Veterinary Entomology and in Forensic Entomology.

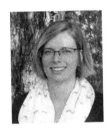

Dr. Amy Murillo is a post-doctoral researcher in the Department of Entomology at the University of California at Riverside where she is currently conducting research to examine impacts of poultry ectoparasites on animal welfare. Her main research interests are developing novel strategies for control of poultry pests and understanding host-parasite interactions.

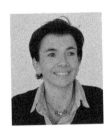

Trees Loncke graduated in 1998 as Veterinarian from the faculty of Veterinary Medicine from Ghent University. She works as CEO of AGROLOGIC, a Belgian company specialized in providing advice on hygiene products for intensive animal production. In 2006 she also founded ALPHATAC a service company specialized in pest control in animal production.

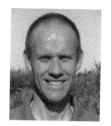 **Prof. Dominiek Maes** is full professor and head of the Unit of Porcine Health Management at the Faculty of Veterinary Medicine at Ghent University Belgium. He is a specialist of the European College of Porcine Health Management. His main research areas include swine reproduction and infectious (mainly respiratory) and non-infectious pig diseases. He has published over 260 papers in international peer-reviewed journals. He is past president of IPVS Belgian branch, the European College of Porcine Health Management, the European Board of Veterinary Specialisation. He is section editor of Livestock Science, and editor in chief of the journal Porcine Health Management.

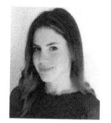 **Dr. Maria Eleni Filippitzi** is a research scientist based at the Veterinary Epidemiology Unit of the Faculty of Veterinary Medicine of Ghent University in Belgium. Her main research interests include the use of quantitative epidemiology methods and tools to prevent and control public health hazards with a focus on antimicrobial use and resistance, the prevention of pig diseases through the application of biosecurity measures and the economic and policy aspects of the One Health approach.

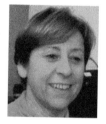 **Dr. Hilde Van Meirhaeghe** DVM, is working as Poultry Consultant for Vetworks, a group of poultry veterinarians giving technical support to the pharmaceutical industry and poultry integrations worldwide. She was involved in study projects on hygiene, food safety and health issues in partnership with the Faculty of Veterinary Medicine in Ghent. As Academic Adviser of the Faculty of Veterinary Medicine – University of Ghent and Course master WVEPAH poultry trainings, she is teaching students and poultry professionals on poultry health issues.

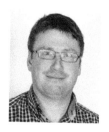 **Maarten De Gussem**, DVM is a poultry veterinarian, partner of Degudap in Belgium and founder of Vetworks, global poultry veterinary consultants for pharmaceutical industry and poultry integrations. He provides support on poultry health topics all over the world, with focus on mycoplasmosis, antibiotic free production, general gut health and coccidiosis. With Vetworks, he audits poultry operations, integrated and non-integrated, on all continents.

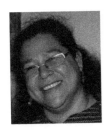

Dr. Véronique Renault is a veterinarian specialised in animal production in the tropics with a master degree in tropical animal health. She worked 15 years in developmental and humanitarian projects related to animal production and health in Africa. She presently works as assistant at the Faculty of Veterinary medicine of Liege in Belgium in Veterinary Epidemiology and Risk Analysis applied to veterinary sciences. Her main research area is on biosecurity in cattle production.

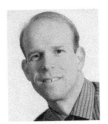

Prof. Weese is a veterinary internist with a focus on infectious diseases, infection control and antimicrobial resistance. He is a Professor at the University of Guelph, holds a Canada Research Chair in zoonotic diseases and is Chief of Infection Control at the Ontario Veterinary College Health Sciences Centre.

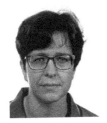

Prof. Dr. Hilde de Rooster is professor in Small Animal Soft Tissue Surgery at the Faculty of Veterinary Medicine of Ghent University in Belgium. She is Diplomate of the European College of Veterinary Surgery. Her main focus is clinical training students, interns, residents and postgraduates in the broad field of soft tissue surgery. Her main research interests are prepubertal gonadectomy, portosystemic shunting and translational oncology.

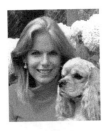

Eline Abma is a PhD student at the Small Animal Department at the Faculty of Veterinary Medicine of Ghent University in Belgium. She is currently investigating novel anticancer treatment modalities and beside a specific interest in canine oncology, she is also interested in canine well-being and epidemiology.

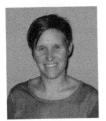

Eline Wydooghe is Diplomat of the European College of Animal Reproduction (ECAR) since 2015. She is working at the clinic of small animal reproduction at the Faculty of Veterinary Medicine of Ghent University in Belgium, where she treats dogs and cats dealing with infertility problems or need assisted reproduction. Furthermore she's doing research on in vitro fertilization of bovine embryos as a model for human.

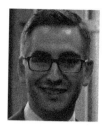

Dr. Steven Sarrazin is working as veterinarian at the Veterinary Epidemiology Unit at the Faculty of Veterinary Medicine of Ghent University in Belgium. His main research interests are quantitative epidemiology and applied statistical data analysis, with a specific emphasis on antimicrobial use in animal production, as well as the application of biosecurity measures in cattle production.

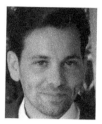

Pierre-Alexandre Dendoncker is a PhD student at Ghent University and Namur University. He is conducting a multidisciplinary research about the welfare, health and behaviour of canine puppies sold in Belgium. Being affiliated to the Epidemiology unit and the laboratory for Ethology of the Faculty of Veterinary Medicine of Ghent University, he has a specific interest in all aspects of the welfare of breeding dogs, including behaviour, husbandry, management and health.

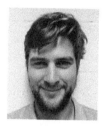

Bert Damiaans is a PhD-student in the Epidemiology Unit at the Faculty of Veterinary Medicine of Ghent University in Belgium. Before starting his PhD, he worked in a veterinary practice in France and Belgium for 4 years. He is involved in a research project on the application of biosecurity in cattle production in Belgium.

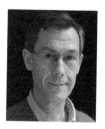

Prof. Dr. Claude Saegerman is full professor of the Liege University in Veterinary Epidemiology and Risk Analysis applied to veterinary sciences and in Biosecurity and good management veterinary practices. Current research is mainly conducted on the development of methods for early clinical detection and understanding dynamics of infection of emerging (vector-borne and/or zoonotic) diseases and rare events, also for prioritizing animal diseases based on an interdisciplinary approach and use of evidence-based medicine, and evaluation of disease control measures (including biosecurity and cost-benefit analysis).

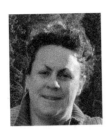 Dr Marie-France Humblet is in charge of biosecurity in the context of students' practical activities, at the Faculty of Veterinary Medicine, University of Liege, Belgium. Her main tasks consist in the assessment of biological risks, the update of Biosecurity SOPs, the elaboration of crisis scenarios and the implementation of biosecurity in the clinics/teaching labs. She implements internal audits to assess the respect of procedures and is also in charge of surveying antimicrobial resistance.

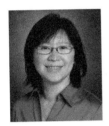 Dr. Patty H. Chen is an assistant professor and clinical veterinarian at Vanderbilt University Medical Center, Department of Pathology, Microbiology, and Immunology, Division of Comparative Medicine. She graduated from the US Army Laboratory Animal Medicine Residency Program in Walter Reed Army Institute of Research, and is a Diplomate of the American College of Laboratory Animal Medicine.

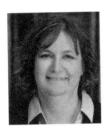 Robin Trundy is an Assistant Director of Vanderbilt Environmental Health & Safety and Institutional Biological Safety Officer for two Vanderbilt University entities. Ms. Trundy holds a Master's degree in Environmental Health Management from Oregon State University and is a certified biological safety professional (CBSP) with 20 years of biosafety experience in academic and contract research settings.

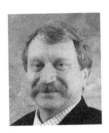 Dr. Scarfe is currently an Extraordinary Professor and the Director of the Center of Excellence for Aquatic Veterinary Education, Diagnostics and Biosecurity Training at the University of Pretoria, Faculty of Veterinary Science (Onderstepoort, S. Africa), and serves as the Associate Director of the International Aquatic Veterinary Biosecurity Consortium, within the Centre of Excellence for Aquatic Veterinary Biosecurity and Education at Ludwig-Maximilians-University (Munich, Germany). He also serves as CEO of Aquatic Veterinary Associates International, LLC (USA), a private veterinary practice that provides aquatic veterinary services to clients and industries

throughout the world, and is a USDA-APHIS Veterinary Medical Officer with the U.S. National Animal Health Response Corps to assist with responses to outbreaks of important foreign animal disease outbreaks in the U.S.

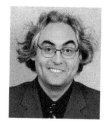

Prof. Dr. Dušan Palić is Chair of Fish Diseases and Fisheries Biology at the Faculty of Veterinary Medicine, Ludwig-Maximilians-University Munich, Germany, and also a Director of International Aquatic Veterinary Biosecurity Consortium. His main research interest is in aquatic animal disease prevention and control, with focus on increasing capacity of veterinary services and students in preparation of biosecurity plans and programs. Prof. Palić is a FAO-UN senior expert for aquatic animal health, and has participated in development of U.S. Department of Agriculture National Veterinary Accreditation Program aquatic animal modules during his tenure at the Iowa State College of Veterinary Medicine and Center for Food Security and Public Health in Ames, Iowa, USA.

Preface on biosecurity in animal production and veterinary medicine

Veterinary medicine is an interdisciplinary field, the goal of which is to minimise the impact of animal diseases through both prevention and treatment. In view of the growing issue of antimicrobial resistance, it has become more important than ever to not only focus on treating disease but also on maintaining the health of animals and avoiding the introduction or development of diseases. Biosecurity is defined in the OIE Terrestrial Animal Health Code as a set of management and physical measures designed to reduce the risk of introduction, establishment and spread of animal diseases, infections or infestations to, from and within an animal population. These preventive, non-medication-based measures are relevant for the maintenance of animal health, and by extension, of food production, food safety, and biodiversity.

Furthermore, the principles of biosecurity are necessary not just for limiting the spread of pathogens *between* animals, but also from animals to humans and from humans to animals. This integrated approach is well known as the 'One Health' concept, which recognises that human health is intrinsically linked to animal health and the environment. In accordance with this concept, biosecurity is a holistic concept, whereby disease prevention strategies applied to the protection of animal health also serves to preserve the environment and protect human health.

Since its creation in 1924, the World Organisation for Animal Health (OIE) has been actively engaged in the prevention and control of animal and zoonotic disease, particularly through the development of standards. As most emerging infectious diseases have the potential to cross national borders with significant inherent trade implications, international collaboration against biological risks is crucial. The OIE promotes transparency and a better understanding of the global animal disease situation by collecting, analysing and disseminating animal health information, strengthening international coordination and cooperation in the control of animal diseases and zoonoses, and ensuring the safety of international trade of animals and their products. The cornerstone of the successful implementation of biosecurity practices within the international community is the compliance of Member Countries with OIE standards and guidelines, which the OIE supports through training where necessary, and through making available appropriate tools and human resources, in particular for developing countries.

The OIE, National Veterinary Services and livestock producers will benefit from the comprehensive information included in the book 'Biosecurity in animal production and veterinary medicine', edited by Profs. Dewulf and Van Immerseel and co-authored by a wide range of international experts from different institutes and industries. It provides a compilation of both the fundamental aspects of biosecurity practices as well as specific and practical information on the application of biosecurity measures in different animal production and animal husbandry settings. In this book, readers will find explanations about the relevance of biosecurity planning for the improvement of animal health and production, as well as for reducing the need for the use of antimicrobials. Practical examples such as those on the implementation of biosecurity that is specially adapted to different animal species will facilitate awareness and motivation among farmers.

The book is a practical guide that can be used by farm and animal facility managers, consultants, veterinarians, animal caretakers, and people with an interest in the prevention of diseases in animals. Academics and students will also benefit from this comprehensive compilation on animal biosecurity. This book contains fundamental information that anyone involved in animal biosecurity should be aware of, and it will contribute to the prevention of diseases in animals and humans while preserving the environment.

Elisabeth Erlacher-Vindel,
Head of the Science and New Technologies Department, OIE

CHAPTER 1

CIRCLES OF DISEASE TRANSMISSION

Magdalena Dunowska

Institute of Veterinary, Animal and Biomedical Sciences
Massey University, University of New Zealand

1 Introduction

A variety of transmissible agents can cause disease in animals. These include viruses, bacteria, fungi and parasites. Within each of these main groups there are hundreds of potential pathogens with unique biological characteristics and life cycles. Our understanding of the causative relationships between infectious agents and disease has evolved over the years. While the canonical Koch's postulates presumed a simple direct relationship between a pathogen and disease, even Koch himself predicted the inadequacy of such an assumption in all situations (Fredericks & Relman, 1996). Today, we have a much better appreciation of the multifactorial nature of many diseases, and the complexity of events that determine not only the outcome of infection for each individual, but also the ability of pathogens to spread within populations. Understanding these complex interactions is necessary for the implementation of effective infection control programs.

New technologies have facilitated advanced molecular research and a sharp increase in our knowledge of the microbial world over the past 20-30 years. At the same time, rapid technological development has also created new challenges. The ever-increasing density of people has led to intensification of agriculture and change of land use through activities such as irrigation, deforestation or urbanisation. These changes have been accompanied by increased international travel, as well as increased international trade of animals and animal-derived products. The association between such anthropogenic activities and the emergence of diseases is fairly well recognised (Mackenzie & Jeggo, 2013). Human encroachment on wildlife habitats has created increased opportunities for cross-species transfer and potential for emergence of new zoonotic diseases, as we have seen with cases of Hendra virus in Australia, Nipah virus in Malaysia or severe acute respiratory syndrome (SARS) virus in China (Plowright et al., 2015). What once may have been confined to a few localised cases of disease now has a potential to spread throughout the world within days. As an example, about 8,000 cases and 900 deaths in 30 countries were traced back to a single SARS-infected person staying overnight at the Metropole hotel in Hong Kong (Mackenzie & Jeggo, 2013). In 2013-2016 we also witnessed an epidemic of Ebola virus infections in West Africa at the unprecedented scale compared to several previous geographically restricted outbreaks (Shultz, Espinel, Espinola, & Rechkemmer, 2016).

Transmission of infectious agents from one host to another is a complex and multi-step process that requires a number of conditions to be fulfilled. Understanding how the pathogens are maintained within individual hosts and within populations enables us to intervene in this process. In a sense, the old saying 'know your enemy' is as applicable to people as it is to microbes. The better we understand the 'offenders' and the methods they adopt in order to survive and perpetuate themselves, the better we are able to effectively target the most relevant stages in their transmission circles.

This chapter provides a short overview of the steps necessary for transmission of microscopic pathogens from one host to another. It is not meant to be a comprehensive review of the topic. Instead, it introduces some basic concept, with an emphasis on common principles that can be exploited for the purpose of infection control.

2 Common steps in transmission of infectious agents

It is important to consider all potential pathogens that may be encountered in a given situation when designing an effective infection control programme (Morley, 2002; Traub-Dargatz, Dargatz, Morley, & Dunowska, 2004). Many of these pathogens have unique biological properties and life cycles. While this needs to be taken into account, it is often practical to focus on commonalities, as opposed to differences. Route of transmission is one of such characteristics that is often shared by several infectious agents and can therefore be exploited in the design of control measures that are effective against a number of different pathogens. For example, the use of disinfectant foot mats or footbaths helps to minimise the spread of pathogens that transmit via the faecal-oral route (Dunowska, Morley, Patterson, Hyatt, & Van Metre, 2006). Similarly, the use of disposable gloves and/or appropriate hand hygiene is an effective control measure against pathogens that can be transmitted through fomites (Neo, Sagha-Zadeh, Vielemeyer, & Franklin, 2016). In contrast, neither hand hygiene nor disinfectant foot mats/footbaths would be particularly effective in controlling arboviral infections such as Bluetongue or African horse sickness. In order to prevent infections with these arboviruses, measures to control vector population (*Culicoides* midges) and to minimise contact between midges and susceptible animals would need to be implemented (Maclachlan & Mayo, 2013). These may include elimination of stagnant water (breeding environment for midges), application of insect repellents, use of screens in stables/barns, or keeping the animals indoors at times when the activity of midges is the greatest (dusk/dawn). Concurrently, minimising the density of susceptible animals, for example via vaccination, could also be implemented.

In general terms, most pathogens have to follow some common steps in order to spread and maintain themselves in populations. These include entry, replication and spread within the host (either locally or systemically), which may or may not be accompanied by disease, and exit to enable infection of the new host (Fig. 1.1). Each of these steps can be targeted by infection control strategies.

Fig. 1.1: Circle of disease transmission: Common steps in a transmission cycle of infectious pathogens and examples of actions that can facilitate breakage of the cycle.

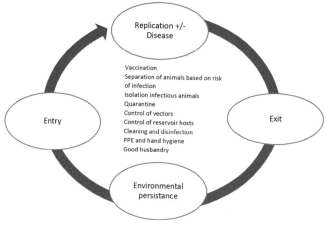

Table 1.1: Routes of entry

Respiratory Tract

Description	Occurs through inhalation of infectious agents.
Protective Mechanisms	Entrapment of pathogens in a blanket of mucous produced by Goblet cells; removal of pathogens by coordinated movement of cilia on epithelial cells; removal of pathogens by specific (secretory antibodies, mainly IgA) or non-specific (phagocytic cells such as neutrophils and macrophages) immunological defences (Antunes & Cohen, 2007; Baskerville, 1981; Fokkens & Scheeren, 2000).
Factors facilitating entry	Concurrent infections e.g. viral infections that destroy ciliary epithelium often predispose subjects to secondary bacterial infections (shipping fever complex); presence of infectious aerosols; poor ventilation combined with crowded environment.
Examples[1]	foot-and-mouth disease, infectious bovine rhinotracheitis, malignant catarrhal fever, anthrax, *Aspergillus* spp, Q fever, tuberculosis

Gastrointestinal Tract

Description	Transmission via ingestion of pathogens. Typically occurs via contamination of feed with faecal material or via contamination of pastures/water supply.
Protective Mechanisms	Peristaltic activity of intestines, low pH of the stomach, presence of digestive enzymes, bile, pancreatic secretions, presence of mucous in the stomach and intestines, specific (mainly IgA) and non-specific (e.g. defensins) immunological defences (Elson & Alexander, 2015)
Factors facilitating spread	Heavy environmental contamination with pathogens that survive outside of their hosts for a prolonged period of time; poor cleaning and disinfection; high density of animals.
Examples[1]	rotaviruses, coronaviruses, parvoviruses, morbilliviruses, bacteria e.g. *Salmonella* or *Campylobacter* species, *Brucella* species, tuberculosis, anthrax, many internal parasites such as coccidia *(e.g. Eimeria* or *Cryptosporidium* species)* or *Giardia* species.

Skin

Description	Pathogens enter the body through the skin barrier.

Protective Mechanisms	Intact skin with a thick layer of cornified epithelium provides an effective barrier against infections with many pathogens. Hence, a break in the integrity of the skin is often necessary for a pathogen to gain an entry via this route, although some pathogens are able to enter through intact skin e.g. hookworms or some fungi (e.g. dermatophytes).
Factors facilitating entry	Presence of skin abrasions, wounds, animal bites, insect bites, etc. Conditions that facilitate trauma (could be minor) to the skin such as presence of abrasive plants on pasture (e.g. thistles), shearing of sheep, or increased activity of biting insects. Use of contaminated needles or surgical equipment.
Examples[1]	arboviruses (e.g. West Nile virus, Bluetongue), or virus and other parapoxviruses, equine infectious anaemia virus, bacteria in contaminated wounds, fungi (e.g. dermatophytes), some parasites (e.g. hookworms of various species)

Reproductive Tract

Description	Sexually transmitted diseases. Transmission can occur through natural mating or via artificial insemination.
Protective Mechanisms	Presence of mucous, innate and acquired immune responses, resident bacterial microbiota (Lepargneur, 2016; Pudney, Quayle, & Anderson, 2005; Tribe, 2015; Wiesenfeld et al., 2002)
Factors facilitating spread	Artificial insemination provides an excellent way of quickly spreading contaminated semen across large geographical areas.
Examples[1]	equine arteritis virus, bovine viral diarrhoea virus, *Trichomonas fetus*, *Brucella* species, *Taylorella equigenitalis* (causative agent of contagious equine metritis)

Others

Description and Examples	Other routes of entry include conjunctiva (e.g. Moraxella bovis – a causative agent for 'pink eye' conjunctivitis in cattle) or placenta (e.g. equid herpesvirus 1, bovine viral diarrhoea virus, porcine parvoviruses).

[1] For more examples see: Diseases and Resources by species available at http://www.cfsph.iastate.edu/

2.1 Entry

Entry of the pathogen can occur via a variety of routes (Table 1.1). Respiratory and gastrointestinal tracts are the most common routes of entry for pathogenic micro-organisms. Some pathogens use one predominant route of entry, while others may use a number of different routes. For example, bovine viral diarrhoea (BVD) virus can enter a new host via a respiratory route (droplet transmission), a venereal route either by natural service or through contaminated equipment used for artificial insemination (fomites). It can also establish infection in a foetus via a transplacental route of entry (Lanyon, Hill, Reichel, & Brownlie, 2014).

2.2 Incubation period

Incubation period is defined as a period between the time of infection (entry) and the development of clinical signs of disease. The length of the incubation period may vary from hours (e.g. rotavirus, influenza viruses), days (e.g. foot-and-mouth disease (FMD) virus) to months (e.g. rabies virus) or even years (e.g. ovine progressive pneumonia lentivirus). The period of infectivity defines a period of time during which the animal is infectious to others. It coincides with shedding of infectious pathogens via various routes (exit). Shedding can start at any point in the infection cycle (Fig. 1.2). For example, clinical signs of Maedi-Visna/ovine progressive pneumonia develop years after primary infection with the causative lentivirus (Perez et al., 2013). Throughout this long incubation period, infected animals can transmit the virus to other susceptible animals. In contrast, the incubation period for FMD is short (1-8 days). None-the-less, shedding of FMD virus may also start before infected animals develop the clinical disease (Alexandersen, Quan, Murphy, Knight, & Zhang, 2003) and the virus may be already widespread by the time infected animals are identified and isolated or destroyed.

The length of the incubation period is important for the development of quarantine guidelines. Animals should be quarantined for a period of time that exceeds the maximum incubation period of the pathogen in question. Knowledge about the length of the incubation period is also useful for back-tracking animals that have been potentially exposed to the infected individuals.

Fig. 1.2: Shedding of a pathogen may start after (A) or before (B) development of clinical signs. Some infected animals may shed the pathogen without any overt clinical disease (C). Pathogens that are shed during the incubation period are more difficult to control than those that are shed only after clinical signs of disease are apparent.

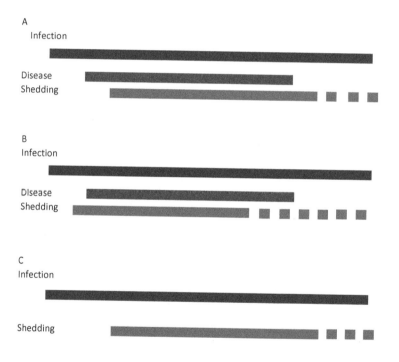

2.3 Spread within the body

Pathogens may remain at the site of entry and cause localised infections, or may use the initial site of entry as a portal for subsequent systemic dissemination throughout the body. Examples of the former include scabby mouth disease in ruminants caused by a parapox virus infection (Buttner & Rziha, 2002), infected wounds, gastrointestinal infections caused by a variety of viral, bacterial and fungal pathogens (Foster & Smith, 2009) or localised upper respiratory tract infections. Systemic spread from the site of entry may occur via the lymphatics, blood vessels or nerves. Following dissemination of pathogens to various tissues, secondary replication in those tissues may lead to generalised systemic disease. The clinical signs observed are dependent on the organ/tissue predilection of the pathogen and on the extent of tissue damage caused by the infection.

2.4 Disease

The severity of disease observed following infection with pathogens varies. It is important to recognise that infection is not synonymous with disease. Diseased animals typically represent the 'tip of the iceberg' of all infected animals (Fig. 1.3). They are reasonably easily recognised by skilled observers such as veterinarians, astute owners, farmers, etc., and should be placed under appropriate containment to prevent transmission of infectious agents to other susceptible hosts (either animals or people). In contrast, sub-clinically infected animals are difficult to recognise. They appear clinically normal, and can be identified only through targeted use of appropriate diagnostic tests. Not surprisingly, sub-clinically infected animals often play an important role in the spread of infectious agents and have been implicated in the introduction of pathogens to new geographical areas or disease-free herds (e.g. introduction of FMD to Europe (Sutmoller & Casas, 2002), equine arteritis virus to New Zealand (Horner, 2004), or equine influenza virus to Australia (Watson, Daniels, Kirkland, Carroll, & Jeggo, 2011)).

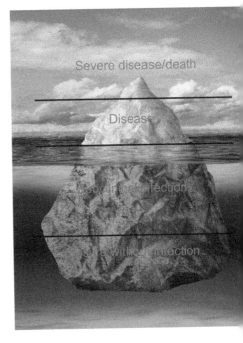

▲

Fig. 1.3: The iceberg concept of the maintenance of pathogens in populations. Only a proportion of animals exposed to an infectious agent become infected. Of those, many develop sub-clinical infections and only some become clinically sick. Severely diseased animals are those most noticeable, but they typically form the 'tip of an iceberg' of all infected animals. Sub-clinically infected animals are difficult to recognise without targeted surveillance. Therefore, they are important sources of infection for other susceptible animals and play a key role in maintaining infectious agents in populations.

2.5 Exit

Pathogens must exit their host in order to initiate infection in a new host. The route of exit is, therefore, inherently linked to the route of entry for many infectious agents. Some pathogens use predominantly, or exclusively, one route of exit. This is particularly true for pathogens that establish localised infections without the systemic spread. Examples include local respiratory tract infections (exit via respiratory secretions), local gastrointestinal tract infections (exit via faeces), or local skin infections (exit via skin). Other pathogens can use several different routes of exit. Pathogens able to cause systemic infections are often shed in various body excretions and secretions. For example, equine arteritis virus (EAV) may be isolated from a variety of tissues and body fluids following infection via a respiratory route (Balasuriya, Go, & MacLachlan, 2013) and classical swine fever virus has been detected in oronasal secretions, conjunctival secretions, urine, faces, semen, and blood from infected pigs (Althouse & Rossow, 2011; E. Weesendorp, A. Stegeman, & W. Loeffen, 2009).

Some pathogens are not shed in secretions/excretions, even though they may still cause disease in the infected animals. Whether or not such pathogens can be transmitted further varies. For example, many vector-borne infections (e.g. West Nile virus or Bluetongue virus) enlist the help of a blood-sucking insect to 'exit' the host through skin. This is also true for Eastern equine encephalitis (EEE) virus when it circulates between mosquitoes and its natural avian hosts. When horses (or people) are bitten by an infected mosquito, they may 'accidentally' become infected with the virus and may develop a neurological disease. However, despite severe clinical signs, the level of viraemia in the horse is usually too low to allow infection by mosquitoes and further transmission of the virus. As such, infected horses are 'dead-end' hosts for EEE – the virus dies together with its aberrant host (Molaei, Armstrong, Graham, Kramer, & Andreadis, 2015).

Pathogenic parasites of th e *Trichinella* species provide an example of yet another way in which infection can be perpetuated in the population in the absence of shedding. This parasitic disease is transmitted via consumption of undercooked meat (common route of infection for people) or carcasses (common route of infection for predatory animals) that contain infectious *Trichinella* cysts (Pozio, 2015).

3 Pathways of pathogen transmission

Traditionally, the transmission of infectious agents has been broken down into three main routes: 1) airborne 2) droplet and 3) contact, each of which requires different infection-control precautions in hospital settings (Siegel, Rhinehart, Jackson, & Committee, 2007). Although these were originally created with human health care settings in mind, the same principles are also applicable to the veterinary field.

3.1 Main routes

3.1.1 Airborne

Conventionally, all respiratory infections were considered to be transmitted via the airborne route. However, to be truly airborne, the infectious agent needs to be dispersed in suspensions of small particles in the air, referred to as infectious aerosols (Fernstrom & Goldblatt, 2013; Gralton, Tovey, McLaws, & Rawlinson, 2011; Seto, 2015). Infectious aerosols are created when pathogens are dispersed in particles smaller than 5 µm, as the particle's settling time is influenced by its size: smaller particles remain suspended in the air for longer periods of time than the larger ones (Gralton et al., 2011; Seto, 2015). Coincidentally, particles within similar size range can be inhaled directly into the lungs, while particles larger than 10 µm are trapped in the mucous of the upper airways and removed by the cilliary action of the respiratory epithelium (Tellier, 2006). Thus, disease transmission is most likely when infectious particles smaller than 10 µm are generated (Gralton et al., 2011; Jones & Brosseau, 2015).

In order to guarantee successful airborne transmission, the pathogen needs not only to be aerosolised, but also to remain infectious in the aerosolised form for a period of time, within which it needs to gain access to the appropriate tissues of the susceptible host(s) (Gralton et al., 2011; Jones & Brosseau, 2015). It is not common for all three conditions to be met. In fact, only three human diseases are currently classified as predominantly airborne: tuberculosis, chicken pox and measles (Seto, 2015). While the ability of other respiratory pathogens to become airborne has been documented (Goyal et al., 2011; Myatt et al., 2004), there is a lack of agreement on the importance of these findings with relation to the likelihood of effective airborne transmission (Jones & Brosseau, 2015). Comparatively few studies looked at the airborne potential of veterinary pathogens, with FMD being a classic example of a veterinary disease with proven airborne transmission (Colenutt et al., 2016; J. Gloster et al., 2009; J. Gloster et al., 2007; Schley, Burgin, & Gloster, 2009). Other economically important veterinary pathogens for which airborne transmission has been documented include porcine respiratory and reproductive syndrome virus and *M. hyopneumoniae* (Alonso, Raynor, Davies, & Torremorell, 2015; Cutler, Wang, Hoff, Kittawornrat, & Zimmerman, 2011; Cutler, Wang, Hoff, & Zimmerman, 2012; Dee, Otake, Oliveira, & Deen, 2009; Otake, Dee, Corzo, Oliveira, & Deen, 2010), classical swine fever virus (Weesendorp, Backer, & Loeffen, 2014; Weesendorp, Stegeman, & Loeffen, 2009), *Rhodococcus equi* (Muscatello et al., 2006) or African swine fever virus (de Carvalho Ferreira, Weesendorp, Quak, Stegeman, & Loeffen, 2013). The importance of airborne transmission of mammalian influenza viruses remains somewhat undetermined (Alonso et al., 2015; Goyal et al., 2011; Jones & Brosseau, 2015; Seto, 2015).

Aerosolised particles containing infectious agents may be dispersed by air currents over considerable distances. For example, transmission of FMD virus has been documented to occur, under suitable conditions, over more than 200 km (Donaldson & Alexandersen, 2002; Gloster et al., 2010). Proximity between infected and susceptible individuals therefore is not an essential condition for infection to occur (Fig. 1.4). This is an important difference between droplet (see below) and true airborne transmission, which makes the latter more difficult to control.

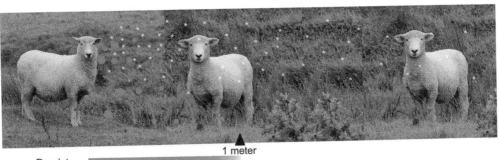

1 meter

Droplet

Airborne

▲

Fig. 1.4: An infected animal generates infectious particles of various sizes. The larger ones (droplets, red circles) settle quickly within approximately 1 metre of the animal. If another susceptible animal is present within that distance, the infectious droplets may fall onto its mucosal surfaces and initiate the infection. Particles smaller than 5 μm in size (infectious aerosol, yellow stars) remain suspended in the air for long periods of time – they may be carried by air currents over considerable distances and be a source of infection to animals at distant locations.

Pathogens present in respiratory secretions may be aerosolised not only through coughing or sneezing, but also through normal breathing (Christensen et al., 2011; Nicas, Nazaroff, & Hubbard, 2005). Infectious aerosol may also be generated from other contaminated sources such as faecal material, dust, or animal bedding during a number of everyday farming activities (Blais Lecours, Veillette, Marsolais, & Duchaine, 2012; Millner, 2009) including the application of animal manure to agricultural land (Jahne, Rogers, Holsen, Grimberg, & Ramler, 2015; Jahne et al., 2016). Hence, pathogens that are shed from sites of the body other than respiratory tract (e.g. faeces) may be accidently aerosolised, which in turn may enable their transmission via the atypical (or opportunistic) route. In this scenario, infection may be initiated when aerosolised gastrointestinal pathogens are deposited on mucosal surfaces of susceptible individuals and subsequently swallowed (Dungan, 2010). To illustrate this concept, porcine epidemic diarrhoea virus has been shown to be present in aerosols around infected animals (Alonso et al., 2015). It has also been proposed that airborne transmission may have contributed to the recent spread of porcine epidemic diarrhoea virus in the USA based on a positive correlation between the spread of disease and the predominant wind direction (Beam et al., 2015). However, as other variables such as the level of physical contact between farms were not available, the authors cautioned against drawing definitive conclusions from the study.

3.1.2 Droplet

Droplet transmission is a common route of transmission of many respiratory pathogens. It occurs via particles that are larger than 5 µm in size. Just like rain drops, such large 'droplets' fall to the ground within a short period of time (Fernstrom & Goldblatt, 2013; Gralton et al., 2011). If a susceptible animal is within a short distance of the source of infectious droplets (e.g. an infectious animal), then the droplets may settle on the susceptible animal's mucosal surfaces, potentially leading to infection (Fig. 1.4). In the case of human infections, the approximate distance within which droplet transmission is likely to occur has been defined as 1 metre (Gralton et al., 2011). While the velocity of particles generated by animals during sneezing or coughing may differ somewhat to that of particles generated by humans, droplet transmission relies on close proximity between the infected animal and a susceptible host, but without the necessity for direct contact between the two.

The separation between airborne and droplet transmission routes is somewhat artificial and considerable overlap exists between these two routes. Many activities generate infectious particles over a broad size range (Gralton et al., 2011). Thus, both infectious aerosols and droplets contribute to the transmission of disease a short distance from the source of infection. At a greater distance (beyond approximately 1 metre), droplet transmission is less likely and airborne transmission becomes more important.

Settled infectious droplets may also be transmitted via fomites such as people's hands, shoes, equipment, etc. The importance of the latter relies on the level of hygiene maintained at premises and on the environmental stability of the pathogen of interest (see indirect contact transmission below).

3.1.3 Contact

Contact transmission results from either direct or indirect contact between infectious and susceptible individuals. Close contact between infected and susceptible individuals (direct transmission, Fig. 1.5) is a pre-requisite for transmission of pathogens that do not survive well outside their hosts (e.g. mammalian influenza viruses, emerging paramyxoviruses Hendra and Nipah). The level of direct contact required for transmission of various pathogens varies and depends on the infectious dose of the pathogen in question, the levels of the pathogen shed by the infected animals, and its typical route of entry.

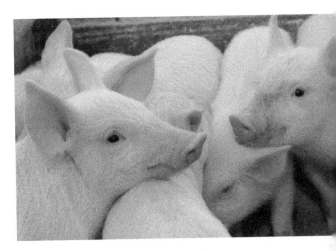

▲
Fig. 1.5: Many pathogens are transmitted by direct contact between infected and susceptible animals. Intensive production systems with high density of animals facilitate such transmission.

Environmental contamination and transmission via fomites (indirect transmission) are important for pathogens that are resistant to adverse environmental conditions. Many gastrointestinal infections are caused by agents that can survive harsh conditions encountered in the gastro-intestinal tract, such as low pH of the stomach or enzymatic action of digestive enzymes. These pathogens can also survive well on inanimate surfaces, sometimes for weeks to months (Kramer, Schwebke, & Kampf, 2006). Examples include rotaviruses, parvoviruses, caliciviruses, enteroviruses, *Salmonella* spp, *Cryptosporidium parvum* and others. Pathogens that show stability under diverse conditions are also often more difficult to disinfect, increasing the likelihood of environmental contamination, particularly in hospital settings. Occasional persistence of *Salmonella* spp in large animal stalls at a veterinary teaching hospital despite rigorous disinfection protocol may serve as an illustration of this point (Dunowska et al., 2007).

3.2 Descriptive terms

From a practical point of view, transmission patterns of infectious agents are often referred to in more descriptive terms, which take into account not only the main route of transmission (one of the three listed above) but also the main source of the infectious agent. The latter is often linked to the main route of exit or the preferred ecological environment for the pathogen in question. We'll discuss 7 commonly used terms.

3.2.1 Faecal-oral transmission

The gastrointestinal tract provides a very efficient route of exit and subsequent spread for many pathogens, particularly if infection is associated with diarrhoea. Voluminous, watery diarrhoea is very difficult to contain, clean and disinfect (Fig. 1.6). The pathogen load in diarrheic faeces can be very high. Watery, diarrheic faeces provide a perfect vehicle for environmental contamination, which facilitates transmission by fomites. Local gastrointestinal infections that manifest themselves as diarrhoea may alter the permeability of the gastrointestinal tract and allow commensal and pathogenic intestinal flora to gain entry into the bloodstream, which negatively impacts the severity of disease and prognosis. In one study (Johns et al., 2009) bacteria were isolated from blood collected from 9 out of 31 mature horses with diarrhoea within 24 hours of admission to the hospital. Horses with bacteraemia were less likely to survive compared to horses with negative blood cultures.

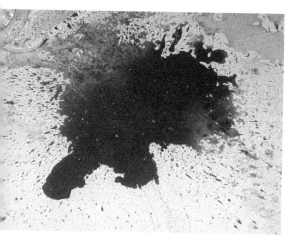

▲
Fig. 1.6: Watery, diarrhoeic faeces often contain a high pathogen load and provide an excellent vehicle for contamination of the environment.

3.2.2 Transmission by fomites

Fomites are inanimate objects that, once contaminated with pathogens, serve as a source of infection in susceptible animals (Fig. 1.7). Examples of fomites include peoples' clothing, boots, vehicles, animal crates, or general farm equipment. To illustrate the importance of this route of transmission, flexible intermediate bulk containers ('feed totes') used for transport of bulk feed were considered to be one of the likely sources of entry of porcine epidemic diarrhoea virus into the United States in 2013 and the subsequent spread of the virus throughout the country (Scott et al., 2016). Permanent structures such as water troughs, fences, gates etc. may also serve as fomites, as may any surface commonly touched by hands including computer keyboards, light switches, phones etc. For example, *Salmonella* species were commonly isolated from hand-contact surfaces in a veterinary teaching hospital whenever a *Salmonella*-shedding animal was hospitalised (Burgess, Morley, & Hyatt, 2004). Transmission via fomites is more likely for pathogens that remain infectious for long periods of time under various environmental conditions than for those that only survive for a short period of time under a narrow range of conditions.

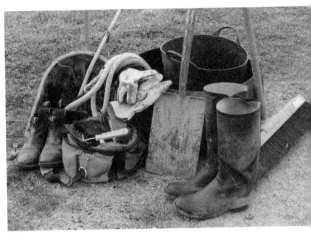

▲

Fig. 1.7: Inanimate objects can become contaminated with pathogens and serve as fomites in indirect contact transmission. Common fomites include footwear, equipment used with animals, contaminated hands, clothing, vehicles, etc.

3.2.3 Vector-borne transmission

This route of transmission relies on the transmission of pathogens from one host to another via vectors. Common vectors include various species of mosquitoes, midges, flies or ticks (Fig. 1.8). The lifecycle of some pathogens involve infection of the vector itself. Examples of such transmissions, referred to as 'biological', include West Nile virus (transmitted by mosquitoes), African horse sickness and Bluetongue viruses (both transmitted by culicoides midges), African swine fever, bovine anaplasmosis, or bovine theileriosis (all three transmitted by ticks). Animals affected by vector-borne diseases are often (but not always) not directly infectious for in-contact susceptible animals, and control of arthropod population is the mainstream for control of the spread of those infections.

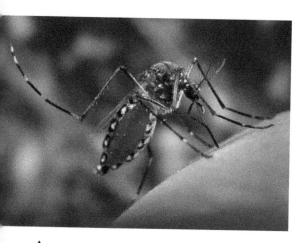

Fig. 1.8: Many diseases are transmitted by arthropod vectors either biologically (the pathogen replicates within the vector) or mechanically.

Other pathogens are transmitted in a purely mechanical manner e.g. equine infectious anaemia is typically transmitted through direct transfer of contaminated blood on the mouth of a biting fly. This is most likely to occur if feeding on an infected horse is interrupted and the fly continues its meal on a nearby uninfected horse. Similarly, *Moraxella bovis* (causative agent for infectious bovine keratoconjunctivitis) is predominantly transmitted within a group of animals via face flies (Kopecky, Pugh, & McDonald, 1986).

The ecology of vector-borne diseases is often complex and influenced by factors such as density of vectors (which is affected by environmental and climatic condition supportive of vector breeding and survival), feeding preference of vectors, or density of susceptible hosts (Marini, Rosa, Pugliese, & Heesterbeek, 2017).

3.2.4 Water-borne transmission

This term refers to indirect transmission via pathogen-contaminated water (Fig. 1.9). This can occur through drinking, but also through other activities such as swimming or using contaminated water for rinsing. Examples of water-borne pathogens include protozoa from *Cryptosporidium*, *Giardia* and *Toxoplasma* species (Dubey, 2004; Moss, 2016), bacteria from *Salmonella*, *Campylobacter*, *E. coli, Pseudomonas* or *Leptospira* species (Aho, Kurki, Rautelin, & Kosunen, 1989; Bayram et al., 2011; Leclerc, Schwartzbrod, & Dei-Cas, 2002; Monahan, Miller, & Nally, 2009; Mughini-Gras et al., 2016; Nohra et al., 2016; Tambalo, Boa, Aryal, & Yost, 2016) and viruses such as avian influenza (Fourment & Holmes, 2015) or noroviruses (Zhou et al., 2016). Although water-borne transmission has been mainly described in relation to epidemics of gastrointestinal disease in people, it can also contribute to the spread of pathogens in veterinary settings. For example, absence of a body of water within 0.5 km of the farm was identified as one of the factors associated with a reduction in the odds of a flock being infected with *Campylobacter species* on Irish low-performance chicken farms (Smith et al., 2016). Infections of sea mammals with parasites typically associated with land animals such as *Toxoplasma gondii, Sarcocystis neurona* or *Neospora caninum* are thought to be a result of contamination of the oceans with water run-offs from land (Dubey et al., 2003; Miller et al., 2002). Of most concern to human health is contamination of drinking water with unfiltered surface water containing faecal pathogens from various wild and farm animals (Ashbolt, 2015; Bowman, 2009; Kuhn et al., 2017; Mughini-Gras et al., 2016; Nohra et al., 2016). It should be noted, however, that the presence of specific pathogens in water supply does not always indicate cross-species

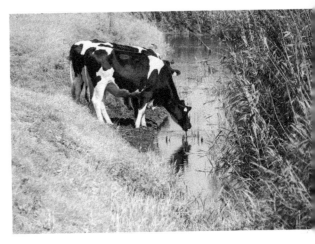

▲
Fig. 1.9: Contamination of drinking water is an efficient way of spreading infections amongst animals that use the same water source. Contaminated water supply has also been linked to epidemics of human gastrointestinal disease.
———

transmission. In one study, no evidence for significant transmission of *Giardia spp* between cattle and people was found despite contamination of water supply with bacterial species present in both human and cattle populations examined (Ehsan et al., 2015). As the quality of water treatment plays a role in preventing water-borne transmission of infectious pathogens, it is not surprising that water-borne diseases in humans are most prevalent in countries with low socio-economic status (Yang et al., 2012).

3.2.5 Sexual transmission

Sexual transmission refers to transmission of pathogens that are shed in reproductive secretions. This may occur during natural mating, but also during artificial reproductive procedures (Lockhart, Thrall, & Antonovics, 1996). Examples include EAV (Balasuriya et al., 2013), *Mycoplasma agalactiae* (causative agent for ovine contagious agalactia) (Prats-van der Ham et al., 2017), BVD virus (Givens & Waldrop, 2004; Grooms, 2004), trichomoniasis (Michi, Favetto, Kastelic, & Cobo, 2016) and others. Pathogens may be transported in contaminated semen over large geographical distances. As an example, EAV was introduced to New Zealand in imported equine semen and subsequently spread throughout the country (Horner, 2004). Introduction of a voluntary control scheme focused on prevention of sexual transmission of the virus eventually lead to the eradication of EAV from New Zealand (McFadden et al., 2013).

3.2.6 Vertical transmission

Vertical transmission relates to transmission of pathogens from mother to her offspring via placenta or during birth. All other transmissions from one animal to another are considered horizontal. Some also regard transmission during the neonatal period as vertical transmission, although technically this represents horizontal spread. For example, small ruminant lentiviruses are transmitted predominantly via ingestion of infected colostrum or milk (Blacklaws et al., 2004; Souza et al., 2015). Examples of pathogens that can be transmitted vertically include BVD virus, bovine leucosis virus (Meas, Usui, Ohashi, Sugimoto, & Onuma, 2002), Bluetongue virus (van der Sluijs et al., 2013) or parvoviruses of various species (Mengeling, Lager, Zimmerman, Samarikermani, & Beran, 1991). Trans-placental infection of the foetus may have different consequences depending on the stage of pregnancy, as can be exemplified by a variety of possible outcomes of BVD virus infection of a pregnant cow, ranging from foetal resorption (early pregnancy), through birth of persistently infected calves or calves with congenital abnormalities (mid-pregnancy) to birth of healthy calves that have cleared the virus and are positive for BVD virus antibodies (late pregnancy) (Lanyon et al., 2014).

3.2.7 Iatrogenic transmission

Iatrogenic transmission refers to man-made transmission. This may occur during surgery or invasive procedures (e.g. injections) via contaminated medical equipment. Blood-borne pathogens can be transmitted in this way not only from one animal to another, but also from animals to humans during needle-stick injuries (Venter & Swanepoel, 2010). While the risk of infection through contaminated medical equipment is limited to individuals undergoing an invasive procedure, contamination of biologicals at the time of productions carries an even greater risk of dissemination of the contaminating pathogen among susceptible populations over large geographical areas. This can be exemplified by an epidemic of scrapie in Italy in 1996/1997, which was traced to a vaccine against *Mycoplasma agalactiae* contaminated with the scrapie agent (Zanusso et al., 2003), or an outbreak of lymphomas in commercial broiler flocks traced to Marek's disease vaccine contaminated with chicken reticuloendotheliosis virus (Fadly et al., 1996).

Some pathogens are transmitted predominantly via one route, while others use several different routes of transmission. For example, rabies is spread nearly exclusively via bites of rabid animals (Crowcroft & Thampi, 2015), while anthrax can be transmitted via inhalation of *Bacillus anthracis* spores, via entry of spores through a break in the skin, or via ingestion of vegetative form of the bacteria in meat from diseased animals (Anonymus, 2012; Bengis & Frean, 2014; Beyer & Turnbull, 2009). However, even diseases that are transmitted predominantly via a single route may, under some circumstances, use alternative routes of transmission. This can be illustrated by several cases of human rabies acquired through organ transplantation (Dutta, 1998; Gibbons, 2002) or the epidemic of mad-cow disease in the UK. The latter was caused by feeding meat and bone meal containing ruminant proteins to ruminants, without adequate precautions to inactivate potentially infectious agents present in the product (Nathanson, Wilesmith, & Griot, 1997). The mad cow disease epidemic would have never occurred in nature, as cows do not normally eat meat-derived proteins of its own species.

---

4 Factors affecting the spread of pathogens within populations

In epidemiological terms, the transmissibility of a pathogen within populations is characterised by a reproductive number R_0. The R_0 denotes the number of secondary infections that would theoretically result from an introduction of one infected individual into a fully susceptible population (Lavine, Poss, & Grenfell, 2008). The same concept can be applied at herd level to illustrate the ability of a pathogen to spread from herd to herd ('herd reproductive number R_H'). Diseases with a R_0/R_H below 1 are not capable of evolving into epidemics and would die on their own even without the implementation of any control efforts. Diseases with a R0/RH greater than 1 have the capability to perpetuate themselves in populations. The higher the R_0/R_H, the more difficult it is to control the spread of the disease.

The R_0/R_H is dependent on a variety of factors, depicted in a traditional epidemiological triangle as those related to the pathogen, the host, and the environment. Determinants of resistance/susceptibility to infection and disease with a particular agent are complex and include not only species, breed, or individual genetic differences, but also factors such as age, nutritional status, or the presence of stressors. The influence of non-pathogen-related factors on R_0/R_H can be illustrated by dynamics of FMD spread among different animal species in various geographical regions. The R_0 during the incubation period of disease in non-vaccinated animals was calculated to be 0.31 for calves, 0.20 for lambs, but as high as 13.20 for piglets and 176 for dairy cows infected with the FMD virus under experimental conditions (Orsel, Bouma, Dekker, Stegeman, & de Jong, 2009). The corresponding R_0 estimates for vaccinated animals were considerably lower and ranged from 1.03 x 10^{-8} to 1.26. These data illustrate that the efficiency of transmission of the FMD virus depends on the species of animals affected, their age and vaccination status. In another study (Estrada, Perez, & Turmond, 2008), it was estimated that the R_H during the FMD outbreak among heavily vaccinated animal populations in Peru decreased from 5.3 at the beginning of the epidemic to 1.31 towards the end. Similar estimates for R_H were reported during the

FMD outbreak among unvaccinated animals in the Netherlands (Bouma et al., 2003), potentially highlighting the importance of other variables (e.g. geography, climate, density of herds, speed of detection of disease and introduction of control measures etc.) affecting the spread of FMD virus between herds.

4.1 The pathogen

Pathogen characteristics that play a role in disease transmission include virulence, survival in the environment, species specificity, ability to persist in the host, or the strength and duration of the induced immune response following infection.

In general, pathogens with broad host range are more difficult to control than species-specific pathogens. This is particularly true for those pathogens that are able to establish infections in domesticated species and in wildlife. For example, outbreaks of highly pathogenic avian influenza outbreaks among chickens have been linked to asymptomatically infected waterfall (Haase et al., 2010; Shin et al., 2015). The source of fatal Nipah and Hendra virus infections in people has been traced to infected horses and pigs, respectively. However, neither horses nor pigs proved to be natural hosts for these viruses, which circulate in nature among flying foxes (Aljofan, 2013; Eaton, Broder, Middleton, & Wang, 2006). As mentioned in the introduction to this chapter, the on-going, human-driven changes in the ecology of many geographical areas are likely to influence the host range of pathogens circulating within those areas.

Pathogens that evoke strong, long-lasting immune responses (e.g. systemic poxviruses, parvoviruses or paramyxoviruses) rely on an on-going supply of young naive individuals to maintain themselves in the population. In contrast, immunity to re-infection with herpesviruses, influenza viruses, or many bacterial pathogens tends to be short-lived, and animals may become re-infected several times in their lifetime.

Some pathogens have evolved sophisticated strategies to evade the immune responses of their hosts, which in turn facilitates their maintenance in populations and hampers any control efforts. Two different examples of such strategies can be provided by influenza viruses and herpesviruses. Influenza viruses may respond fairly quickly to pressures generated by the host's immune response through antigenic drift (slow change in antigenicity due to accumulation of mutations at the antigenic sites of the virus) or antigenic shift (a sudden change in antigenicity due to exchange of whole segments of the genome between two different viruses) (Bouvier & Palese, 2008; Epstein & Price, 2010). This creates a constant supply of new viral variants that may be partially recognised, or not recognised at all, by the immune responses raised to their progenitors, which in turn has obvious implications for the level of immunity in the population and for the efficacy of available vaccines. In contrast, herpesviruses are comparatively antigenically stable, but renowned for their ability to establish life-long infections in their hosts. This is accomplished by establishing latency (van der Meulen, Favoreel, Pensaert, & Nauwynck, 2006). During latency, the viral genome undergoes very limited transcription and infectious viruses are not produced. This means that latently infected animals are not infectious. They are also usually clinically normal. Under certain conditions (e.g. stress or immunosuppression), the latent virus may undergo re-activation, which leads to the establishment of productive infection and subsequent transmission to a new host. As it may be difficult to detect (and therefore control) all latently infected animals, they may become a source of infection to others. For example, re-activation of the virus is the most likely explanation for sporadic cases of abortion or neurological disease due to equine herpesvirus type 1 infection in a closed group of horses.

4.2 The host

Host factors that are important in the transmission of infectious agents include nutritional status, age, presence of concurrent infections, level of immunity or individual genetic predispositions. All of these combined determine the level of resistance/susceptibility to infection with a given pathogen. Host-related factors that are important for the transmission of infectious agents in populations include density of susceptible hosts and availability of carrier/intermediate hosts, when applicable.

Animals may remain healthy following exposure to an infectious agent either because they are resistant to infection with that pathogen (e.g. horses are resistant to infection with the FMD virus) or because they have some level of pathogen-specific immunity. Immune animals exposed to the pathogen may still become infected with that pathogen, but they mount a fast, effective immune response, which controls the infection. In other words, they are susceptible to infection, but resistant to disease. Shedding of pathogens by immune animals, where it occurs, is typically of a much lower level and duration than shedding observed following infection of fully susceptible animals. Immune animals are therefore unlikely to constitute an important source of infection for other animals, although vaccination should not be regarded as a sole infection control strategy in the absence of other preventive measures. Under some circumstances (e.g. 'poor responders'), vaccinated animals may still play a role in transmission of infectious agents, as has been the case in several equine influenza outbreaks (Powell, Watkins, Li, & Shortridge, 1995; van Maanen, van Essen, Minke, Daly, & Yates, 2003; Yamanaka, Niwa, Tsujimura, Kondo, & Matsumura, 2008).

Some pathogens may cause overt clinical disease in animals from one species, but only sub-clinical infections in other animals. Sub-clinically infected animals constitute reservoir hosts for such pathogens. They are excellent sources of infection for susceptible animals (of the same or different species), as they are difficult to detect without specific surveillance programmes, which are usually costly to run. Awareness of the presence and distribution of potential reservoir hosts for pathogens of interest is important in implementing effective infection control programmes in any given area. For example, healthy reptiles are a common source of *Salmonella* infection (Bertrand et al., 2008), rodents are a source of hantavirus infections for people and cattle may act as carriers for *E.coli* 0157 infection in children (David et al., 2004; Warshawsky et al., 2002). Many pathogens need a constant supply of susceptible hosts in order to maintain themselves in populations.

For pathogens that require complex transmission cycles involving vectors, maintenance or intermediate hosts, the availability of such hosts is an important factor in the spread of infection. Consequently, elimination of those hosts helps control diseases in a given area. This is particularly important for viruses and some parasites, which cannot multiply outside of their hosts, and less important for free-living organisms such as bacteria.

The higher the density of susceptible hosts, the easier it is for a pathogen to maintain the cycle of infections. Intensification of animal production systems in developed countries has brought challenges linked to enhanced transmission of infectious agents within dense populations of young animals with various levels of immunity.

A high level of immunity (more than 70% of resistant animals) in any given population is believed to minimise, or break altogether, the ability of the pathogen to be maintained in such population. This is the basis for the concept of 'herd immunity', and the goal of many vaccination-based control programmes. Examples of successful disease eradication efforts based on maintenance of high level of immunity in populations include global eradiation of smallpox (Strassburg, 1982) and rinderpest (Roeder, Mariner, & Kock, 2013), or local eradication of rabies in several countries (Flamand et al., 1992).

4.3 The environment

Environmental conditions play an important role in maintaining or breaking transmission cycles of infectious agents. Conditions that cause stress in animals (e.g. extreme temperatures, overcrowding, unsettled social structure) facilitate the establishment of infections. It is well recognised that transported animals are prone to developing respiratory disease (Earley, Buckham Sporer, & Gupta, 2017; Oikawa, Takagi, Anzai, Yoshikawa, & Yoshikawa, 1995). Similarly, calves kept in larger groups were more likely to develop respiratory disease than those kept in smaller groups, although there was no difference in the risk of developing diarrhoea between different sized groups in the same study

(Svensson & Liberg, 2006). Thus, the dynamics of disease spread and presentation varies between different populations of animals. Any activity that changes the established balance between hosts and their pathogens (including availability of the vectors or reservoir hosts) is likely to result in altered disease transmission patterns as has been observed following deforestation, irrigation or urbanisation (Mackenzie & Jeggo, 2013).

5 Summary

A number of steps are necessary for the transmission of an infectious agent from the infected individual to another susceptible host. Common steps include entry, development of disease (may be sub-clinical), exit and transmission of the pathogen to a new host. In terms of control, spread of infectious pathogens between infected and susceptible individuals can be divided into airborne, droplet and contact (direct and indirect) transmission. Of these, airborne transmission is most difficult to control, but it is not as common as the other two. Some pathogens have a preference for one specific route of transmission while others may be transmitted equally well via different routes. Knowledge of main transmission patterns and factors associated with these patterns is important in establishing effective control strategies. The outcome of infection and the ability of the pathogen to be maintained in a given population depends on several factors, including those related to the pathogen, the host and the environment. Pathogens are able to adapt to changing conditions. As such, established transmission patterns may not remain static. Anthropomorphic activities that influence climatic and geographic conditions are likely to drive such changes, for example by their impact on availability of susceptible hosts and vectors.

References

Aho, M., Kurki, M., Rautelin, H., & Kosunen, T. U. (1989). Water-borne outbreak of Campy-lobacter enteritis after outdoor infantry drill in Utti, Finland. *Epidemiology and Infection, 103*(1), 133-141.

Alexandersen, S., Quan, M., Murphy, C., Knight, J., & Zhang, Z. (2003). Studies of quantitative parameters of virus excretion and transmission in pigs and cattle experimentally infected with foot-and-mouth disease virus. *Journal of Comparative Pathology, 129*(4), 268-282.

Aljofan, M. (2013). Hendra and Nipah infection: emerging paramyxoviruses. *Virus Research, 177*(2), 119-126. doi: 10.1016/j.virusres.2013.08.002

Alonso, C., Raynor, P. C., Davies, P. R., & Torremorell, M. (2015). Concentration, Size Distribution, and Infectivity of Airborne Particles Carrying Swine Viruses. *PLoS One, 10*(8), e0135675. doi: 10.1371/journal.pone.0135675

Althouse, G. C., & Rossow, K. (2011). The potential risk of infectious disease dissemination via artificial insemination in swine. *Reproduction in Domestic Animals, 46 Suppl 2*, 64-67. doi: 10.1111/j.1439-0531.2011.01863.x

Anonymus. (2012). *Anthrax*. Ministry of Health. Retrieved from http://www.health.govt.nz/system/files/documents/publications/cd-manual-anthrax-may2012.pdf

Antunes, M. B., & Cohen, N. A. (2007). Mucociliary clearance--a critical upper airway host defense mechanism and methods of assessment. *Curr Opin Allergy Clin Immunol, 7*(1), 5-10. doi: 10.1097/ACI.0b013e3280114eef

Ashbolt, N. J. (2015). Microbial Contamination of Drinking Water and Human Health from Community Water Systems. *Curr Environ Health Rep, 2*(1), 95-106. doi: 10.1007/s40572-014-0037-5

Balasuriya, U. B., Go, Y. Y., & MacLachlan, N. J. (2013). Equine arteritis virus. *Veterinary Microbiology, 167*(1-2), 93-122. doi: 10.1016/j.vetmic.2013.06.015

Baskerville, A. (1981). Mechanisms of infection in the respiratory tract. *New Zealand Veterinary Journal, 29*(12), 235-238.

Bayram, Y., Guducuoglu, H., Otlu, B., Aypak, C., Gursoy, N. C., Uluc, H., & Berktas, M. (2011). Epidemiological characteristics and molecular typing of Salmonella enterica serovar Typhi during a waterborne outbreak in Eastern Anatolia. *Annals of Tropical Medicine and Parasitology, 105*(5), 359-365. doi: 10.1179/1364859411Y.0000000024

Beam, A., Goede, D., Fox, A., McCool, M. J., Wall, G., Haley, C., & Morrison, R. (2015). A Porcine Epidemic Diarrhea Virus Outbreak in One Geographic Region of the United States: Descriptive Epidemiology and Investigation of the Possibility of Airborne Virus Spread. *PLoS One, 10*(12), e0144818. doi: 10.1371/journal.pone.0144818

Bengis, R. G., & Frean, J. (2014). Anthrax as an example of the One Health concept. *Revue Scientifique et Technique, 33*(2), 593-604.

Bertrand, S., Rimhanen-Finne, R., Weill, F. X., Rabsch, W., Thornton, L., Perevoscikovs, J., ... Heck, M. (2008). Salmonella infections associated with reptiles: the current situation in Europe. *Euro Surveill, 13*(24).

Beyer, W., & Turnbull, P. C. (2009). Anthrax in animals. *Molecular Aspects of Medicine, 30*(6), 481-489. doi: 10.1016/j.mam.2009.08.004

Blacklaws, B. A., Berriatua, E., Torsteinsdottir, S., Watt, N. J., de Andres, D., Klein, D., & Harkiss, G. D. (2004). Transmission of small ruminant lentiviruses. *Veterinary Microbiology*, 101(3), 199-208. doi: 10.1016/j.vetmic.2004.04.006

Blais Lecours, P., Veillette, M., Marsolais, D., & Duchaine, C. (2012). Characterization of bioaerosols from dairy barns: reconstructing the puzzle of occupational respiratory diseases by using molecular approaches. *Applied and Environmental Microbiology*, 78(9), 3242-3248. doi: 10.1128/AEM.07661-11

Bouma, A., Elbers, A. R., Dekker, A., de Koeijer, A., Bartels, C., Vellema, P., ... de Jong, M. C. (2003). The foot-and-mouth disease epidemic in The Netherlands in 2001. *Preventive Veterinary Medicine*, 57(3), 155-166.

Bouvier, N. M., & Palese, P. (2008). The biology of influenza viruses. *Vaccine, 26 Suppl 4*, D49-53.

Bowman, D. D. (2009). Essential veterinary education in water-borne transmission of disease. *Revue Scientifique et Technique*, 28(2), 589-596.

Burgess, B. A., Morley, P. S., & Hyatt, D. R. (2004). Environmental surveillance for Salmonella enterica in a veterinary teaching hospital. *J Am Vet Med Assoc*, 225(9), 1344-1348.

Buttner, M., & Rziha, H. J. (2002). Parapoxviruses: from the lesion to the viral genome. *J Vet Med B Infect Dis Vet Public Health*, 49(1), 7-16.

Christensen, L. S., Brehm, K. E., Skov, J., Harlow, K. W., Christensen, J., & Haas, B. (2011). Detection of foot-and-mouth disease virus in the breath of infected cattle using a hand-held device to collect aerosols. *Journal of Virological Methods*, 177(1), 44-48. doi: 10.1016/j.jviromet.2011.06.011

Colenutt, C., Gonzales, J. L., Paton, D. J., Gloster, J., Nelson, N., & Sanders, C. (2016). Aerosol transmission of foot-and-mouth disease virus Asia-1 under experimental conditions. *Veterinary Microbiology*, 189, 39-45. doi: 10.1016/j.vetmic.2016.04.024

Crowcroft, N. S., & Thampi, N. (2015). The prevention and management of rabies. *BMJ, 350*, g7827. doi: 10.1136/bmj.g7827

Cutler, T. D., Wang, C., Hoff, S. J., Kittawornrat, A., & Zimmerman, J. J. (2011). Median infectious dose (ID(5)(0)) of porcine reproductive and respiratory syndrome virus isolate MN-184 via aerosol exposure. *Veterinary Microbiology*, 151(3-4), 229-237. doi: 10.1016/j.vetmic.2011.03.003

Cutler, T. D., Wang, C., Hoff, S. J., & Zimmerman, J. J. (2012). Effect of temperature and relative humidity on ultraviolet (UV 254) inactivation of airborne porcine respiratory and reproductive syndrome virus. *Veterinary Microbiology*, 159(1-2), 47-52. doi: 10.1016/j.vetmic

David, S. T., MacDougall, L., Louie, K., McIntyre, L., Paccagnella, A. M., Schleicher, S., & Hamade, A. (2004). Petting zoo-associated Escherichia coli 0157:h7--secondary transmission, asymptomatic infection, and prolonged shedding in the classroom. *Canada Communicable Disease Report*, 30(20), 173-180.

de Carvalho Ferreira, H. C., Weesendorp, E., Quak, S., Stegeman, J. A., & Loeffen, W. L. (2013). Quantification of airborne African swine fever virus after experimental infection. *Veterinary Microbiology*, 165(3-4), 243-251. doi: 10.1016/j.vetmic.2013.03.007

Dee, S., Otake, S., Oliveira, S., & Deen, J. (2009). Evidence of long distance airborne transport of porcine reproductive and respiratory syndrome virus and Mycoplasma hyopneumoniae. *Veterinary Research*, 40(4), 39. doi: 10.1051/vetres/2009022

Donaldson, A. I., & Alexandersen, S. (2002). Predicting the spread of foot and mouth disease by airborne virus. *Revue Scientifique et Technique, 21*(3), 569-575.

Dubey, J. P. (2004). Toxoplasmosis – a waterborne zoonosis. *Veterinary Parasitology, 126*(1-2), 57-72. doi: 10.1016/j.vetpar.2004.09.005

Dubey, J. P., Zarnke, R., Thomas, N. J., Wong, S. K., Van Bonn, W., Briggs, M., ...Thulliez, P. (2003). Toxoplasma gondii, Neospora caninum, Sarcocystis neurona, and Sarcocystis canis-like infections in marine mammals. *Veterinary Parasitology, 116*(4), 275-296.

Dungan, R. S. (2010). BOARD-INVITED REVIEW: fate and transport of bioaerosols associated with livestock operations and manures. *Journal of Animal Science, 88*(11), 3693-3706. doi: 10.2527/jas.2010-3094

Dunowska, M., Morley, P. S., Patterson, G., Hyatt, D. R., & Van Metre, D. C. (2006). Evaluation of the efficacy of a peroxygen disinfectant-filled foot mat for reduction of bacterial load on footwear in a large animal hospital setting. *J Am Vet Med Assoc, 228*(12), 1935-1939.

Dunowska, M., Morley, P. S., Traub-Dargatz, J. L., Davis, M. A., Patterson, G., Frye, J. G., . . . Dargatz, D. A. (2007). Comparison of Salmonella enterica serotype Infantis isolates from a veterinary teaching hospital. *J Appl Microbiol, 102*(6), 1527-1536.

Dutta, J. K. (1998). Rabies transmission by oral and other non-bite routes. *Journal of the Indian Medical Association, 96*(12), 359.

Earley, B., Buckham Sporer, K., & Gupta, S. (2017). Invited review: Relationship between cattle transport, immunity and respiratory disease. *Animal, 11*(3), 486-492. doi: 10.1017/S1751731116001622

Eaton, B. T., Broder, C. C., Middleton, D., & Wang, L. F. (2006). Hendra and Nipah viruses: different and dangerous. *Nat Rev Microbiol, 4*(1), 23-35. doi: 10.1038/nrmicro1323

Ehsan, A. M., Geurden, T., Casaert, S., Parvin, S. M., Islam, T. M., Ahmed, U. M., ...Claerebout, E. (2015). Assessment of zoonotic transmission of Giardia and Cryptosporidium between cattle and humans in rural villages in Bangladesh. *PLoS One, 10*(2), e0118239. doi: 10.1371/journal.pone.0118239

Elson, C. O., & Alexander, K. L. (2015). Host-microbiota interactions in the intestine. *Digestive Diseases, 33*(2), 131-136. doi: 10.1159/000369534

Epstein, S. L., & Price, G. E. (2010). Cross-protective immunity to influenza A viruses. *Expert Rev Vaccines, 9*(11), 1325-1341. doi: 10.1586/erv.10.123

Estrada, C., Perez, A. M., & Turmond, M. C. (2008). Herd reproduction ratio and time-space analysis of a foot-and-mouth disease epidemic in Peru in 2004. *Transboundary and Emerging Diseases, 55*(7), 284-292. doi: 10.1111/j.1865-1682.2008.01023.x

Fadly, A. M., Witter, R. L., Smith, E. J., Silva, R. F., Reed, W. M., Hoerr, F. J., & Putnam, M. R. (1996). An outbreak of lymphomas in commercial broiler breeder chickens vaccinated with a fowlpox vaccine contaminated with reticuloendotheliosis virus. *Avian Pathol, 25*(1), 35-47.

Fernstrom, A., & Goldblatt, M. (2013). Aerobiology and its role in the transmission of infectious diseases. *J Pathog, 2013*, 493960. doi: 10.1155/2013/493960

Flamand, A., Coulon, P., Lafay, F., Kappeler, A., Artois, M., Aubert, M., ...Wandeler, A. J. (1992). Eradication of rabies in Europe. *Nature, 360*(6400), 115-116. doi: 10.1038/360115a0

Fokkens, W. J., & Scheeren, R. A. (2000). Upper airway defence mechanisms. *Paediatr Respir Rev, 1*(4), 336-341.

Foster, D. M., & Smith, G. W. (2009). Pathophysiology of diarrhea in calves. *Veterinary Clinics of North America. Food Animal Practice, 25*(1), 13-36, xi.

Fourment, M., & Holmes, E. C. (2015). Avian influenza virus exhibits distinct evolutionary dynamics in wild birds and poultry. *BMC Evol Biol, 15*, 120. doi: 10.1186/s12862-015-0410-5

Fredericks, D. N., & Relman, D. A. (1996). Sequence-based identification of microbial pathogens: a reconsideration of Koch's postulates. *Clinical Microbiology Reviews, 9*(1), 18-33.

Gibbons, R. V. (2002). Cryptogenic rabies, bats, and the question of aerosol transmission. *Annals of Emergency Medicine, 39*(5), 528-536.

Givens, M. D., & Waldrop, J. G. (2004). Bovine viral diarrhea virus in embryo and semen production systems. *Veterinary Clinics of North America. Food Animal Practice, 20*(1), 21-38.

Gloster, J., Jones, A., Redington, A., Burgin, L., Sorensen, J. H., Turner, R., ...Paton, D. (2009). Airborne spread of foot-and-mouth disease – Model intercomparison. *Veterinary Journal.*

Gloster, J., Jones, A., Redington, A., Burgin, L., Sorensen, J. H., Turner, R., ...Paton, D. (2010). Airborne spread of foot-and-mouth disease--model intercomparison. *Veterinary Journal, 183*(3), 278-286. doi: 10.1016/j.tvjl.2008.11.011

Gloster, J., Williams, P., Doel, C., Esteves, I., Coe, H., & Valarcher, J. F. (2007). Foot-and-mouth disease – quantification and size distribution of airborne particles emitted by healthy and infected pigs. *Veterinary Journal, 174*(1), 42-53.

Goyal, S. M., Anantharaman, S., Ramakrishnan, M. A., Sajja, S., Kim, S. W., Stanley, N. J., ... Raynor, P. C. (2011). Detection of viruses in used ventilation filters from two large public buildings. *American Journal of Infection Control, 39*(7), e30-38. doi: 10.1016/j.ajic.2010.10.036

Gralton, J., Tovey, E., McLaws, M. L., & Rawlinson, W. D. (2011). The role of particle size in aerosolised pathogen transmission: a review. *Journal of Infection, 62*(1), 1-13. doi: 10.1016/j.jinf.2010.11.010

Grooms, D. L. (2004). Reproductive consequences of infection with bovine viral diarrhea virus. *Veterinary Clinics of North America. Food Animal Practice, 20*(1), 5-19. doi: 10.1016/j.cvfa.2003.11.006

Haase, M., Starick, E., Fereidouni, S., Strebelow, G., Grund, C., Seeland, A., ...Harder, T. (2010). Possible sources and spreading routes of highly pathogenic avian influenza virus subtype H5N1 infections in poultry and wild birds in Central Europe in 2007 inferred through likelihood analyses. *Infect Genet Evol, 10*(7), 1075-1084. doi: 10.1016/j.meegid.2010.07.005

Horner, G. W. (2004). Equine viral arteritis control scheme: a brief review with emphasis on laboratory aspects of the scheme in New Zealand. *New Zealand Veterinary Journal, 52*(2), 82-84.

Jahne, M. A., Rogers, S. W., Holsen, T. M., Grimberg, S. J., & Ramler, I. P. (2015). Emission and Dispersion of Bioaerosols from Dairy Manure Application Sites: Human Health Risk Assessment. *Environ Sci Technol, 49*(16), 9842-9849. doi: 10.1021/acs.est.5b01981

Jahne, M. A., Rogers, S. W., Holsen, T. M., Grimberg, S. J., Ramler, I. P., & Kim, S. (2016). Bioaerosol Deposition to Food Crops near Manure Application: Quantitative Microbial Risk Assessment. *J Environ Qual, 45*(2), 666-674. doi: 10.2134/jeq2015.04.0187

Johns, I., Tennent-Brown, B., Schaer, B. D., Southwood, L., Boston, R., & Wilkins, P. (2009). Blood culture status in mature horses with diarrhoea: a possible association with survival. *Equine Vet J, 41*(2), 160-164.

Jones, R. M., & Brosseau, L. M. (2015). Aerosol transmission of infectious disease. *Journal of Occupational and Environmental Medicine, 57*(5), 501-508. doi: 10.1097/JOM.0000000000000448

Kopecky, K. E., Pugh, G. W., Jr., & McDonald, T. J. (1986). Infectious bovine keratoconjunctivitis: contact transmission. *American Journal of Veterinary Research, 47*(3), 622-624.

Kramer, A., Schwebke, I., & Kampf, G. (2006). How long do nosocomial pathogens persist on inanimate surfaces? A systematic review. *BMC Infect Dis, 6*, 130.

Kuhn, K. G., Falkenhorst, G., Emborg, H. D., Ceper, T., Torpdahl, M., Krogfelt, K. A., ...Molbak, K. (2017). Epidemiological and serological investigation of a waterborne Campylobacter jejuni outbreak in a Danish town. *Epidemiology and Infection, 145*(4), 701-709. doi: 10.1017/S0950268816002788

Lanyon, S. R., Hill, F. I., Reichel, M. P., & Brownlie, J. (2014). Bovine viral diarrhoea: pathogenesis and diagnosis. *Veterinary Journal, 199*(2), 201-209. doi: 10.1016/j.tvjl.2013.07.024

Lavine, J. S., Poss, M., & Grenfell, B. T. (2008). Directly transmitted viral diseases: modeling the dynamics of transmission. *Trends in Microbiology, 16*(4), 165-172.

Leclerc, H., Schwartzbrod, L., & Dei-Cas, E. (2002). Microbial agents associated with waterborne diseases. *Critical Reviews in Microbiology, 28*(4), 371-409. doi: 10.1080/1040-840291046768

Lepargneur, J. P. (2016). Lactobacillus crispatus as biomarker of the healthy vaginal tract. *Annales de Biologie Clinique, 74*(4), 421-427. doi: 10.1684/abc.2016.1169

Lockhart, A. B., Thrall, P. H., & Antonovics, J. (1996). Sexually transmitted diseases in animals: ecological and evolutionary implications. *Biological Reviews of the Cambridge Philosophical Society, 71*(3), 415-471.

Mackenzie, J. S., & Jeggo, M. (2013). Reservoirs and vectors of emerging viruses. *Curr Opin Virol, 3*(2), 170-179. doi: 10.1016/j.coviro.2013.02.002

Maclachlan, N. J., & Mayo, C. E. (2013). Potential strategies for control of bluetongue, a globally emerging, Culicoides-transmitted viral disease of ruminant livestock and wildlife. *Antiviral Research, 99*(2), 79-90. doi: 10.1016/j.antiviral.2013.04.021

Marini, G., Rosa, R., Pugliese, A., & Heesterbeek, H. (2017). Exploring vector-borne infection ecology in multi-host communities: A case study of West Nile virus. *Journal of Theoretical Biology, 415*, 58-69. doi: 10.1016/j.jtbi.2016.12.009

McFadden, A. M., Pearce, P. V., Orr, D., Nicoll, K., Rawdon, T. G., Pharo, H., & Stone, M. (2013). Evidence for absence of equine arteritis virus in the horse population of New Zealand. *New Zealand Veterinary Journal, 61*(5), 300-304. doi: 10.1080/00480169.2012.755664

Meas, S., Usui, T., Ohashi, K., Sugimoto, C., & Onuma, M. (2002). Vertical transmission of bovine leukemia virus and bovine immunodeficiency virus in dairy cattle herds. *Veterinary Microbiology, 84*(3), 275-282.

Mengeling, W. L., Lager, K. M., Zimmerman, J. K., Samarikermani, N., & Beran, G. W. (1991). A current assessment of the role of porcine parvovirus as a cause of fetal porcine death. *Journal of Veterinary Diagnostic Investigation, 3*(1), 33-35. doi: 10.1177/104063879100300107

Michi, A. N., Favetto, P. H., Kastelic, J., & Cobo, E. R. (2016). A review of sexually transmitted bovine trichomoniasis and campylobacteriosis affecting cattle reproductive health. *Theriogenology, 85*(5), 781-791. doi: 10.1016/j.theriogenology.2015.10.037

Miller, M. A., Gardner, I. A., Kreuder, C., Paradies, D. M., Worcester, K. R., Jessup, D. A., ... Conrad, P. A. (2002). Coastal freshwater runoff is a risk factor for Toxoplasma gondii infection of southern sea otters (Enhydra lutris nereis). *International Journal for Parasitology, 32*(8), 997-1006.

Millner, P. D. (2009). Bioaerosols associated with animal production operations. *Bioresour Technol, 100*(22), 5379-5385. doi: 10.1016/j.biortech.2009.03.026

Molaei, G., Armstrong, P. M., Graham, A. C., Kramer, L. D., & Andreadis, T. G. (2015). Insights into the recent emergence and expansion of eastern equine encephalitis virus in a new focus in the Northern New England USA. *Parasit Vectors, 8*, 516. doi: 10.1186/s13071-015-1145-2

Monahan, A. M., Miller, I. S., & Nally, J. E. (2009). Leptospirosis: risks during recreational activities. *Journal of Applied Microbiology*.

Morley, P. S. (2002). Biosecurity of veterinary practices. *Veterinary Clinics of North America. Food Animal Practice, 18*(1), 133-155, vii.

Moss, J. A. (2016). Waterborne Pathogens: The Protozoans. *Radiologic Technology, 88*(1), 27-48.

Mughini-Gras, L., Penny, C., Ragimbeau, C., Schets, F. M., Blaak, H., Duim, B., ...van Pelt, W. (2016). Quantifying potential sources of surface water contamination with Campylobacter jejuni and Campylobacter coli. *Water Res, 101*, 36-45. doi: 10.1016/j.watres.2016.05.069

Muscatello, G., Gerbaud, S., Kennedy, C., Gilkerson, J. R., Buckley, T., Klay, M., ...Browning, G. F. (2006). Comparison of concentrations of Rhodococcus equi and virulent R. equi in air of stables and paddocks on horse breeding farms in a temperate climate. *Equine Veterinary Journal, 38*(3), 263-265.

Myatt, T. A., Johnston, S. L., Zuo, Z., Wand, M., Kebadze, T., Rudnick, S., & Milton, D. K. (2004). Detection of airborne rhinovirus and its relation to outdoor air supply in office environments. *American Journal of Respiratory and Critical Care Medicine, 169*(11), 1187-1190. doi: 10.1164/rccm.200306-760OC

Nathanson, N., Wilesmith, J., & Griot, C. (1997). Bovine spongiform encephalopathy (BSE): causes and consequences of a common source epidemic. *American Journal of Epidemiology, 145*(11), 959-969.

Neo, J. R., Sagha-Zadeh, R., Vielemeyer, O., & Franklin, E. (2016). Evidence-based practices to increase hand hygiene compliance in health care facilities: An integrated review. *American Journal of Infection Control, 44*(6), 691-704. doi: 10.1016/j.ajic.2015.11.034

Nicas, M., Nazaroff, W. W., & Hubbard, A. (2005). Toward understanding the risk of secondary airborne infection: emission of respirable pathogens. *J Occup Environ Hyg, 2*(3), 143-154.

Nohra, A., Grinberg, A., Midwinter, A. C., Marshall, J. C., Collins-Emerson, J. M., & French, N. P. (2016). Molecular epidemiology of C. coli isolated from different sources in New Zealand between 2005 and 2014. *Applied and Environmental Microbiology*. doi: 10.1128/AEM.00934-16

Oikawa, M., Takagi, S., Anzai, R., Yoshikawa, H., & Yoshikawa, T. (1995). Pathology of equine respiratory disease occurring in association with transport. *Journal of Comparative Pathology, 113*(1), 29-43.

Orsel, K., Bouma, A., Dekker, A., Stegeman, J. A., & de Jong, M. C. (2009). Foot and mouth disease virus transmission during the incubation period of the disease in piglets, lambs, calves, and dairy cows. *Preventive Veterinary Medicine, 88*(2), 158-163.

Otake, S., Dee, S., Corzo, C., Oliveira, S., & Deen, J. (2010). Long-distance airborne transport of infectious PRRSV and Mycoplasma hyopneumoniae from a swine population infected with multiple viral variants. *Veterinary Microbiology, 145*(3-4), 198-208. doi: 10.1016/j.vetmic.2010.03.028

Perez, M., Munoz, J. A., Biescas, E., Salazar, E., Bolea, R., de Andres, D., ...Lujan, L. (2013). Successful Visna/maedi control in a highly infected ovine dairy flock using serologic segregation and management strategies. *Preventive Veterinary Medicine, 112*(3-4), 423-427. doi: 10.1016/j.prevetmed.2013.07.019

Plowright, R. K., Eby, P., Hudson, P. J., Smith, I. L., Westcott, D., Bryden, W. L., ...McCallum, H. (2015). Ecological dynamics of emerging bat virus spillover. *Proc Biol Sci, 282*(1798), 20142124. doi: 10.1098/rspb.2014.2124

Powell, D. G., Watkins, K. L., Li, P. H., & Shortridge, K. F. (1995). Outbreak of equine influenza among horses in Hong Kong during 1992. *Veterinary Record, 136*(21), 531-536.

Pozio, E. (2015). Trichinella spp. imported with live animals and meat. *Veterinary Parasitology, 213*(1-2), 46-55. doi: 10.1016/j.vetpar.2015.02.017

Prats-van der Ham, M., Tatay-Dualde, J., de la Fe, C., Paterna, A., Sanchez, A., Corrales, J. C., ...Gomez-Martin, A. (2017). Detecting asymptomatic rams infected with Mycoplasma agalactiae in ovine artificial insemination centers. *Theriogenology, 89*, 324-328 e321. doi: 10.1016/j.theriogenology.2016.09.014

Pudney, J., Quayle, A. J., & Anderson, D. J. (2005). Immunological microenvironments in the human vagina and cervix: mediators of cellular immunity are concentrated in the cervical transformation zone. *Biology of Reproduction, 73*(6), 1253-1263. doi: 10.1095/biolreprod.105.043133

Roeder, P., Mariner, J., & Kock, R. (2013). Rinderpest: the veterinary perspective on eradication. *Philosophical Transactions of the Royal Society of London. Series B: Biological Sciences, 368*(1623), 20120139. doi: 10.1098/rstb.2012.0139

Schley, D., Burgin, L., & Gloster, J. (2009). Predicting infection risk of airborne foot-and-mouth disease. *J R Soc Interface, 6*(34), 455-462.

Scott, A., McCluskey, B., Brown-Reid, M., Grear, D., Pitcher, P., Ramos, G., ...Singrey, A. (2016). Porcine epidemic diarrhea virus introduction into the United States: Root cause investigation. *Preventive Veterinary Medicine, 123*, 192-201. doi: 10.1016/j.prevetmed.2015.11.013

Seto, W. H. (2015). Airborne transmission and precautions: facts and myths. *Journal of Hospital Infection, 89*(4), 225-228. doi: 10.1016/j.jhin.2014.11.005

Shin, J. H., Woo, C., Wang, S. J., Jeong, J., An, I. J., Hwang, J. K., ...Kim, S. H. (2015). Prevalence of avian influenza virus in wild birds before and after the HPAI H5N8 outbreak in 2014 in South Korea. *J Microbiol, 53*(7), 475-480. doi: 10.1007/s12275-015-5224-z

Shultz, J. M., Espinel, Z., Espinola, M., & Rechkemmer, A. (2016). Distinguishing epidemiological features of the 2013-2016 West Africa Ebola virus disease outbreak. *Disaster Health, 3*(3), 78-88. doi: 10.1080/21665044.2016.1228326

Siegel, J. D., Rhinehart, E., Jackson, M., & Committee, t. H. I. C. P. A. (2007). 2007 Guideline for Isolation Precautions: Preventing Transmission of Infectious Agents in Healthcare Settings. Retrieved from http://www.cdc.gov/ncidod/dhqp/pdf/isolation2007.pdf

Smith, S., Messam, L. L., Meade, J., Gibbons, J., McGill, K., Bolton, D., & Whyte, P. (2016). The impact of biosecurity and partial depopulation on Campylobacter prevalence in Irish broiler flocks with differing levels of hygiene and economic performance. *Infect Ecol Epidemiol, 6*, 31454. doi: 10.3402/iee.v6.31454

Souza, T. S., Pinheiro, R. R., Costa, J. N., Lima, C. C., Andrioli, A., Azevedo, D. A., ...Costa Neto, A. O. (2015). Interspecific transmission of small ruminant lentiviruses from goats to sheep. *Braz J Microbiol, 46*(3), 867-874. doi: 10.1590/S1517-838246320140402

Strassburg, M. A. (1982). The global eradication of smallpox. *American Journal of Infection Control, 10*(2), 53-59.

Svensson, C., & Liberg, P. (2006). The effect of group size on health and growth rate of Swedish dairy calves housed in pens with automatic milk-feeders. *Preventive Veterinary Medicine, 73*(1), 43-53.

Tambalo, D. D., Boa, T., Aryal, B., & Yost, C. K. (2016). Temporal variation in the prevalence and species richness of Campylobacter spp. in a prairie watershed impacted by urban and agricultural mixed inputs. *Canadian Journal of Microbiology, 62*(5), 402-410. doi: 10.1139/cjm-2015-0710

Traub-Dargatz, J. L., Dargatz, D. A., Morley, P. S., & Dunowska, M. (2004). An overview of infection control strategies for equine facilities, with an emphasis on veterinary hospitals. *Veterinary Clinics of North America. Equine Practice, 20*(3), 507-520, v.

Tribe, R. M. (2015). Small Peptides with a Big Role: Antimicrobial Peptides in the Pregnant Female Reproductive Tract. *American Journal of Reproductive Immunology, 74*(2), 123-125. doi: 10.1111/aji.12379

van der Meulen, K. M., Favoreel, H. W., Pensaert, M. B., & Nauwynck, H. J. (2006). Immune escape of equine herpesvirus 1 and other herpesviruses of veterinary importance. *Veterinary Immunology and Immunopathology, 111*(1-2), 31-40.

van der Sluijs, M. T., Schroer-Joosten, D. P., Fid-Fourkour, A., Vrijenhoek, M. P., Debyser, I., Moulin, V., ...de Smit, A. J. (2013). Transplacental transmission of Bluetongue virus serotype 1 and serotype 8 in sheep: virological and pathological findings. *PLoS One, 8*(12), e81429. doi: 10.1371/journal.pone.0081429

van Maanen, C., van Essen, G. J., Minke, J., Daly, J. M., & Yates, P. J. (2003). Diagnostic methods applied to analysis of an outbreak of equine influenza in a riding school in which vaccine failure occurred. *Veterinary Microbiology, 93*(4), 291-306.

Venter, M., & Swanepoel, R. (2010). West Nile virus lineage 2 as a cause of zoonotic neurological disease in humans and horses in southern Africa. *Vector Borne Zoonotic Dis, 10*(7), 659-664. doi: 10.1089/vbz.2009.0230

Warshawsky, B., Gutmanis, I., Henry, B., Dow, J., Reffle, J., Pollett, G., ...Rodgers, F. (2002). Outbreak of Escherichia coli O157:H7 related to animal contact at a petting zoo. *Can J Infect Dis, 13*(3), 175-181.

Watson, J., Daniels, P., Kirkland, P., Carroll, A., & Jeggo, M. (2011). The 2007 outbreak of equine influenza in Australia: lessons learned for international trade in horses. *Revue Scientifique et Technique, 30*(1), 87-93.

Weesendorp, E., Backer, J., & Loeffen, W. (2014). Quantification of different classical swine fever virus transmission routes within a single compartment. *Veterinary Microbiology, 174*(3-4), 353-361. doi: 10.1016/j.vetmic.2014.10.022

Weesendorp, E., Stegeman, A., & Loeffen, W. (2009). Dynamics of virus excretion via different routes in pigs experimentally infected with classical swine fever virus strains of high, moderate or low virulence. *Veterinary Microbiology, 133*(1-2), 9-22. doi: 10.1016/j.vetmic.2008.06.008

Weesendorp, E., Stegeman, A., & Loeffen, W. L. (2009). Quantification of classical swine fever virus in aerosols originating from pigs infected with strains of high, moderate or low virulence. *Veterinary Microbiology, 135*(3-4), 222-230. doi: 10.1016/j.vetmic.2008.09.073

Wiesenfeld, H. C., Heine, R. P., Krohn, M. A., Hillier, S. L., Amortegui, A. A., Nicolazzo, M., & Sweet, R. L. (2002). Association between elevated neutrophil defensin levels and endometritis. *Journal of Infectious Diseases, 186*(6), 792-797. doi: 10.1086/342417

Yamanaka, T., Niwa, H., Tsujimura, K., Kondo, T., & Matsumura, T. (2008). Epidemic of equine influenza among vaccinated racehorses in Japan in 2007. *Journal of Veterinary Medical Science, 70*(6), 623-625.

Yang, K., LeJeune, J., Alsdorf, D., Lu, B., Shum, C. K., & Liang, S. (2012). Global distribution of outbreaks of water-associated infectious diseases. *PLoS Negl Trop Dis, 6*(2), e1483. doi: 10.1371/journal.pntd.0001483

Zanusso, G., Casalone, C., Acutis, P., Bozzetta, E., Farinazzo, A., Gelati, M., ...Caramelli, M. (2003). Molecular analysis of iatrogenic scrapie in Italy. *Journal of General Virology, 84*(Pt 4), 1047-1052. doi: 10.1099/vir.0.18774-0

Zhou, N., Zhang, H., Lin, X., Hou, P., Wang, S., Tao, Z., ...Xu, A. (2016). A waterborne norovirus gastroenteritis outbreak in a school, eastern China. *Epidemiology and Infection, 144*(6), 1212-1219. doi: 10.1017/S0950268815002526

Photo credits

CDC Public Health Image Library, James Gathany: figure 1.8

Colurbox: figures 1.3, 1.5, 1.9

Magda Dunowska: figure 1.7

Quentin Roper: figure 1.6

CHAPTER 2

GENERAL PRINCIPLES OF BIOSECURITY IN ANIMAL PRODUCTION AND VETERINARY MEDICINE

Jeroen Dewulf[1]

Filip Van Immerseel[2]

[1] Faculty of Veterinary Medicine, Department of Obstetrics, Reproduction and Herd Health, Veterinary Epidemiology Unit, University of Ghent, 9820 Merelbeke, Belgium
[2] Faculty of Veterinary Medicine, Department of Pathology, Bacteriology and Avian Diseases, University of Ghent, 9820 Merelbeke, Belgium

1 What is biosecurity?

Biosecurity, as defined in this book, refers to the combination of all the different measures implemented to reduce the risk of introduction and spread of disease agents (Barceló and Marco, 1998; Amass and Clark, 1999). Biosecurity measures can be implemented at different levels such as country, region, herd or flock, and even individual animals. Implementing biosecurity involves adopting a set of attitudes and behaviour to reduce risk in all activities involving animal production or animal care. Biosecurity is based on the prevention of and protection against infectious agents. The measures to be established should not be seen as constraints but rather as part of a process aimed at improving the health of animals, people and the environment. Biosecurity can be subdivided in two main components: external biosecurity or sometimes also called bio-exclusion which is aimed at keeping pathogens out of the herd; and internal biosecurity or bio-management which focuses on preventing the spread of pathogens within the herd. Bio-containment (avoiding the spread of pathogens from herd to herd) is mainly associated with external biosecurity.

2 Why is biosecurity important?

Biosecurity is considered as the foundation of all disease control programmes. The aim of combining all biosecurity measures is to prevent both the introduction as well as the spread of infectious agents in a group of animals. As such it targets reducing the infection pressure exerted upon the animals. Effective biosecurity is the foundation of disease prevention, which can be complemented by additional preventive measures such as vaccination or use of feed additives. Biosecurity is important both in controlling exotic as well as endemic diseases. If biosecurity and disease prevention measures are well implemented it is possible to reduce curative treatment of diseased animals to an absolute minimum (Fig. 2.1). If biosecurity is well established then additional preventive measures will have a greater impact and the need for curative treatment can be kept to a minimum.

Fig. 2.1: Biosecurity as the foundation of all disease prevention programmes

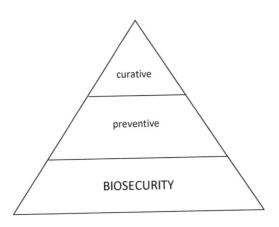

curative

preventive

BIOSECURITY

Improving biosecurity, and by consequence reducing infection pressure, may also result in substantial improvements in production results as well as reduced antimicrobial use as discussed in detail in chapter 3 that covers the relation between biosecurity and animal health/performance and the use of antimicrobials. In a recent study by Laanen et al. (2014) over 550 farmers were asked what motivated them to take disease prevention measures. The top 5 answers were: 1) to improve profit via higher productivity, 2) to obtain farm stability, 3) to improve quality and safety of their products, 4) to improve animal welfare and 5) to fulfil their duty to keep their animals healthy.

3 Biosecurity and disease transmission

As we describe in detail in Chapter 1 of this book (circles of disease transmission) infectious diseases can spread through many different transmission routes. The relative importance of the different routes depends greatly on the epidemiology of the pathogen in question. Transmission of some pathogens may be airborne, some may be transmitted through vectors and some may be spread through semen, etc. The goal of biosecurity measures is generally to prevent these different transmission routes in an attempt to break the infection cycle. When designing biosecurity measures one can either approach the topic from the point of view of one specific pathogen and design measures that are specifically adapted to the epidemiology of that pathogen. Alternatively, a biosecurity plan can be made much more generic (not disease specific) and include the majority of the transmission routes with a focus on those that are more important because they play a crucial role in the transmission routes of many different pathogens or because they are of importance in the transmission pathways of the most prevalent or damaging diseases. In the species-specific chapters of this book (pigs, poultry, cattle, horses, dogs, etc.) we will focus in general on generic biosecurity measures rather than disease-specific plans, as they are of greater general relevance and can be applied more widely.

4 The principles of biosecurity

When designing biosecurity programmes, there are some general principles that are of value in all different environments.

4.1 Separation of high- and low-risk animals and environments

To avoid disease transmission it is important to try to keep the sources of infection (e.g. animals, persons, vermin) separate from the susceptible contacts as much as possible. This can be achieved by preventing direct contact between high-risk (infectious) and low-risk (susceptible) animals as well as by preventing indirect contact (Fig. 2.2).

Fig. 2.2: The general aim of biosecurity measures is to prevent direct (e.g. animal to animal contact) and indirect (e.g. persons, vermin, vehicles) disease transmission ▼

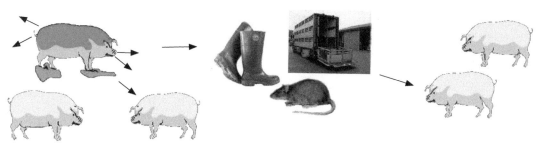

Whenever contact between the high- and low-risk animas or compartments cannot be avoided (e.g. buying new breeding stock, entrance of professional visitors, etc.) precautionary measures should be implemented (e.g. quarantine period, change of clothing and footwear, see further).

4.2 Reduction of the general infection pressure

Even with the best possible biosecurity it is not always possible, and probably not even desirable, to keep animals in sterile conditions. It is very hard therefore to prevent all contact with potential harmful infectious agents? However, the goal of biosecurity measures is to keep infection pressure below a level which allows the natural immunity of the animals to cope with the infections. Consequently, biosecurity is not a matter of 'all or nothing' but a matter of controlling the infection pressure as much as possible.

4.3 Not all transmission routes are of equal importance

As mentioned before some transmission routes may be highly efficient in spreading a wide range of different pathogens (e.g. direct animal contact), whereas other transmission routes (e.g. feed) are less efficient (Fig. 2.3). Therefore, when designing biosecurity control programmes, it is important to focus first on high-risk transmission routes and only subsequently on the lower-risk transmission routes. Emphasis is frequently and erroneously placed on wrong measures and a great deal of energy is put into preventing low-risk transmission routes and ignoring high-risk routes. This depends on the pathogen involved of course, because some are specifically associated with these so-called low transmission routes (e.g. some *Salmonella* serotypes in feed for poultry).

Fig. 2.3: Theoretical ranking of different routes for disease transmission from low- to high-risk (after Boklund et al., 2008)

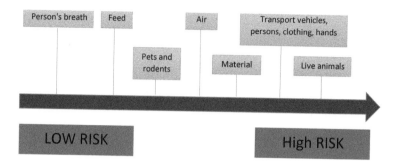

4.4 Risk is a combination of probability of transmission and frequency of occurrence of transmission routes

In addition to the probability of pathogen transmission via the different transmission routes, the frequency of occurrence of the transmission route is also highly significant. If a certain transmission route (e.g. transmission via the hand of animal carers) has a low probability of occurrence but the handling is repeated very frequently (e.g. animal carer touches the animals several times a day without precautionary measures), the risk of disease transmission ends up being very substantial. Therefore, when designing biosecurity programmes, one also has to focus on actions that are repeated very regularly as even if they are low-risk they will become important due to the frequency with which they are carried out.

4.5 Larger animal groups pose higher risks

The larger the herds or flocks, the more important the biosecurity measures will be. Large groups of animals obviously have more animals that may be infected and maintain an infection cycle and increase the infection pressure over the limit that the animals can cope with. Larger herds or flocks also have more frequent contact with the outside world (e.g. movement of animals, feed transport, professional visitors, etc.) all of which carry a certain risk of disease introduction. Also, in larger and more productive herds, high-producing animals may be more susceptible and the consequences of disease introduction may be more severe compared to smaller herds. We often see that farms gradually increase in size without fundamentally adapting the implemented biosecurity measures. In these cases the managers reason that they have worked according to a certain number of customs for many years without problem and do not understand why they should adapt. And yet, the risks related to disease introduction and spread are much more important in large herds.

5 The components of biosecurity

The main components of external and internal biosecurity are discussed below in general terms. In the species-specific or risk-specific chapters of this book all the different components are discussed in much greater detail and with references to the scientific literature describing all the measures and their impact.

5.1 External biosecurity

External biosecurity or bio-exclusion includes all measures taken to prevent the introduction of infectious agents into farms as well as the prevention of the spread of infectious agents from farms (bio-containment). External biosecurity measures are associated with all actions where there is contact between the farm and the outside world such as infrastructure aspects such as organisation of the farm buildings, presence of entrance restriction for animals and persons (e.g. hygiene lock, quarantine pen). They also include measures imposed upon others (e.g. restrictions of visitors, hygiene of transport vehicles, feed safety). In many instances external biosecurity is better understood and implemented by farmers than internal biosecurity. This is probably because external biosecurity measures received more attention in the past as they were promoted as a way of controlling epidemic diseases such as foot-and-mouth disease, classical swine fever and highly pathogenic avian influenza. As a result, countries with minimum legal requirements governing biosecurity focus in the main on external biosecurity measures.

Following are the main components of external biosecurity.

5.1.1 Purchase of animals and animal products

Any introduction of new animals or animal products (e.g. sperm, embryo's) involves the risk of unintended introduction of pathogens against which no farm immunity exists. As a consequence, the primary aim should be to avoid the purchase of animals or genetic material wherever possible. Direct contact between animals from different farms, through pasture contact for instance, should also be avoided. Moreover, in addition to the risk of disease introduction, the frequent addition of 'naïve' animals may also favour the continuous circulation of herd-specific pathogens. This may hamper the control and eradication of certain pathogens in groups of animals. If the introduction of new animals is unavoidable general rules state that the number of introductions should be limited, and even more importantly, the number of source herds or flocks should be limited. The latter should also have a documented (high) health status to avoid the introduction of at least a number of diseases. Upon arrival the new animals should always go straight to a quarantine stable completely separate from the rest of the farm buildings (this applies to pig herds for example, but not poultry flocks where an all-in, all-out principle is applied). The quarantine period should be sufficiently long to allow for the detection of clinical symptoms and the adaptation of new animals to their new environment (e.g. through vaccination).

5.1.2 Transport of animals, removal of manure and carcasses

Pathogens may spread through the transport of live animals and/or the removal of cadavers or manure. Animal transport vehicles should always be empty therefore, cleaned and disinfected before entering the premises. The premises should preferably also be split up into a clean and a dirty section. All inbound and outbound traffic that serves multiple companies and therefore carries a high risk should be directed via the dirty road. The clean road should be preserved for intra-farm movements and potential supply of animals – but only in fully cleaned and disinfected lorries – and for supply of harmless products. Manure should also be transported via the dirty road. Cadavers should always be treated as likely sources of infection and handled with specific attention therefore (e.g. use gloves when manipulating cadavers) and stored in a cooled and closed place. After pick-up the storage place should be thoroughly cleaned and disinfected.

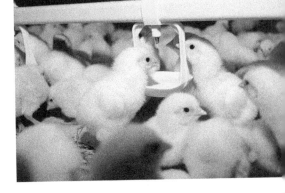

Fig. 2.4: Clean and safe water is of huge importance for the health of the animals

▼

5.1.3 Supply of fodder, water and equipment

Pathogens can be introduced and spread efficiently in herds through feed and especially through drinking water. Thorough management of the feed and drinking water facilities and regular quality and safety checks are highly advisable therefore (see chapter 9) (Fig. 2.4). Equipment that comes into contact with animals should also be disinfected before introduction and should not be exchanged between farms.

5.1.4 Access of personnel and visitors

Humans may act as a mechanical vector if they have been in contact with infected animals and then have contact with susceptible animals without taking precautionary measures. The first measure therefore is to keep the number of people with access to animal facilities to a minimum.

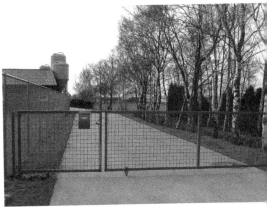

▲

Fig. 2.5: Provision of clear entrance control to avoid unwanted visitors

When visitors and personnel enter stables, they should always wear clean and herd- or flock-specific clothing and footwear and should wash their hands thoroughly. Hygiene locks should be available for this purpose that ensure a clear separation between the dirty and clean area.

A good hygiene lock should include a walk through concept in which the first area is the dirty part where clothing and footwear can be removed and hands can be washed. A bench should separate this area from the clean area where clean and herd-specific clothing and footwear are provided and which provides access to the stables (Fig. 2.6).

Fig. 2.6: Design of a hygiene lock

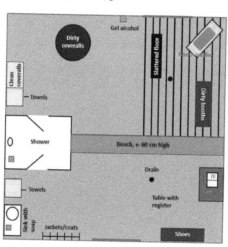

5.1.5 Vermin and bird control

A number of pathogens may be transmitted directly or indirectly by rodents, birds, dogs and cats, from outside the farm or between different compartments of the farm. They may also act as reservoirs for herd- or flock-specific pathogens that continue to circulate in the farm. All farms should have an efficient vermin control programme therefore. Their aim is to prevent vermin taking up residence in the barn surroundings. This can be achieved by removing different hiding places in the vicinity of the barns (e.g. plants, piles of dirt). Feed should also be stored in well closed rooms that vermin cannot access. Birds can be prevented from entering barns by covering all air inlets with nets that prevent entry. More info on insect and rodent control can be found in chapters 10 and 11.

5.1.6 Location and environment

Some diseases are spread via airborne transmission or through vectors. In these cases, the location of the farm is important and the proximity of neighbouring farms or slaughterhouses may be a risk. Wild animals may also be a source of diseases if they come into contact with farm animals. Good fencing to avoid contact between animals should be installed therefore in regions where wild animals are present. Airborne transmission can be avoided through air filtration which might be considered for high health farms (see chapter 7).

5.2 Internal biosecurity

Internal biosecurity or bio-management consists of all the measures taken to prevent spread of infectious agents within the farm from one age category to another or from one production group to another (and even within groups). Internal biosecurity measures are strongly linked to farm management and daily practice of animal carers (e.g. hygienic measures between compartments, working lines, cleaning and disinfection practices, etc.). Unlike external biosecurity measures, these are much more oriented towards controlling endemic infectious diseases. It was only more recently that attention started focusing on internal biosecurity measures. This is probably the result of the intensification of animal production where animal groups have become larger and more vulnerable, and where production efficacy is becoming more critical. Increased focus on reduced and responsible antimicrobial use in animal production has also drawn attention to internal biosecurity measures (see chapter 3. Biosecurity and its relation with animal health/performance and the use of antimicrobials).

These are the main components of internal biosecurity.

5.2.1 Disease management

To ensure good health among animals it is important to have a proper disease management strategy which includes correct han-

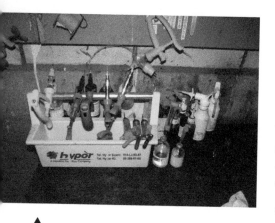

▲
Fig. 2.7: Badly stored needles, syringes and medicines may be a source of infection

dling and treatment of diseased animals, including proper diagnostics, isolation and disease registration as well as improving the immunity status of susceptible animals, particularly through vaccination. Diseased animals should be isolated in a sickbay in order to prevent other animals being exposed to pathogens. Treatment of animals should be performed carefully to avoid iatrogenic disease transmission. Needles for instance may become contaminated by a host of environmental germs through usage and storage and as such become efficient disease transmitters.

5.2.2 All in / All out (AI/AO)

The AI/AO principle helps to prevent cross-contamination between consecutive production batches and makes it possible to clean and disinfect the barns between different production batches. Strict application of the all-in/all-out principle is a very important measure in breaking the infection cycle between subsequent production batches. Slower growing animals in a batch (e.g. piglets, calves) should not be held back and added to the next batch of younger animals as these are likely to be carriers of one or more infectious diseases that will cause retarded growth and a source of infection among a younger susceptible age group.

5.2.3 Stocking density

High stocking density induces stress which results in an increased susceptibility to infections and an increased excretion of germs. Moreover high stocking density will also probably result in animal welfare issues. In general the legislative norms should be considered as minimum requirements rather than ideal values.

5.2.4 Compartmentalisation and working lines

Animals of different ages may have different degrees of susceptibility to certain pathogens and it is crucial therefore to keep different age groups apart and to work according to strict working lines starting at the youngest animals and ending with the oldest animals and finally the quarantine stable and sick bay. In order to avoid transferring germs on footwear, boot washers and disinfection baths can be placed between production units. For risk-bearing groups (e.g. quarantine stables, sickbay), an additional hygiene lock for changing clothing, footwear and washing hands is recommended in order to avoid pathogen spread between different age groups.

5.2.5 Cleaning and disinfecting

In order to break the infection cycle between consecutive production rounds, pens should be thoroughly cleaned and disinfected (C&D). This consists of seven steps: 1) dry cleaning and removal of all organic material; 2) soaking of all surfaces to loosen any remaining organic material; 3) high-pressure cleaning with water to remove all dirt; 4) drying the stable to avoid dilution of the disinfectant applied in the next step; 5) disinfection of the stable to further reduce the concentration of germs; 6) drying of the stable to ensure that animals cannot come into contact with pools of remaining disinfectant and 7) testing the efficiency of the procedure through surface sampling. This is discussed in detail in chapter 6.

6 Conclusions

There is no doubt that biosecurity is the foundation of any successful disease control programme. When designing biosecurity programs there are a number of general principles that should be taken into account irrespective of the animal species. Both external and internal biosecurity measures are of utmost importance in preventing the introduction of pathogens on farms and avoiding disease spread between animal populations on farms. Once a biosecurity programme has been developed, it implementation will only be successful if all the partners involved (farmers, veterinarians, authorities, advisors, et.) cooperate and are sufficiently motivated to adhere to the rules.

References

Boklund, A., 2008. Exotic disease in swine: Evaluation of biosecurity and control of strategies for classical swine fever. PhD Thesis, Denmark.

Barceló, J. and Marco, E., 1998. On-farm biosecurity. In: Proceedings of the 15th IPVS Congress, Birmingham, England, 5-9 July, 129-133.

Amass, S.F. and Clark, L.K., 1999. Biosecurity considerations for pork production units. *Journal of Swine Health and Production* 7, 217-228

CHAPTER 3

BIOSECURITY AND ITS RELATIONSHIP WITH HEALTH, PRODUCTION AND ANTIMICROBIAL USE

Merel Postma[1]

Jeroen Dewulf[1]

[1] Faculty of Veterinary Medicine, Department of Reproduction, Veterinary Epidemiology Unit, University of Ghent, 9820 Merelbeke, Belgium

1 Introduction

It is very often argued that improving biosecurity in animal production has many positive effects on animal health and production, and although this is rarely disputed, until recent relatively little quantitative data was available to support these statements. Yet in the last decade we have seen a substantial increase in interest in this topic resulting in more and better insights. In this chapter therefore, we try to summarise the current scientific data available on the relationship between biosecurity and health, production and antimicrobial use. The latter is an increasingly important aspect as it is linked to the selection of antimicrobial resistance and therefore forms a risk both for animal and human health. Moreover, describing the benefits of implementing biosecurity measures may also provide strong motivation for those who have to implement these measures on a daily basis.

2 Biosecurity and health

As discussed in chapter 2, the basic principles of biosecurity are 1) the separation of infected and diseased animals through the prevention of direct and indirect contact and 2) the reduction of the general infection pressure. Improvements in biosecurity aim at reducing the introduction and spread of disease, resulting in reduced morbidity and mortality rates, making biosecurity a tool in eradication programmes as well as in daily herd health management (Maes et al., 2008; Lambert et al., 2012a; Zhang et al., 2013; Gillespie et al., 2015; Postma et al., 2015b; Postma et al., 2016a; Postma et al., 2016c; Postma et al., 2017). The study by Postma et al. (2016a) revealed that the number of treatments against certain disease symptoms (e.g. respiratory, gastrointestinal, etc.) was significantly lower in farms with higher internal and external biosecurity. Laanen et al. (2013) and Postma et al. (2016b) described a positive association between biosecurity and reduced antimicrobial use, suggesting a reduced need for the use of antibiotics, possibly due to a higher health status in herds benefiting from a higher biosecurity level. In the case of ruminants, several publications, describing the opinions of farmers and experts, emphasise the importance of biosecurity in improving health (Hoe and Ruegg, 2006; Laanen et al., 2014; Sahlström et al., 2014; Postma et al., 2016c; Shortall et al., 2017). Shortall et al. (2017) for example described that keeping a closed herd was rated as the most effective measure for preventing disease-causing agents from entering or leaving any place where farm animals are present. The *Salmonella* status in ruminants can be influenced by biosecurity measures as well, as shown by Ågren et al. (2017). They reported that the presence of *Salmonella* test-positive herds within a 5-km radius or the presence of rodents presented important risk factors (Ågren et al., 2017). Velkers et al. (2017) described the importance of biosecurity in poultry production for the prevention of *Campylobacter* and Avian Influenza. With emerging diseases threatening horses in the European Union, the implementation of biosecurity measures in the equine sector has been stimulated as well (Nixon, 2015). Descriptions of the importance of implementing biosecurity measures in sheep (Sahlström et al., 2014; Schimmer et al., 2014) and goat production (Bond et al., 2015) have also appeared, in relation to the prevention of *Coxiella burnetii* (Q fever) infections for example.

It has been noted that farmers perceive biosecurity as a tool for reducing disease. An online questionnaire, conducted in Belgium among 218 pig, 279 cattle and 61 poultry farmers, found that approximately half of the respondents were convinced of the positive effect of biosecurity on the reduction of disease at their farms (Laanen et al., 2014). At the same time many scientific publications described important shortcomings in on-farm levels of biosecurity (Brennan and Christley, 2012; Ssematimba et al., 2013; Gosling et al., 2014; Sarrazin et al., 2014; Backhans et al., 2015; Pritchard et al., 2015; Hernández-Jover et al., 2016; Postma et al., 2016a; Millman et al., 2017) suggesting that there is still much room for improvement.

Results of intervention studies showing the effect of improved biosecurity on animal health are scarcer. Improved biosecurity in pig production was proven to be beneficial, as a single intervention or in combination with vaccinations for instance, in reducing problems with porcine reproductive and respiratory syndrome virus (PRRSV) (Rathkjen and Dall, 2017), *Mycoplasma hyopneumoniae* (Maes et al., 2008), *Salmonella spp.* (Taker and Bilkei, 2007; Fraser et al., 2010; Gotter et al., 2012; Andres and Davies, 2015), *Yersinia spp.* (Vanantwerpen et al., 2017) or even parasitic infections (Kungu et al., 2017). In ruminants improvements in the level of biosecurity have been described in relation to Johne's disease (Ritter et al., 2016). In beef suckler farms in the United Kingdom a significant drop in the probability of seropositivity was seen for bovine viral diarrhoea virus (BVDV) and *Leptospira hardjo* in intervention farms with improved biosecurity measures compared to control farms (Cardwell et al., 2016). In poultry the positive effect of improved biosecurity is mainly described for *Campylobacter spp.* (Georgiev et al., 2016; Smith et al., 2016) and *Salmonella spp.* (Fraser et al., 2010). The study of Georgiev et al. (2016) describes that enhanced biosecurity reduces the odds of colonisation with *Campylobacter* at partial depopulation (OR= 0.25) and final depopulation (OR= 0.47). Another intervention study in poultry production resulted in a 50% reduction in *Campylobacter* colonisation thanks to biosecurity measures such as disinfection baths for boots or changing boots and washing hands (Gibbens et al., 2001). In some cases the focus merely on biosecurity in itself resulted in a reduction of pathogens as illustrated in the study by Sandberg et al. (2017), that revealed that by simply enhancing the focus on compliance with mandatory biosecurity it was possible to reach a reduction of *Campylobacter jejuni* in poultry.

Improvements in biosecurity in animal production could also reduce the risk of the transmission of zoonotic pathogens. Vanantwerpen et al. (2017), for example, described that the seropositivity of pigs to *Yersinia spp.* was associated with an increasing number of piglet suppliers, a high pig density in the area, the use of semi-slatted floors in the fattening unit and the possibility of snout contact. The importance of both internal and external biosecurity was shown by Pletinckx et al. (2013) in relation to the prevalence of methicillin-resistant *Staphylococcus aureus* (MRSA) in poultry, dairy cattle, pigs and humans. Significant risk factors for the seroprevalence of *Coxiella burnetii* in Dutch dairy and non-dairy sheep farms were the location, the number of supplying farms, goat density in the area and wearing farm-specific clothing and boots (Schimmer et al., 2014). As mentioned above, the risk of introduction and spread of zoonotic poultry pathogens *Campylobacter* and *Salmonella* could also be reduced by implementing biosecurity measures (Gibbens et al., 2001; Fraser et al., 2010; Georgiev et al., 2016). Osimani et al. (2017) specifically described the implementation of biosecurity measures such as rodent control and drinking water hygiene in relation to zoonotic campylobacteriosis. Many papers, such as one by Ssematimba et al. (2013), describe the importance of biosecurity in relation to Avian Influenza. Moran et al. (2017) studied the risk of zoonotic pathogen transmission, e.g. *Salmonella*, *Leptospira*, *Escherichia coli* or intestinal parasites, between dogs, livestock and people. The results of this study highlight the importance of keeping pet animals out of the stables (Moran et al., 2017). Furthermore an expert survey by Léger et al. (2017) highlighted the importance of biosecurity measures in relation to (re) emerging (zoonotic) diseases such as Blue Tongue virus, Classical Swine Fever and Rabies.

3 Biosecurity and production

A study carried out in Belgium, France, Germany and Sweden found a positive association between a higher level of external biosecurity and the number of weaned piglets per sow per year (Fig. 3.1) (Postma et al., 2016a). Furthermore, there was a strong association between internal and external biosecurity, possibly suggesting an indirect link between biosecurity and other parameters as shown in figure 3.1. The results obtained in this study concurred with a study by Dors et al. (2013), that described a higher number of pigs born per sow per year and sold per year in herds with a proper level of biosecurity. Using the same data as the studies by Postma et al. (2016a), Collineau et al. (2017a) described the profile of 'top-farms' that manage to combine both high technical performance and low antimicrobial use. The top-farms had fewer gastro-intestinal symptoms in suckling piglets and fewer respiratory symptoms in finishers, partly explaining their reduced need for antimicrobials and higher performance. On the other hand the top-farms' biosecurity level was higher and the herds were mainly located in sparsely populated pig areas. Internal biosecurity acquired a higher score in the top-farms thanks in particular to better compartmentalisation of the production units and appropriate use of equipment. Disease management (e.g. diseased animal were isolated and consistently handled after healthy animals) was also better in the top-farms. The top-farms furthermore showed a tendency towards better biosecurity practices for personnel and visitors (Collineau et al., 2017a). However a word of caution is required as one needs to remain cautious when interpreting these results as these associations do not prove a direct causal relationship and other potentially related factors such as overall herd management, genetics, feeding, etc. may have influenced the observed association.

Fig. 3.1: Causal pathway with statistically significant associations in the multivariable models between several herd management, production variables and internal and external biosecurity scores in farrow-to-finish pig herds. Gender person farrowing = gender of the person responsible for taking care of the pigs in the farrowing unit, #= number. Black lines represent the result of a multi-variable linear regression analysis based on data from 4 EU countries. The light grey dotted lines indicate a significant effect between these parameters exclusively through interaction with the country. The p-values correspond to the multi-variable model. All models were corrected for the country effect by placing country as a fixed variable in the model, hence the circle around the Figure. Source: Postma et al. (2016a).

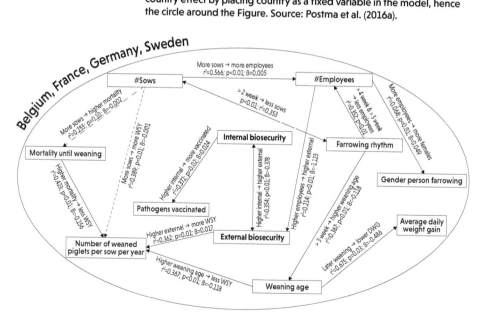

Nevrkla et al. (2014) described a study in which a sow herd was repopulated with minimum disease gilts in a decontaminated stable. This resulted in a higher numbers of piglets produced. An intervention study in Belgium (Postma et al., 2017) describes the improvement in the level of biosecurity and herd management without jeopardising the production parameters and at the same time reducing antimicrobial use. Biosecurity levels were improved by 3.8% for external biosecurity and 14.2% for internal biosecurity based on the biocheck.ugent scoring system (see chapter 5 on measuring biosecurity). Some technical parameters, e.g. number of weaned piglets per sow per year (+1.1), daily weight gain (+5.9 g/day) and mortality in the finisher period (-0.6%), were even positively influenced in the intervention period of +/- 8 months. In an earlier study in Belgium, Laanen et al. (2013) found that the biosecurity variables of 'removal of animals, manure and cadavers', 'vermin and bird control', 'fattening unit' and 'cleaning and disinfection' were positively associated with the daily weight gain in finishers.

Although more research into several animal species would be needed in order to further elaborate on the positive effects of biosecurity on animal production, the above-mentioned results suggest that improvements in the level of biosecurity would be highly likely to result in the better technical performance of a herd.

4 Biosecurity and antimicrobial use

When experts in pig health were asked to rank alternatives to antimicrobial agents based on their perceived effectiveness, feasibility and return on investment, biosecurity ranked first for internal and second for external biosecurity, suggesting that improvements in biosecurity are perceived as the most promising alternative to antimicrobial use in pig production (Postma et al., 2015b).

Several other studies have also demonstrated this relationship. Fertner et al. (2015) described that Danish weaner farms using a lower volume of antimicrobials than the national median, had shown similarities relating to separating sections on farms and using all in / all out procedures with subsequent cleaning, which are two important biosecurity measures. Moreover, in breeder-finisher pig herds in Belgium it was found that herds with higher internal bio-security scores had lower antimicrobial treatment incidences, suggesting that improved biosecurity might help in reducing the use of antimicrobials (Laanen et al., 2013). A significant association was found between disinfection of the loading area, gilt quarantine and adaptation, farm structure/working lines and all in / all out practices and lower antimicrobial use in French breeder-finishers herds (Lannou et al., 2012). A recent study in four European countries revealed a significant association between higher weaning age, a week system of five weeks or more and external biosecurity and a lower antimicrobial treatment incidence (Fig. 3.2) (Postma et al., 2016b). This finding was confirmed by Collineau et al. (2017a) who studied the profile of top-farmers. In this study a particularly positive association was discovered between the level of internal biosecurity and a better control of infectious diseases and a reduced need for antimicrobials (Collineau et al., 2017a).

Fig. 3.2: Causal pathway associations for TI 200 days and TI Breeding. Causal pathway with statistically significant associations in the multivariable models for the TI 200 days and the TI Breeding associated with production, management or biosecurity variables. TI= treatment incidence (antimicrobial use quantification), WSY= number of weaned piglets per sow per year. Black lines represent the result of a multivariable linear regression analysis based on data from 4 EU countries. The light grey line indicates 0.05 < p < 0.10. The p-values and ß-values correspond to the multi-variable model. All models were corrected for the country effect by placing country as a fixed variable in the model, hence the circle around the Figure. Source: Postma et al. (2016b).

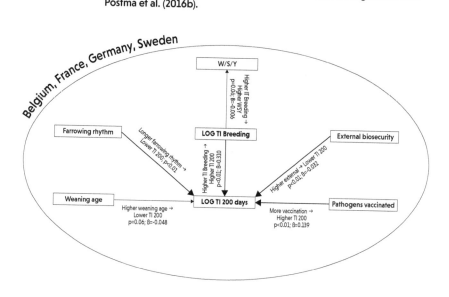

External and internal biosecurity are shown to be highly corre-
lated to each other (Postma et al., 2016a). Given this correlation
it is possible that the effects observed to result from internal biosecurity improvement, could generate similar effects on antimicrobial use from birth until slaughter if external biosecurity is also
improved, or vice versa. Since improving internal biosecurity level
can be a rather simple intervention (e.g. strict hygiene protocols,
correct use of working lines) at herd level, it could be an important
consideration in the reduction of antimicrobial use.

In Denmark an investigation was carried out into which measures implemented by farmers and their veterinarians resulted in
a reduction in their annual antimicrobial consumption of ≥10%
following the introduction of the 'Yellow Card system'. Amongst
others, they found that cleaning procedures, adequate action
regarding diseased animals (e.g. earlier decision to euthanize) and
all-in/all-out are all regarded by farmers and veterinarians as good
measures to reduce antimicrobial use (Dupont et al., 2017). A
study by Dohmen et al. (2017) concluded that improved biosecurity, especially the presence of a hygiene lock and pest control by a
professional, were associated with a lower likelihood of extended-
spectrum beta-lactamase (ESBL)-*Escherichia coli*-positive farms.
Tests for methicillin-resistant *Staphylococcus aureus* (MRSA) in
animals and personnel in dairy herds with closely related pig herds
revealed that a high MRSA prevalence in milk samples was associated with poor hygiene during milking routines (e.g. milkers not
wearing gloves) (Locatelli et al., 2017).

An intervention study carried out in Flanders, Belgium, succeeded
in reducing antimicrobial use from birth to slaughter by 52% and
in the sows by 32% by improving herd management and biosecurity levels in combination with antimicrobial stewardship (Fig. 3.3)
(Postma et al., 2017). In this study, the management and biosecurity interventions that were implemented by the farmers were
generally relatively simple to implement. They involved changing
the working habits and routines of the farmer himself (e.g. changing needles, hand and personal hygiene, analysis of water quality). Interventions incurring high costs and/or more pronounced

changes, such as introducing a new hygiene lock to change clothes/ boots and wash hands, were implemented less frequently. An important focus of the suggested advice was a good and early registration of disease symptoms in order to be able to take proper and timely control measures (e.g. biosecurity, vaccination, climate changes) and to create awareness about the importance of the 'prevention is better than cure' principle. An important success factor of the Postma et al. (2017) study was the order of action: 'check, improve and reduce'. This implies that herd counselling always started with a thorough evaluation of the herd management, biosecurity and health situation followed by tailored advice with specific suggestions for improvement. In this process it is important that an advisor/coach helps the farmer by explaining what he/she could improve along with outlining the risk when certain practices are not performed correctly. In addition, follow up and feedback on the agreed and implemented improvements is of great importance in order to retain levels of motivation. Only after implementation

Fig. 3.3: Graphical visualisation of reduction in antimicrobial usage in breeding animals (sows), piglets, finishers or over the total period from birth to slaughter after 61 herds were given recommendations to improve herd management, biosecurity and to use antimicrobials more prudently. The values in the bars represent the antimicrobial use for prophylactic use (red) or curative use (green) and lighter colours represent the results of antimicrobial use after carrying out the interventions. The percentage above the bars represents the reduction in antimicrobial use that was achieved over all participating herds. Standard = (routine) prophylactic antimicrobial use.

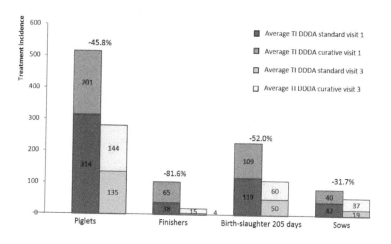

of these improvements, can changes and reductions in antimicrobial use be suggested. By taking this approach, farmers are able to maintain control of the health situation and are less reluctant to change certain antimicrobial treatment procedures.

A comparable type of intervention study performed in Belgium on 15 broiler farms resulted in an average reduction of 29% in antimicrobial use, by improving the level of biosecurity by 5% for external biosecurity and 4% for internal biosecurity according to the biocheck.ugent scoring system (see chapter 5 on measuring biosecurity) (Gelaude et al., 2013).
Studies into other animal species describing the associations between biosecurity and antimicrobial usage are scarce. However, the results obtained in pig production could be applied to other (farm) animals. Improvements in the level of biosecurity should be an essential cornerstone in the effort to reduce antimicrobial use in herds or flocks.

5 Economic impact of improved biosecurity

Farmers do not always perceive improvement in biosecurity as feasible or cost-effective, mainly because they lack information about the cost and in particular the revenues (Fraser et al., 2010; Laanen et al., 2014). Research and field experiments showing that improvement in the biosecurity status is beneficial for farm performances and that it could be economically feasible were described therefore as being of utmost importance in convincing farmers according to several authors (Casal et al., 2007; Valeeva et al., 2011; Laanen et al., 2014). Corrégé I. et al. (2012) made an inventory of the application of biosecurity measures in 77 breeder-finisher herds in France. They showed that the difference in standardised margins between farms with high biosecurity and those with lower levels were estimated at around € 200/sow per year (Corrégé I. et al., 2012).
In the case of African swine fever, Fasina et al. (2012) described a model resulting in a cost-benefit ratio of 29 obtained by the implementation of biosecurity measures and the monitoring thereof. An

economic evaluation based on the results of the study by Postma et al. (2017) has shown, that on average the participating herds achieved a financial gain or overall benefit (including labour costs of all persons involved: coach, veterinarian, farmer, etc.) of € 2.67/ finisher pig per year by partaking in this 'team effort' approach to improve herd management and biosecurity and reduce antimicrobial use (Rojo-Gimeno C. and Postma M. et al., 2016). In a comparable study carried out in four European Union countries, an economic evaluation of proposed interventions in biosecurity among others, resulted in a median change in net farm profit among Belgian and French farms estimated at € 4.46 and € 1.23 per sow per year, respectively (Collineau et al., 2017b).

Although it is tempting to try to deduce a list of most influential or promising biosecurity measures from all the above, it assumed that this is impossible as effective biosecurity advice has to be tailored to the specific herd. In some herds or situations one type of measurement will be the most important and influential whereas in other herds a totally different measure is required. This is simply due to the fact that all herds are different and require different levels of implementation of the different biosecurity measures.

6 Conclusions

Based on the literature review presented we can conclude that there is sufficient data available revealing that good biosecurity in animal production does result in improved animal health and subsequent improvements in technical performances. A very important additional effect is the fact that biosecurity is also an important tool in the reduction of antimicrobial use and the fight against antimicrobial resistance. Finally very recent publications have also shown that all of this is also economically beneficial which should motivate farmers to implement even more biosecurity measures.

References

Ågren, E.C.C., Frössling, J., Wahlström, H., Emanuelson, U., Sternberg Lewerin, S., 2017. A questionnaire study of associations between potential risk factors and salmonella status in Swedish dairy herds. Preventive Veterinary Medicine 143, 21-29.

Alarcon, P., Rushton, J., Nathues, H., Wieland, B., 2013. Economic efficiency analysis of different strategies to control post-weaning multi-systemic wasting syndrome and porcine circovirus type 2 subclinical infection in 3-weekly batch system farms. Preventive Veterinary Medicine 110, 103-118.

Andres, V.M., Davies, R.H., 2015. Biosecurity Measures to Control Salmonella and Other Infectious Agents in Pig Farms: A Review. Comprehensive Reviews in Food Science and Food Safety 14, 317-335.

Arruda, A.G., Poljak, Z., Friendship, R., Carpenter, J., Hand, K., 2015. Descriptive analysis and spatial epidemiology of porcine reproductive and respiratory syndrome (PRRS) for swine sites participating in area regional control and elimination programs from 3 regions of Ontario. Canadian Journal of Veterinary Research-Revue Canadienne De Recherche Veterinaire 79, 268-278.

Backhans, A., Sjölund, M., Lindberg, A., Emanuelson, U., 2015. Biosecurity level and health management practices in 60 Swedish farrow-to-finish herds. Acta Veterinaria Scandinavica 57, 14.

Boerlage, A.S., Dung, T.T., Hoa, T.T.T., Davidson, J., Stryhn, H., Hammell, K.L., 2017. Production of red tilapia (Oreochromis spp.) in floating cages in the Mekong Delta, Vietnam: mortality and health management. Diseases of Aquatic Organisms 124, 131-144.

Boklund, A., Alban, L., Mortensen, S., Houe, H., 2004. Biosecurity in 116 Danish fattening swineherds: descriptive results and factor analysis. Preventive Veterinary Medicine 66, 49-62.

Bond, K.A., Vincent, G., Wilks, C.R., Franklin, L., Sutton, B., Stenos, J., Cowan, R., Lim, K., Athan, E., Harris, O., Macfarlane-Berry, L., Segal, Y., Firestone, S.M., 2015. One Health approach to controlling a Q fever outbreak on an Australian goat farm. Epidemiology & Infection FirstView, 1-13.

Brennan, M.L., Christley, R.M., 2012. Biosecurity on cattle farms: A study in North West England. PLoS ONE 7, e28139.

Brennan, M.L., Christley, R.M., 2013. Cattle producers' perceptions of biosecurity. BMC Veterinary Journal 9, 71.

Cardwell, J.M., Van Winden, S., Beauvais, W., Mastin, A., De Glanville, W.A., Hardstaff, J., Booth, R.E., Fishwick, J., Pfeiffer, D.U., 2016. Assessing the impact of tailored biosecurity advice on farmer behaviour and pathogen presence in beef herds in England and Wales. Preventive Veterinary Medicine 135, 9-16.

Casal, J., De Manuel, A., Mateu, E., Martín, M., 2007. Biosecurity measures on swine farms in Spain: Perceptions by farmers and their relationship to current on-farm measures. Preventive Veterinary Medicine 82, 138-150.

Collineau, L., Backhans, A., Dewulf, J., Emanuelson, U., grosse Beilage, E., Lehébel, A., Lösken, S., Okholm Nielsen, E., Postma, M., Sjölund, M., Stärk, K.D.C., Belloc, C., 2017a. Profile of pig farms combining high performance and low antimicrobial use within four European countries. Veterinary Record In press.

Collineau, L., Rojo-Gimeno, C., Léger, A., Backhans, A., Loesken, S., Nielsen, E.O., Postma, M., Emanuelson, U., Beilage, E.g., Sjölund, M., Wauters, E., Stärk, K.D.C., Dewulf, J., Belloc, C., Krebs, S., 2017b. Herd-specific interventions to reduce antimicrobial use in pig production without jeopardising technical and economic performance. Preventive Veterinary Medicine 144, 167-178.

Corrégé I., Fourchon P., Le Brun, T., Berthelot, N., 2012. Biosécurité et hygiène en élevage de porcs : état des lieux et impact sur les performances technico-économiques. Journées Recherche Porcine 44, 101-102.

Dohmen, W., Dorado-García, A., Bonten, M.J.M., Wagenaar, J.A., Mevius, D., Heederik, D.J.J., 2017. Risk factors for ESBL-producing Escherichia coli on pig farms: A longitudinal study in the context of reduced use of antimicrobials. PLOS ONE 12, e0174094.

Dors, A., Czyzewska, E., Pomorska-Mól, M., Kolacz, R., Pejsak, Z., 2013. Effect of various husbandry conditions on the production parameters of swine herds in Poland. Polish Journal of Veterinary Sciences 16, 707-713.

Dupont, N., Diness, L.H., Fertner, M., Kristensen, C.S., Stege, H., 2017. Antimicrobial reduction measures applied in Danish pig herds following the introduction of the 'Yellow Card' antimicrobial scheme. Preventive Veterinary Medicine 138, 9-16.

East, I.J., Davis, J., Sergeant, E.S.G., Garner, M.G., 2014. Structure, dynamics and movement patterns of the Australian pig industry. Australian Veterinary Journal 92, 52-57.

Fasina, F.O., Lazarus, D.D., Spencer, B.T., Makinde, A.A., Bastos, A.D.S., 2012. Cost Implications of African Swine Fever in Smallholder Farrow-to-Finish Units: Economic Benefits of Disease Prevention Through Biosecurity. Transboundary and Emerging Diseases 59, 244-255.

Fertner, M., Boklund, A., Dupont, N., Enoe, C., Stege, H., Toft, N., 2015. Weaner production with low antimicrobial use: a descriptive study. Acta Veterinaria Scandinavica 57, 38.

Figi, R., Goldinger, F., Fuschini, E., Hartnack, S., Sidler, X., 2014. Modifizierte Dysenterie-Teilsanierung in einem Kernzuchtschweinebetrieb. Schweizer Archiv für Tierheilkunde 156, 373-380.

Fraser, R.W., Williams, N.T., Powell, L.F., Cook, A.J.C., 2010. Reducing Campylobacter and Salmonella Infection: Two Studies of the Economic Cost and Attitude to Adoption of On-farm Biosecurity Measures. Zoonoses and Public Health 57, e109-e115.

Gelaude, P., Postma, M., Schlepers, M., Vanderhaeghen, W., Maes, D., J., D., 2013. Eindverslag van het project RED AB pluimvee. Ghent University, Merelbeke, Belgium, 29.

Georgiev, M., Beauvais, W., Guitian, J., 2016. Effect of enhanced biosecurity and selected on-farm factors on Campylobacter colonization of chicken broilers. Epidemiology and Infection 145, 553-567.

Gibbens, J.C., Pascoe, S.J.S., Evans, S.J., Davies, R.H., Sayers, A.R., 2001. A trial of biosecurity as a means to control Campylobacter infection of broiler chickens. Preventive Veterinary Medicine 48, 85-99.

Gillespie, A.V., Grove-White, D.H., Williams, H.J., 2015. Husbandry, health and biosecurity of the smallholder and pet pig population in England. Veterinary Record 177, 47.

Gosling, R.J., Martelli, F., Wintrip, A., Sayers, A.R., Wheeler, K., Davies, R.H., 2014. Assessment of producers' response to Salmonella biosecurity issues and uptake of advice on laying hen farms in England and Wales. British Poultry Science 55, 559-568.

Gotter, V., Klein, G., Koesters, S., Kreienbrock, L., Blaha, T., Campe, A., 2012. Main risk factors for Salmonella infections in pigs in north-western Germany. Preventive Veterinary Medicine 106, 301-307.

Hernández-Jover, M., Higgins, V., Bryant, M., Rast, L., McShane, C., 2016. Biosecurity and the management of emergency animal disease among commercial beef producers in New South Wales and Queensland (Australia). Preventive Veterinary Medicine 134, 92-102.

Hoe, F.G.H., Ruegg, P.L., 2006. Opinions and Practices of Wisconsin Dairy Producers About Biosecurity and Animal Well-Being. Journal of Dairy Science 89, 2297-2308.

Hybschmann, G.K., Ersbøll, A.K., Vigre, H., Baadsgaard, N.P., Houe, H., 2011. Herd-level risk factors for antimicrobial demanding gastrointestinal diseases in Danish herds with finisher pigs: A register-based study. Preventive Veterinary Medicine 98, 190-197.

Ikwap, K., Erume, J., Owiny, D.O., Nasinyama, G.W., Melin, L., Bengtsson, B., Lundeheim, N., Fellström, C., Jacobson, M., 2014. Salmonella species in piglets and weaners from Uganda: Prevalence, antimicrobial resistance and herd-level risk factors. Preventive Veterinary Medicine 115, 39-47.

Julio Pinto, C., Santiago Urcelay, V., 2003. Biosecurity practices on intensive pig production systems in Chile. Preventive Veterinary Medicine 59, 139-145.

Kungu, J.M., Dione, M.M., Ejobi, F., Ocaido, M., Grace, D., 2017. Risk factors, perceptions and practices associated with Taenia solium cysticercosis and its control in the smallholder pig production systems in Uganda: a cross-sectional survey. BMC Infectious Diseases 17, 1.

Laanen, M., Maes, D., Hendriksen, C., Gelaude, P., De Vliegher, S., Rosseel, Y., Dewulf, J., 2014. Pig, cattle and poultry farmers with a known interest in research have comparable perspectives on disease prevention and on-farm biosecurity. Preventive Veterinary Medicine 115, 1-9.

Laanen, M., Persoons, D., Ribbens, S., de Jong, E., Callen, B., Strubbe, M., Maes, D., Dewulf, J., 2013. Relationship between biosecurity and production/antimicrobial treatment characteristics in pig herds. The Veterinary Journal 198, 508-512.

Lambert, M.-È., Arsenault, J., Poljak, Z., D'Allaire, S., 2012a. Epidemiological investigations in regard to porcine reproductive and respiratory syndrome (PRRS) in Quebec, Canada. Part 2: Prevalence and risk factors in breeding sites. Prev Vet Med 104.

Lambert, M.-È., Arsenault, J., Poljak, Z., D'Allaire, S., 2012b. Epidemiological investigations in regard to porcine reproductive and respiratory syndrome (PRRS) in Quebec, Canada. Part 2: Prevalence and risk factors in breeding sites. Preventive Veterinary Medicine 104, 84-93.

Lambert, M.È., Poljak, Z., Arsenault, J., D'Allaire, S., 2012c. Epidemiological investigations in regard to porcine reproductive and respiratory syndrome (PRRS) in Quebec, Canada. Part 1: Biosecurity practices and their geographical distribution in two areas of different swine density. Preventive Veterinary Medicine 104, 74-83.

Lannou, J., Hémonic A., Delahaye, A.-C., Guinaudeau, J., Corrégé I., Morvan, R., Gueguen, F., Lewandowski, E., Adam, M., 2012. Antibiotiques en elevage porcin: modalites d'usage et relation avec les pratiques d'elevage. Association Française de Médecine Vétérinaire Porcine.

Léger, A., De Nardi, M., Simons, R., Adkin, A., Ru, G., Estrada-Peña, A., Stärk, K.D.C., 2017. Assessment of biosecurity and control measures to prevent incursion and to limit spread of emerging transboundary animal diseases in Europe: An expert survey. Vaccine.

Leslie, E.E.C., Geong, M., Abdurrahman, M., Ward, M.P., Toribio, J., 2015. A description of smallholder pig production systems in eastern Indonesia. Preventive Veterinary Medicine 118, 319-327.

Locatelli, C., Cremonesi, P., Caprioli, A., Carfora, V., Ianzano, A., Barberio, A., Morandi, S., Casula, A., Castiglioni, B., Bronzo, V., Moroni, P., 2017. Occurrence of methicillin-resistant Staphylococcus aureus in dairy cattle herds, related swine farms, and humans in contact with herds. Journal of Dairy Science 100, 608-619.

Maes, D., Segales, J., Meyns, T., Sibila, M., Pieters, M., Haesebrouck, F., 2008. Control of Myco-plasma hyopneumoniae infections in pigs. Veterinary Microbiology 126, 297-309.

Meunier, M., Guyard-Nicodème, M., Dory, D., Chemaly, M., 2015. Control Strategies against Campylobacter at the Poultry Production Level: Biosecurity Measures, Feed Additives and Vaccination. Journal of Applied Microbiology, n/a-n/a.

Millman, C., Christley, R., Rigby, D., Dennis, D., O'Brien, S.J., Williams, N., 2017. 'Catch 22': Biosecurity awareness, interpretation and practice amongst poultry catchers. Preventive Veterinary Medicine 141, 22-32.

Moran, N.E., Ferketich, A.K., Wittum, T.E., Stull, J.W., 2017. Dogs on livestock farms: A cross-sectional study investigating potential roles in zoonotic pathogen transmission. Zoonoses and Public Health, https://www.ncbi.nlm.nih.gov/pubmed/28677886.

Nantima, N., Ocaido, M., Ouma, E., Davies, J., Dione, M., Okoth, E., Mugisha, A., Bishop, R., 2015. Risk factors associated with occurrence of African swine fever outbreaks in smallholder pig farms in four districts along the Uganda-Kenya border. Tropical Animal Health and Pro-duction 47, 589-595.

Nevrkla, P., Cechova, M., Hadas, Z., 2014. Use of repopulation for optimizing sow reproductive performance and piglet loss. Acta Veterinaria Brno 83, 321-325.

Nieuwenhuis, N., Duinhof, T.F., van Nes, A., 2012. Economic analysis of outbreaks of porcine reproductive and respiratory syndrome virus in nine sow herds. Veterinary Record 170, 225.

Nixon, J., 2015. Learning about equine biosecurity. Veterinary Record 176, i-ii.

Olofsson, E., Noremark, M., Lewerin, S.S., 2014. Patterns of between-farm contacts via profes-sionals in Sweden. Acta Veterinaria Scandinavica 56.

Osimani, A., Aquilanti, L., Pasquini, M., Clementi, F., 2017. Prevalence and risk factors for ther-motolerant species of Campylobacter in poultry meat at retail in Europe. Poultry Science 96, 3382-3391.

Pletinckx, L.J., Verhegghe, M., Crombé, F., Dewulf, J., De Bleecker, Y., Rasschaert, G., Butaye, P., Goddeeris, B.M., De Man, I., 2013. Evidence of possible methicillin-resistant Staphylococcus aureus ST398 spread between pigs and other animals and people residing on the same farm. Preventive Veterinary Medicine 109, 293-303.

Postma, M., Stärk, K.D.C., Sjölund, M., Backhans, A., Beilage, E.G., Lösken, S., Belloc, C., Col-lineau, L., Iten, D., Visschers, V., Nielsen, E.O., Dewulf, J., 2015a. Alternatives to the use of antimicrobial agents in pig production: A multi-country expert-ranking of perceived effective-ness, feasibility and return on investment. Preventive Veterinary Medicine 118, 457-466.

Postma, M., Backhans, A., Collineau, L., Loesken, S., Sjölund, M., Belloc, C., . . . Dewulf, J. (2016). The biosecurity status and its associations with production and management characteristics in farrow-to-finish pig herds. Animal, 10(3), 478-489. doi:10.1017/S1751731115002487.

Postma, M., Backhans, A., Collineau, L., Loesken, S., Sjölund, M., Belloc, C., Emanuelson, U., grosse Beilage, E., Nielsen, E.O., Stärk, K.D.C., Dewulf, J., 2016b. Evaluation of the relationship between the biosecurity status, production parameters, herd characteristics and antimicrobial use in farrow-to-finish pig production in four EU countries. Porcine Health Management 2, 9.

Postma, M., Speksnijder, D.C., Jaarsma, A.D.C., Verheij, T.J.M., Wagenaar, J.A., Dewulf, J., 2016c. Opinions of veterinarians on antimicrobial use in farm animals in Flanders and the Netherlands. Veterinary Record 179, 68-68.

Postma, M., Vanderhaeghen, W., Sarrazin, S., Maes, D., Dewulf, J., 2017. Reducing Antimicrobial Use in Pig Production without Jeopardising Production Parameters. Zoonoses and Public Health 64, 63-74.

Pritchard, K., Wapenaar, W., Brennan, M.L., 2015. Cattle veterinarians' awareness and understanding of biosecurity. Veterinary Record 176, 546.

Rathkjen, P.H., Dall, J., 2017. Control and eradication of porcine reproductive and respiratory syndrome virus type 2 using a modified-live type 2 vaccine in combination with a load, close, homogenise model: an area elimination study. Acta Veterinaria Scandinavica 59, 4.

Ribbens, S., Dewulf, J., Koenen, F., Mintiens, K., De Sadeleer, L., de Kruif, A., Maes, D., 2008. A survey on biosecurity and management practices in Belgian pig herds. Preventive Veterinary Medicine 83, 228-241.

Ritter, C., Jansen, J., Roth, K., Kastelic, J.P., Adams, C.L., Barkema, H.W., 2016. Dairy farmers' perceptions toward the implementation of on-farm Johne's disease prevention and control strategies. Journal of Dairy Science 99, 9114-9125.

Rojo-Gimeno C. and Postma M., Dewulf J., Hogeveen H., Lauwers L., Wauters E., 2016. Farm-economic analysis of reducing antimicrobial use whilst adopting good management strategies on farrow-to-finish pig farms. Preventive Veterinary Medicine Accepted 5 May 2016, 74-87 http://www.sciencedirect.com/science/article/pii/S0167587716301313?via%3Dihub.

Sahlström, L., Virtanen, T., Kyyrö, J., Lyytikäinen, T., 2014. Biosecurity on Finnish cattle, pig and sheep farms – results from a questionnaire. Preventive Veterinary Medicine 117, 59-67.

Sandberg, M., Dahl, J., Lindegaard, L.L., Pedersen, J.R., 2017. Compliance/non-compliance with biosecurity rules specified in the Danish Quality Assurance system (KIK) and Campylobacter-positive broiler flocks 2012 and 2013. Poultry Science 96, 184-191.

Sarrazin, S., Cay, A.B., Laureyns, J., Dewulf, J., 2014. A survey on biosecurity and management practices in selected Belgian cattle farms. Preventive Veterinary Medicine 117, 129-139.

Schembri, N., Hernandez-Jover, M., Toribio, J.A.L.M.L., Holyoake, P.K., 2015. On-farm characteristics and biosecurity protocols for small-scale swine producers in eastern Australia. Preventive Veterinary Medicine 118, 104-116.

Schimmer, B., Lange, M.M.A.d., Hautvast, J.L.A., Vellema, P., Duynhoven, Y.T.H.P.v., 2014. Coxiella burnetii seroprevalence and risk factors on commercial sheep farms in The Netherlands. Veterinary Record 175, 17.

Shortall, O., Green, M., Brennan, M., Wapenaar, W., Kaler, J., 2017. Exploring expert opinion on the practicality and effectiveness of biosecurity measures on dairy farms in the United Kingdom using choice modeling. Journal of Dairy Science 100, 2225-2239.

Simon-Grifé, M., Martín-Valls, G.E., Vilar, M.J., García-Bocanegra, I., Martín, M., Mateu, E., Casal, J., 2013. Biosecurity practices in Spanish pig herds: Perceptions of farmers and veterinarians of the most important biosecurity measures. Preventive Veterinary Medicine 110, 223-231.

Smith, S., Messam, L.L.M., Meade, J., Gibbons, J., McGill, K., Bolton, D., Whyte, P., 2016. The impact of biosecurity and partial depopulation on Campylobacter prevalence in Irish broiler flocks with differing levels of hygiene and economic performance. Infection Ecology & Epidemiology 6, 10.3402/iee.v3406.31454.

Ssematimba, A., Hagenaars, T.J., de Wit, J.J., Ruiterkamp, F., Fabri, T.H., Stegeman, J.A., de Jong, M.C.M., 2013. Avian influenza transmission risks: Analysis of biosecurity measures and contact structure in Dutch poultry farming. Preventive Veterinary Medicine 109, 106-115.

Taker, M.Y.C., Bilkei, G., 2007. Successful salmonella eradication in a South-Hungarian growing-finishing unit. Tieraerztliche Umschau 62, 314-318.

Twomey, D.F., Miller, A.J., Snow, L.C., Armstrong, J.D., Davies, R.H., Williamson, S.M., Featherstone, C.A., Reichel, R., Cook, A.J.C., 2010. Association between biosecurity and Salmonella species prevalence on English pig farms. Veterinary Record 166, 722-724.

Valeeva, N.I., van Asseldonk, M.A.P.M., Backus, G.B.C., 2011. Perceived risk and strategy efficacy as motivators of risk management strategy adoption to prevent animal diseases in pig farming. Preventive Veterinary Medicine 102, 284-295.

Vanantwerpen, G., Berkvens, D., De Zutter, L., Houf, K., 2017. Assessment of factors influencing the within-batch seroprevalence of human enteropathogenic Yersinia spp. of pigs at slaughter age and the analogy with microbiology. Preventive Veterinary Medicine 137, 93-96.

Velkers, F.C., Blokhuis, S.J., Veldhuis Kroeze, E.J.B., Burt, S.A., 2017. The role of rodents in avian influenza outbreaks in poultry farms: a review. Veterinary Quarterly 37, 182-194.

Zhang, Y.-h., Li, C.-S., Liu, C.-C., Chen, K.Z., 2013. Prevention of losses for hog farmers in China: Insurance, on-farm biosecurity practices, and vaccination. Research in Veterinary Science 95, 819-824.

CHAPTER 4

HOW TO MOTIVATE FARMERS TO IMPLEMENT BIOSECURITY MEASURES

Lucie Collineau[1]

Katharina D.C. Stärk[1,2]

[1] SAFOSO AG, CH-3097 Liebefeld, Switzerland
[2] Royal Veterinary College, North Mymms, UK, AL9 7TA

1 Introduction

International organisations and national governments use a range of policies and mechanisms to ensure a harmonized, effective and efficient approach to the prevention and management of infectious diseases in animals, plants and humans. However, because of the rising costs resulting from policies, the increasing number of challenges presented by regulations and the accepted responsibility of primary producers, the implementation of biosecurity measures is commonly devolved to the private sector, particularly the farming industries and farmers (Higgins et al., 2016a). In the European Union (EU) in particular, the 'Animal Health Law' clearly states that the implementation of biosecurity measures comes under the responsibility of farm operators and professionals (European Parliament and EU Council, 2016). This type of approach assumes that farmers are willing to take responsibility for biosecurity and have the necessary knowledge and resources to do so (Higgins et al., 2016a). Previous research however has shown that despite reported concerns about the threat of disease and the high level of awareness about the risk of disease, farmers are not always committed to implementing biosecurity to the level expected by competent authorities (Garforth et al., 2013; Brennan & Christley, 2013).

Improving farm-level biosecurity does indeed require farmers to change their daily routine and it is well-known that adapting practices presents a challenge (Kristensen & Jakobsen, 2011); farmers are strongly influenced by practice and tend to implement what is most familiar to them (Casal et al., 2007). Increased biosecurity can also incur extra costs or extra labour which is likely to discourage farmers from implementing recommended measures (Alarcon et al., 2014). Moreover, the benefits of biosecurity measures are not always tangible; any potential cost-effectiveness depends on the context of each specific farm, i.e. needs to be assessed in relation to the risk of the occurrence of a diseases. It is therefore not a fixed but a variable benefit. While the uptake of biosecurity measures by farmers increases in the case of an outbreak (Brennan et al., 2016), routinely maintaining high levels of biosecurity, even during apparent 'silent' periods of disease transmission, is especially challenging (Garforth et al., 2013). Farmers are also sometimes reluctant to adopt biosecurity measures to control food-borne zoonoses, e.g. *Salmonella* spp. or *Campylobacter* spp. that have little or no impact on animal health or production. Indeed, these are more likely to benefit society than the individual farmer, and can lead to a 'social dilemma' with conflicting private and collective interests in what can be seen as a public good (Fraser et al., 2010; Kristensen & Jakobsen, 2011).

In this context, motivation among farmers for implementing biosecurity measures becomes a key pre-requisite to assuring the resilience of the sector. But what is the best way to achieve and maintain a high level of motivation? To answer this question it is critical to identify the motivators and barriers to the adoption of biosecurity measures on farms. In other words, one needs to understand why farmers behave the way they do and what factors influence their decision as to whether to implement recommended biosecurity measures or not (Garforth, 2015). We address this question following the so-called 'Theory of Planned Behaviour' that has been used by many of the psycho-social studies carried out in the farming sector as part of an investigation into farmer behaviour (Ajzen, 1991).

2 Principles of the Theory of Planned Behaviour

The Theory of Planned Behaviour is based on the Theory of Reasoned Action developed in the 1970's by Fishbein and Ajzen (Fishbein and Ajzen, 1975). To summarise, the Theory of Planned Behaviour assumes that the actual behaviour of an individual may be predicted by the strength of his or her intention to engage in that behaviour (Fig. 4.1.). The intention itself reflects the individual's motivation towards that behaviour, and is believed to be influenced simultaneously by i) the attitude, ii) subjective norm and iii) perceived behavioural control of the individual (Ajzen, 1991). Attitude refers to the individual's personal disposition towards engaging in the behaviour. It captures whether the individual has positive or negative beliefs about the impact of the behaviour on producing the outcome of interest, as well as his or her evaluation of this outcome. Subjective norm reflects the individual's perceptions on whether 'significant others' want him or her to engage in such behaviour and on the individual's motivation to satisfy such external expectations. Perceived behavioural control takes into account the individual's perception of his or her ability to execute and sustain the behaviour, as well as the factors he or she perceives as hindering or facilitating the achievement of the behaviour (Ajzen, 1991). To the extent that perceived behavioural control is realistic, it can also be used to predict actual behaviour.

Fig. 4.1: Schematic representation of the Theory of Planned Behaviour (Ajzen, 2005)

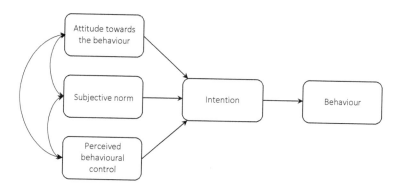

The Theory of Planned Behaviour has been successfully applied to explain or predict individual behaviour in diverse contexts such as health behaviour or eco-citizenship (Armitage & Conner, 2001), as well as to develop interventions aimed at changing an individual's behaviour (Hardeman et al., 2002). In the farming sector, it has been commonly used as a tool to explore farmers' decision making processes and to inform knowledge transfer (Edwards-Jones, 2006), including in the field of livestock disease management (Garforth et al., 2013; Alarcon et al., 2014). It was also applied to understanding the process used by small animal veterinarians when making decisions about antimicrobials (Mateus et al., 2014).

Below we present and discuss key components of farmers' attitudes, subjective norms and perceived behavioural control that are likely to influence intentions as well as associated behaviour in the context of biosecurity measures at their farm. The understanding of these drivers should support governments, veterinarians and other relevant advisors in increasing motivation among farmers for implementing and sustain biosecurity measures.

3 Farmers' attitude towards the implementation of biosecurity measures

The attitude of farmers towards the implementation of biosecurity measures reflects their positive or negative beliefs about the effectiveness of biosecurity to prevent disease on their farm, as well as their evaluation of how important disease prevention is in the particular context of their farm.

3.1 Perceived risk of disease occurrence

Previous literature has shown that a farmer's decision to implement biosecurity measures is partly based on his/her own judgment of the risk of a certain disease affecting his/her farm (Brennan et al., 2016). Risk averse farmers are particularly likely to show more specific farm-protection behaviour (Valeeva et al., 2011). The notion of 'risk' includes both the likelihood of a disease occurring and the severity of the consequences (i.e. the impact) of the disease should it occur. The likelihood of disease occurrence is usually perceived to be higher in the wake of an epidemic in the region or the country. For example, the interest and willingness among farmers to implement biosecurity measures was shown to increase significantly following the first outbreak of porcine reproductive and respiratory syndrome (PRRS) that appeared in Sweden in 2007 (Nöremark et al., 2009), or during the influenza pandemic H1N1/09 outbreak in Australia in 2009 (Hernández-Jover et al., 2012a). Farmers from densely populated pig areas were also reported as implementing stricter biosecurity practices, probably because they perceive the risk of the transmission of diseases from neighbouring farms as a more immediate threat (Simon-Grifé et al., 2013).

The perceived potential impact of the disease also plays a role, with epidemic or exotic diseases being perceived as having a higher impact than endemic diseases (Valeeva et al., 2011). This may explain why farmers attribute greater importance to external biosecurity measures (e.g. measures applied to visitors or external vehicles that could act as carriers of infectious agents not already present in the farm) when compared with internal biosecurity measures (Casal et al., 2007). Larger farms were shown to be more willing to implement biosecurity measures than smaller ones, probably because they would suffer a higher impact should a disease outbreak occur at their farm (Nöremark et al., 2009; Simon-Grifé et al., 2013).

3.2 Perceived cost-effectiveness of biosecurity measures

Believing in the cost-effectiveness of a biosecurity measure also appears to be one of the essential requirements behind a farmer's decision to implement the measure; farmers may decide not to comply with the recommended measure if they do not believe that they will obtain positive return on investment (Alarcon et al., 2014). An interview conducted among 56 cattle farmers in North-West England showed that the majority believed that biosecurity was more cost-effective (75%, n = 42) and more time-efficient (66%, n = 37) than treating disease on-farm; most farmers (64%, n = 36) also believed that benefits could be attained by implementing even a small number of biosecurity measures (Brennan & Christley, 2013). The interview revealed that the preferred information channels for cost-effectiveness of biosecurity measures were primarily private veterinarians (93%, n = 52) followed by research papers / professional press (77%, n = 43) and finally government information (52%, n = 29) (Brennan & Christley, 2013). Breeding companies, feed representatives and peer farmers are deemed to be relevant and trusted external sources of information (Alarcon et al., 2014).

Farmers were shown to prioritise familiar biosecurity measures, i.e. biosecurity measures already implemented on their farm, although some discrepancies exist between reported importance of biosecurity measures and the actual degree of implementation thereof (Casal et al., 2007). Other biosecurity measures are regarded as common sense or part of good husbandry practices, e.g. proper cleaning and disinfection, selectiveness with regards sourcing new animals or keeping new animals separate from existing stock upon arrival; the evaluation of their cost-effectiveness seems unnecessary as farmers are willing to implement them as part of their desire to be a 'good farmer' operating a 'clean farm' (Alarcon et al., 2014; Higgins et al., 2016a).

In many situations, however, farmers lack evidence of the cost-effectiveness of biosecurity measures, making them less likely to implement such measures (Alarcon et al., 2014). For example, while considering the potential effectiveness of *Salmonella* spp. control measures, an English pig farmer reported that he was sceptical and had to see it working: 'I would feel it necessary to actually see it working before I did anything' (Marier et al., 2016). The issue of questionable or unproven efficacy of biosecurity measures is partly shared by veterinary practitioners (Gunn et al., 2008). Even if general evidence is present, farmers have to deal with the uncertainty about the effectiveness of a measure if applied on their particular farm. They reported that regardless of the actions carried out on a farm, there were occasions when biosecurity measures were not going to be effective or time-efficient (Brennan et al., 2016).

4 Subjective norm

The subjective norm among farmers towards implementing biosecurity measures reflects their perceptions about whether 'significant others' – e.g. governments, farmer unions, local administration, colleagues – want them commit to implement biosecurity measures at their farm, and whether farmers are motivated to comply with this perceived external pressure.

4.1 Perceived influence from governments and research institutions

National governments, backed up by research institutions, have developed a range of policies, guidelines and mechanisms to persuade farmers to commit to implementing biosecurity measures (Moore et al., 2008). Some approaches were shown to be more successful than others. For example, pig farmers reported having implemented specific biosecurity measures (e.g. changing their farrowing system) to comply with the *Salmonella* spp. control programme conducted by the UK government (Alarcon et al., 2014). In many cases however, the achieved level of biosecurity does not reach the level expected by national competent authorities (Garforth, 2015). For example, in 2008, the Danish government introduced a legal requirement for larger dairy farms to develop and implement a farm-specific biosecurity plan. One year later, a survey conducted among 25 farmers showed that none of them had set up the mandatory biosecurity plan or implemented any procedures comparable to a systematic biosecurity programme (Kristensen & Jakobsen, 2011).

Despite a lower-than-expected implementation of biosecurity measures, farmers report doing all they reasonably can to minimise the risk of disease (Garforth et al., 2013) and are very satisfied with the measures they are applying on their own farms (Casal et al., 2007). The recommendations that are not implemented are either seen as irrelevant or impractical for individuals (Garforth et al., 2013). For example, Bennett and Cooke (2005) reported a strong reluctance among UK cattle farmers to follow any biosecurity guidelines recommended by the government as part of the national bovine tuberculosis (bTB) control programme, even among farmers who had experienced bTB outbreaks in the past. Over 50% of farmers stated that they would never implement any of the recommended measures for five out of nine proposed biosecurity categories, even if they received financial support, because they perceived them as impractical or time-consuming (Bennett & Cooke, 2005).

Lack of trust in government agencies and associated scientific institutions may affect farmers' decisions to implement on-farm biosecurity practices (Higgins et al., 2016a). For example, in-depth interviews conducted with 37 sheep and cattle farmers in Australia showed that scientific institutions linked to the government suffered from a lack of trust and credibility, which threatens the success of the biosecurity and surveillance system for infectious livestock diseases in the country (Palmer et al., 2009). Lack of trust in governmental agencies can be related, among others, to a perceived failure by the government to control epidemics in the past. This was the case following the 2001 foot-and-mouth disease epidemic in the UK: 'The handling of the last FMD epidemic was completely wrong; it shouldn't have spread the way it did' (Heffernan et al., 2008; Donaldson, 2008).

While farmers recognise that they are responsible for controlling endemic diseases that occur on their farm, many attribute the responsibility for implementing proper biosecurity measures to governments as part of the prevention of epidemic or exotic threats (Higgins et al., 2016a). Such measures include adequate border control, as well as the establishment of effective policies and regulations (Heffernan et al., 2008). Higgings et al. (2016b) argued that such views reflect a particular agricultural institutional logic in which governments have a 'moral responsibility to support farmers and family farming' (Higgins et al., 2016b). Another reason for farmers to delegate biosecurity back to governments could relate to the fact that biosecurity measures also benefit society as whole, rather than individual farmers who incur the implementation costs (Kristensen & Jakobsen, 2011). In other words, because biosecurity serves collective interests such as the control of zoonoses, access to international markets or maintenance of high animal welfare standards, farmers also expect governments to accept part of the responsibility for biosecurity.

4.2 Perceived influence of veterinarians, farm advisors and peer farmers

Veterinarians are commonly seen by farmers as being the most credible and reliable sources of information about biosecurity and disease risk management (Garforth et al., 2013; Brennan & Christley, 2013; Alarcon et al., 2014). Because recommendations from central sources are not always relevant to their particular context, farmers expect their veterinarian to interpret and contextualise information and to translate it into advice based on his or her scientific expertise and knowledge of the local epidemiological situation (Garforth et al., 2013). However, veterinarians do not always see themselves as prime providers of biosecurity information to farmers (Gunn et al., 2008). Indeed, many of them feel that their clients are not willing, or cannot afford to invest in biosecurity measures. Some also admit that they are not fully convinced of the benefits of biosecurity measures, or that they do not have enough resources or expertise to provide biosecurity advice to clients (Gunn et al., 2008). However, the ability of veterinarians to convince farmers of the logic in the recommended measures was reported as a key factor in ensuring compliance with external recommendations (Racicot et al., 2012; Laanen et al., 2014). The previous confidence and trust of farmers in the advice of veterinarian, as well as the acknowledgement of their professional competence, were also identified as critical requirements among farmers when it came to implementing measures recommended by their veterinarian (Alarcon et al., 2014).

In addition to the advice they receive from their veterinarian, farmers also consider recommendations from other advisors before deciding to implement biosecurity measures, particularly when a substantial financial investment is involved. Breeding companies, feed company representatives, livestock dealers, transporters and agricultural consultants, among others were reported as auxiliary industries with relevant influence on decisions about biosecurity (Gunn et al., 2008; Alarcon et al., 2014). Nonetheless, as with veterinarians, these advisors appear to be sceptical about the cost-effectiveness and practicality of biosecurity; they also feel that farmers are not sufficiently motivated to provide the facilities and competences needed for the maintenance of good biosecurity (Gunn et al., 2008). Farm assurance schemes could provide another channel for convincing farmers to commit to implementing high biosecurity standards. However, a survey conducted among sheep and pig farmers in the UK revealed that assurance scheme members did not perceive enhanced biosecurity or disease control as a benefit of the assurance scheme; they just saw a set of rules or recommendations with which they had to comply in order to sell their products (Garforth et al., 2013).

Groups of farmers were also mentioned as another opportunity for exchanging ideas and information about biosecurity and disease control (Garforth et al., 2013). For example success 'stable schools' have been organised with success in Denmark to encourage mutual advice and shared learning among organic dairy farmers willing to phase out the use of antimicrobial drugs at their farms by increasing disease prevention and improved animal health management (Vaarst et al., 2007). However, the lack of social cohesion among the farming community, as well as the perceived excessive need for confidentiality within the livestock industry were described as major barriers to farmer group initiatives, with farmers 'only telling the good things and not the bad things' about problems of disease at their farms (Heffernan et al., 2008; Alarcon et al., 2014).

5 Perceived behavioural control

Even among those farmers with a positive attitude towards biosecurity measures, we often note a gap between farmers' reported beliefs about biosecurity measures (e.g. perceived importance or cost-effectiveness) and the measures actually implemented on the farm (Casal et al., 2007). It means that other factors, including very practical ones such as the cost or practicality of biosecurity measures, have an impact on final implementation. Farmers' perceived behavioural control describes the belief among farmers in their ability to implement biosecurity measures (also known as 'self-efficacy'), as well as factors perceived as hindering or facilitating the implementation of biosecurity measures.

5.1 Influence of the farm's financial circumstances

Many farmers are optimistic about the ability to control disease prevention using biosecurity measures on their farm (Brennan et al., 2016). However, one of the main barriers to actual implementation is the financial circumstance of the farm. Frazer et al. (2010) showed a clear inverse relationship between the willingness of farmers to adopt a biosecurity measure and the estimated cost (Fraser et al., 2010). For example, when it comes to implementing biosecurity measures to control *Salmonella* spp. in pig production in England, most of the farmers (79%) agreed that the greatest barrier was the cost or a lack of benefit from implementing a measure of uncertain efficacy – 'There are all sorts of things I would love to do if I had the money but most of them have to be cost-efficient' (Marier et al., 2016). Some farmers have also reported that difficult financial circumstances prevent them from making major investments that would contribute to improved biosecurity, e.g. renovating or constructing new buildings, or that it impedes the employment of staff required to ensure the effective implementation of biosecurity measures (Alarcon et al., 2014).

Given the major influence that financial circumstances have on the implementation of biosecurity measures, using economic incentives or penalties was suggested as a way of facilitating the adoption of such measures (Alarcon et al., 2014; Niemi et al., 2016). Benett (2012) argued that financial support from governments to increase biosecurity could be economically profitable, especially when we consider the negative external factors of infectious diseases among animals, e.g. impact on the health of the livestock of other producers, public health and animal welfare. Public–private partnership cost-sharing schemes could also be considered as a way of ensuring that responsibility and costs of epidemic livestock diseases are appropriately shared (Bennett, 2012).

5.2 Feasibility of biosecurity measures

The feasibility of recommended measures was mentioned as a key driver in farmers' perceived behavioural control over the implementation of biosecurity measures. Many farmers refer to a particular feature of their farm such as geographical location, layout of buildings or lack of space, when explaining why they think it is impractical to adopt a proposed measure (Garforth et al., 2013). Running an outdoor farm is perceived as being particularly incompatible with the implementation of certain biosecurity measures to control wildlife or airborne diseases for instance (Brennan et al., 2016). By way of an example, all of the nine sheep farmers interviewed in England by Garforth et al. (2013) reported that they were unable to reduce contact with wildlife – 'No you can't. Unless you shoot all the wildlife you can't do anything about it' (Garforth et al., 2013). They also stated that outdoor farming also seriously compromised *Salmonella* spp. control in pig production – 'My vet would repeat exactly what I've just said to you, there is very little you can do about it, you are outdoors and that's it' (Marier et al., 2016).

Another practical aspect influencing the implementation of biosecurity measures is the amount of extra labour required (Alarcon et al., 2014). For example, a survey on the willingness of pig farmers to adopt biosecurity measures to control for *Salmonella* spp. in the UK showed that they were much more likely to implement good rodent control rather than strict between-batch biosecurity, as this was perceived as much easier and less time consuming (Fraser et al., 2010). The extra workload associated with *Salmonella* spp. biosecurity measures was also reported as an issue among English pig farmers – 'If it was relatively easy to implement and didn't require a lot of time and costs, and if it was going to help our *Salmonella* spp. scores then we would be interested in doing it' (Marier et al., 2016).

Non-compliance with biosecurity measures is also associated with poor training of farm personnel and lack of communications between the personnel working on the farm and the technical services (Vaillancourt & Carver, 1998). Larger farms, in particular, with high turnover of farm personnel face difficulties in the routine application of a strict biosecurity plan. Explaining the meaning of each measure in relation to the transmission of diseases to this type of staff can be quite challenging.

6 Practical recommendations

Fig. 4.2: Summary of the main motivators and barriers affecting the adoption of biosecurity measures by farmers. These can be used as a basis for formulating practical recommendations directed at governments, veterinarians and other relevant farm advisors with the aim of motivating farmers to implement biosecurity measures.

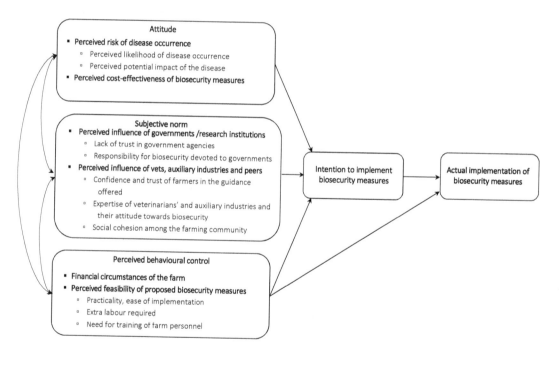

1) Intensified communications about risk

Farmers should be made aware of the level of risk to which their animals are exposed, so that they can consider applying more or different measures, or applying measures more strictly in those instances where they perceive the level of risk to be high. Because risk perception is influenced by recent disease incidence, effective surveillance activities to provide early warning and up-to-date epidemiological information about disease threats should be put in place both locally and nationally (Garforth et al., 2013).

The potential impact of both exotic and endemic animal diseases should also be made clear to farmers (Valeeva et al., 2011). Local veterinarians, who are perceived by farmers as being their main partner for interpreting and contextualising information from national sources, as well as the farming press should be used as the preferred communication channels to enhance communications about risk to farmers (Garforth et al., 2013).

2) Evidence of the benefits of biosecurity measures

Additional data should be provided about the benefits of implementing biosecurity measures, e.g. showing practical examples of farms where implementation was successful. Farmers as well as their key advisors, including veterinarians, reported having doubts about the potential cost-effectiveness and relevance of certain biosecurity measures (Gunn et al., 2008). Practical aspects such as extra labour or training should also be quantified so that farmers can make evidence-based decisions about whether to implement certain measures on their farm. Veterinarians should improve their skills and expertise so that they can provide biosecurity advice to their clients. Although they are not necessarily aware of it, farmers do consider them as the prime source of information about biosecurity.

3) Targeted advice on biosecurity measures

Biosecurity recommendations provided by central sources are often rejected out of hand as being irrelevant to or impractical for individual farmers because they are too generic. When it comes to the actual implementation of biosecurity measures, it is not possible to use a 'one size fits all' approach. If recommended measures are to have credibility among farmers, advice should be adjusted and tailored to the features of their particular farm, considering the animal species produced, the type of production (e.g. indoor vs outdoor) or the farm size (e.g. number of employees). Veterinarians and other farm advisors can also play a key role in interpreting and adapting national recommendations to the particular context of their clients' farms.

4) Improved collaboration between relevant stakeholders

The successful implementation of on-farm biosecurity measures will benefit from an improved collaboration and communications between all the stakeholders. Farmers receive information from a great many sources so there is a risk of confusion if messages are inconsistent or contradictory (Moore et al., 2008). Successful biosecurity management also depends on building up trust among stakeholders (Hernández-Jover et al., 2012b). For example, knowledge of biosecurity and practices among farmers is not always readily acknowledged by competent authorities, or even researchers (Higgins et al., 2016a). Farmers may see biosecurity recommendations as a set of external rules with which they have to comply rather than an opportunity to capitalise on their ability to control diseases occurring at their farm. Strengthening and acknowledging the expertise of farmers will encourage them to take responsibility for biosecurity and in turn improve their commitment to implementing sustained biosecurity measures.

References

Ajzen, I. (1991). The theory of planned behavior. *Organizational Behavior and Human Decision Processes, 50*(2), 179-211.

Ajzen, I. (2005). *Attitudes, personality and behaviour*. Open University Press. McGraw-Hill Education. Second edition.

Alarcon, P., Wieland, B., Mateus, A. L. P., & Dewberry, C. (2014). Pig farmers' perceptions, attitudes, influences and management of information in the decision-making process for disease control. *Preventive Veterinary Medicine, 116*(3), 223-242.

Armitage, C. J., & Conner, M. (2001). Efficacy of the Theory of Planned Behaviour: A meta-analytic review. *British Journal of Social Psychology, 40*(4), 471-499.

Bennett, R. (2012). Economic rationale for interventions to control livestock disease. *Euro-Choices, 11*(2), 5-11.

Bennett, R., & Cooke, R. (2005). Control of bovine TB: preferences of farmers who have suffered a TB breakdown. *Veterinary Record, 156*, 143-145.

Brennan, M. L., & Christley, R. M. (2013). Cattle producers' perceptions of biosecurity. *BMC Veterinary Research, 9*(1), 71.

Brennan, M., Wright, N., Wapenaar, W., Jarratt, S., Hobson-West, P., Richens, I., Kaler, J., et al. (2016). Exploring attitudes and beliefs towards implementing cattle disease prevention and control measures: a qualitative study with dairy farmers in Great Britain. *Animals, 6*(10), 61.

Casal, J., De Manuel, A., Mateu, E., & Martín, M. (2007). Biosecurity measures on swine farms in Spain: Perceptions by farmers and their relationship to current on-farm measures. *Preventive Veterinary Medicine, 82*(1), 138-150.

Donaldson, A. (2008). Biosecurity after the event: risk politics and animal disease. *Environment and Planning A, 40*(7), 1552-1567.

Edwards-Jones, G. (2006). Modelling farmer decision-making: concepts, progress and challenges. *Animal Science, 82*(06), 783.

European Parliament and EU Council. (2016). Regulation (Eu) 2016/429 of the European Parliament and of the Council of 9 March 2016 on transmissible animal diseases and amending and repealing certain acts in the area of animal health ('Animal Health Law'). *Official Journal of the European Union, 59*, L 84/1-208.

Fishbein, M., & Ajzen, I. (1975). *Belief, Attitude, Intention, and Behavior: An Introduction to Theory and Research*. Reading, MA. Addison-Wesley.

Fraser, R. W., Williams, N. T., Powell, L. F., & Cook, A. J. C. (2010). Reducing campylobacter and salmonella infection: two studies of the economic cost and attitude to adoption of on-farm biosecurity measures. *Zoonoses and Public Health, 57*(7-8), e109-e115.

Garforth, C. (2015). Livestock keepers' reasons for doing and not doing things which governments, vets and scientists would like them to do. *Zoonoses and Public Health, 62*, 29-38.

Garforth, C. J., Bailey, A. P., & Tranter, R. B. (2013). Farmers' attitudes to disease risk management in England: A comparative analysis of sheep and pig farmers. *Preventive Veterinary Medicine, 110*(3-4), 456-466.

Gunn, G. J., Heffernan, C., Hall, M., McLeod, A., & Hovi, M. (2008). Measuring and comparing constraints to improved biosecurity amongst GB farmers, veterinarians and the auxiliary industries. *Preventive Veterinary Medicine, 84*(3), 310-323.

Hardeman, W., Johnston, M., Johnston, D., Bonetti, D., Wareham, N., & Kinmonth, A. L. (2002). Application of the Theory of Planned Behaviour in Behaviour Change Interventions: A Systematic Review. *Psychology & Health, 17*(2), 123-158.

Heffernan, C., Nielsen, L., Thomson, K., & Gunn, G. (2008). An exploration of the drivers to biosecurity collective action among a sample of UK cattle and sheep farmers. *Preventive Veterinary Medicine, 87*(3), 358-372.

Hernández-Jover, M., Taylor, M., Holyoake, P., & Dhand, N. (2012a). Pig producers' perceptions of the Influenza Pandemic H1N1/09 outbreak and its effect on their biosecurity practices in Australia. *Preventive Veterinary Medicine, 106*(3), 284-294.

Hernández-Jover, M., Gilmour, J., Schembri, N., Sysak, T., Holyoake, P. K., Beilin, R., & Toribio, J.-A. L. M. L. (2012b). Use of stakeholder analysis to inform risk communication and extension strategies for improved biosecurity amongst small-scale pig producers. *Preventive Veterinary Medicine, 104*(3), 258-270.

Higgins, V., Bryant, M., Hernández-Jover, M., Rast, L., & McShane, C. (2016a). Devolved responsibility and on-farm biosecurity: practices of biosecure farming care in livestock production. *Sociologia Ruralis*, doi: 10.1111/soru.12155.

Higgins, V., Bryant, M., Hernandez-Jover, M., McShane, C., & Rast, L. (2016b). Harmonising devolved responsibility for biosecurity governance: The challenge of competing institutional logics. *Environment and Planning A, 48*(6), 1133-1151.

Kristensen, E., & Jakobsen, E. B. (2011). Danish dairy farmers' perception of biosecurity. *Preventive Veterinary Medicine, 99*(2), 122-129.

Laanen, M., Maes, D., Hendriksen, C., Gelaude, P., De Vliegher, S., Rosseel, Y., & Dewulf, J. (2014). Pig, cattle and poultry farmers with a known interest in research have comparable perspectives on disease prevention and on-farm biosecurity. *Preventive Veterinary Medicine, 115*(1), 1-9.

Marier, E., Piers Smith, R., Ellis-Iversen, J., Watson, E., Armstrong, D., Hogeveen, H., & Cook, A. J. C. (2016). Changes in perceptions and motivators that influence the implementation of on-farm Salmonella control measures by pig farmers in England. *Preventive Veterinary Medicine, 133*, 22-30.

Mateus, A. L. P., Brodbelt, D. C., Barber, N., & Stärk, K. D. C. (2014). Qualitative study of factors associated with antimicrobial usage in seven small animal veterinary practices in the UK. *Preventive Veterinary Medicine, 117*, 68-78.

Moore, D. A., Merryman, M. L., Hartman, M. L., & Klingborg, D. J. (2008). Comparison of published recommendations regarding biosecurity practices for various production animal species and classes. *Journal of the American Veterinary Medical Association, 233*(2), 249-256.

Niemi, J. K., Sahlström, L., Kyyrö, J., Lyytikäinen, T., & Sinisalo, A. (2016). Farm characteristics and perceptions regarding costs contribute to the adoption of biosecurity in Finnish pig and cattle farms. *Review of Agricultural, Food and Environmental Studies*, 1-9.

Nöremark, M., Lindberg, A., Vågsholm, I., & Sternberg Lewerin, S. (2009). Disease awareness, information retrieval and change in biosecurity routines among pig farmers in association with the first PRRS outbreak in Sweden. *Preventive Veterinary Medicine, 90*(1), 1-9.

Palmer, S., Fozdar, F., & Sully, M. (2009). The effect of trust on West Australian farmers' responses to infectious livestock diseases. *Sociologia Ruralis, 49*(4), 360-374.

Racicot, M., Venne, D., Durivage, A., & Vaillancourt, J.-P. (2012). Evaluation of the relationship between personality traits, experience, education and biosecurity compliance on poultry farms in Quebec, Canada. *Preventive Veterinary Medicine, 103*(2), 201-207.

Simon-Grifé, M., Martín-Valls, G. E., Vilar, M. J., García-Bocanegra, I., Martín, M., Mateu, E., & Casal, J. (2013). Biosecurity practices in Spanish pig herds: Perceptions of farmers and veterinarians of the most important biosecurity measures. *Preventive Veterinary Medicine, 110*(2), 223-231.

Vaarst, M., Nissen, T. B., Østergaard, S., Klaas, I. C., Bennedsgaard, T. W., & Christensen, J. (2007). Danish Stable Schools for Experiential Common Learning in Groups of Organic Dairy Farmers. *Journal of Dairy Science, 90*(5), 2543-2554.

Vaillancourt, J. P., & Carver, D. K. (1998). Biosecurity: perception is not reality. *Poultry Digest, 57*(6), 28-36.

Valeeva, N. I., van Asseldonk, M. A. P. M., & Backus, G. B. C. (2011). Perceived risk and strategy efficacy as motivators of risk management strategy adoption to prevent animal diseases in pig farming. *Preventive Veterinary Medicine, 102*(4), 284-295.

4

CHAPTER 5

HOW TO MEASURE BIOSECURITY AND THE HYGIENE STATUS OF FARMS

Jeroen Dewulf[1]

Merel Postma[1]

Filip Van Immerseel[2]

Bo Vanbeselaere[1,3]

Kaat Luyckx[1]

[1] Faculty of Veterinary Medicine, Department of Obstetrics, Reproduction and Herd Health, Veterinary Epidemiology Unit, University of Ghent, 9820 Merelbeke, Belgium
[2] Faculty of Veterinary Medicine, Department of Pathology, Bacteriology and Avian Diseases, University of Ghent, 9820 Merelbeke, Belgium
[3] CID LINES NV, 8900 Ieper, Belgium

1 Introduction

"You need to be able to measure, to be able to improve." This is one of the most famous quotes of William Thomson (better known as Lord Kelvin), a famous British mathematician of the 19th century. This is certainly true of biosecurity and hygiene. The inability to measure accurately and reproducibly the biosecurity and hygiene status of farms has long been one of the main obstacles in the pursuit of improvements in both. If farm managers need to be motivated to enhance the biosecurity or hygiene status of their farm, it is essential to provide them with quantitative goals and benchmarks, which can be used to position the farm with respect to its biosecurity and hygiene status, so that the measures required for improvements can be identified and their impact subsequently measured, if possible quantitatively.

2 How to measure on-farm biosecurity

Several systems have been designed for making inventories of biosecurity measures taken in animal production. They are often developed as checklists or as manuals either by independent advisory organisations or as support material for marketing specific disease prevention products (e.g. vaccines). An example of the latter is the recently launched COMBAT system of Boehringer Ingelheim that helps to identify biosecurity hazards in relation to the PRRS infections in pig production. Like the COMBAT PRRS system, many of these systems were developed with a view to controlling a specific disease. The dichotomous checklist of Wageningen University for example was developed to gain an insight in the risks factors associated with the introduction and spread of *Streptococcus suis* in herds (Wageningen University, 2008). The American Association of Swine Veterinarians (AASV) (2007) in collaboration with Iowa State University (Holtkamp et al., 2010), designed a system (PADRAP) that evaluates the biosecurity protocols used in breeding or growing pig herds and identifies possible risk factors for PRRSV infection, along with benchmarking of the herd compared to other herds. Other countries published fact sheets on the principles of biosecurity, to reduce the risk of introduction and spread of classical swine fever for instance (Defra, 2007). In Australia, information on biosecurity is also available for pig producers via the Australian Pork Industry (2003). They also recently developed manuals for pig producers that includes an internal audit system called APIQ√® which stands for Australian Pork Industry Quality Assurance Programme (www.apiq.com.au). This system enables producers to demonstrate that their on-farm practices reflect good farming practice with regards management, animal welfare, food safety, biosecurity and traceability.

At Ghent University, the Biocheck.UGent™ biosecurity scoring system was developed and is currently available for use in pig herds and poultry flocks and is under development for dairy, beef and veal herds (release expected beginning 2018) (www.biocheck. ugent.be). The Biocheck.UGent™ system is a risk-based scoring system to quantify on-farm biosecurity (Laanen et al., 2010; Gelaude et al., 2014; Ghent University, 2015). It does not start from a specific disease but rather approaches biosecurity in general and focuses on those aspects that are common to the transmission of many different types of infectious diseases (see chapter 1 on circles of disease transmission). The Biocheck.UGent™ system for pig and broiler production includes 109 (pig) and 79 (broiler) questions respectively. The mainly di- or trichotomous questions are divided into several subcategories for internal and external biosecurity. Every subcategory consists of 2 to 19 questions. The answer to every question results in a score between zero (when this measure is not implemented at all) and one (when the measure is fully implemented). Depending on the importance of a particular biosecurity measure the score per question is multiplied by a weight factor (Laanen et al., 2013; Gelaude et al., 2014). The subcategories also have a specific weight factor equal to their determined relative importance for disease transmission as determined by a large group of pig and poultry specialists (Laanen et al., 2013; Gelaude et al., 2014). The Biocheck.UGent™ scoring system thus provides a risk-based score which takes into account the relative importance of all different biosecurity measures. The final score for both internal and external biosecurity can range from zero, indicating a total absence of the described biosecurity measures, to 100, indicating a full application of the described measures. The average of internal and external biosecurity scores provides the overall biosecurity score. The Biocheck.UGent™ scoring tool is accessible to everybody and there is no charge to use it.

After filling in the Biocheck.UGent™ questionnaire, the results are presented in a report and spider diagram. The personal scores allow evaluation of the strong and weak points of the biosecurity on a particular farm and provide a basis for improvements. The report shows where efforts can be made to improve the biosecurity aspects that are weakly implemented on the farm.

Fig. 5.1: Example of a Biocheck.UGent™ report for a broiler flock

GHENT
UNIVERSITY

BIOCHECK.UGENT

POULTRY

Nr	Description	Score	Country average
External biosecurity			
A	Purchase of one day old chicks	90 %	54 %
B	Exports of live animals	58 %	63 %
C	Feed and water supply	71 %	50 %
D	Removal of manure and dead animals	56 %	68 %
E	Entrance of visitors and personnel	70 %	70 %
F	Supply of materials	56 %	49 %
G	Infrastructure and biological vectors	76 %	83 %
H	Location of the farm	61 %	65 %
	Subtotal External biosecurity:	*68 %*	*64 %*
Internal biosecurity			
A	Disease management	63 %	79 %
B	Cleaning and disinfection	55 %	56 %
C	Materials and measures between compartments	29 %	58 %
	Subtotal Internal biosecurity:	*52 %*	*64 %*
N/A = Not applicable	**Total:**	63 %	**64 %**

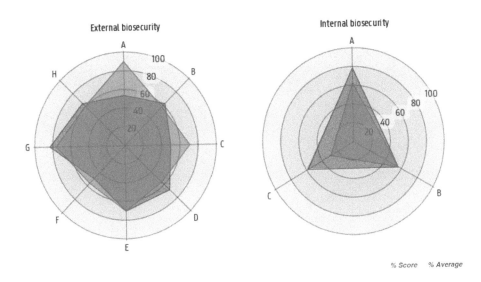

To use the Biocheck.UGent™ scoring system, it is strongly advised to first visit the specific herd or flock in order to make a visual assessment of the situation at the farm and to then fill in the questionnaire together with the farm manager. This method (visiting before completing the Biocheck.UGent™), simplifies the task of filling in the questionnaire as the answer to many of the questions will already be available due to the visual inspection. In these conditions, it generally takes no longer than 30 minutes to complete the questionnaire.

Since its introduction, Biocheck.UGent™ has been used in over 5000 farms scattered over about 40 countries (Fig. 5.3 and 5.4). Furthermore, the Biocheck.UGent™ has already been used in several scientific studies as a tool to determine on-farm biosecurity levels (Table 5.1).

Fig. 5.3: Use of the Biocheck.UGent™ – PIGS in the world (August 2017)

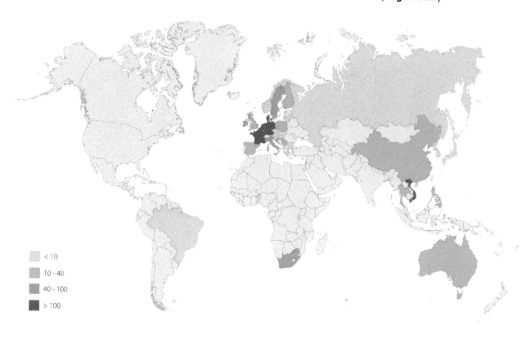

Fig. 5.4: Use of the Biocheck.UGent™ – POULTRY in the world (August 2017)

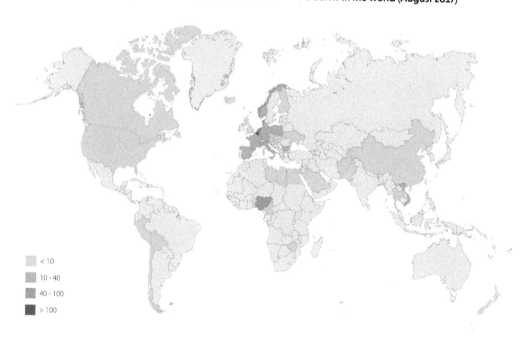

BIOSECURITY IN ANIMAL PRODUCTION AND VETERINARY MEDICINE

Table 5.1: List of the scientific publications in which the Biocheck.UGent™ has been used

PUBLICATION	AUTHORS
Biosecurity level and health management practices in 60 Swedish farrow-to-finish herds.	Backhans et al., 2015
Antimicrobial use in Swedish farrow-to-finish pig herds is related to farmer characteristics.	Backhans et al., 2016
Evaluation of the relationship between the biosecurity status, production parameters, herd characteristics and antimicrobial usage in farrow-to-finish pig production in four EU countries.	Postma et al., 2016a
Farm-economic analysis of reducing antimicrobial use whilst adopting good management strategies on farrow-to-finish pig farm.	Rojo Gimeno et al., 2016
Reducing Antimicrobial Usage in Pig Production without Jeopardizing Production Parameters.	Postma et al., 2017
Relationship between biosecurity and production/antimicrobial treatment characteristics in pig herds.	Laanen et al., 2013
Review of transmission routes of 24 infectious diseases preventable by biosecurity measures and comparison of the implementation of these measures in pig herds in six European countries.	Filippitzi et al., 2017
Vurdering af smittebeskyttelse I 140 danske svinebesaetninger (Assessment of biosecurity in 140 Danish pig herds).	Ramvad et al., 2017
Scoring biosecurity in European conventional broiler production.	Van Limbergen et al., 2017

3 How to measure hygiene status

After cleaning and disinfection (C&D), hygiene status should be monitored in order to evaluate the quality of the cleaning and disinfection protocol. Several methods for carrying outhygiene controls, either as a routine control or after a sanitary crisis, have been used and described, i.e. agar contact plates (ACP), swab samples, air samples, ATP analysis and visual inspection). The hygiene status is mainly analysed by monitoring the level of bacteriological contamination surface and air samples.

3.1 Bacteriological monitoring

Bacteriological monitoring after C&D often focuses on total aerobic bacterial counts (Corrégé et al., 2003; Hancox et al., 2013; Ward et al., 2006) and/or specific pathogens (Carrique-Mas et al., 2009; Merialdi et al., 2013; Mueller-Doblies et al., 2010; L J Pletinckx et al., 2013; Rose et al., 1999). In addition to the total aerobic bacterial counts, various specific microbiological indicator organisms such as *Escherichia coli, Enterococcus* spp., *Salmonella* and methicillin resistant *Staphylococcus aureus* have also been used to evaluate the hygiene status of animal houses. *Escherichia coli* has been shown to be a suitable indicator organism for monitoring the possible presence of *Salmonella* (Dewaele et al., 2011; Gradel et al., 2004a; Winfield and Groisman, 2003). Indicator organisms should be easy to culture and identify, and be present at higher levels at the sample location than the pathogen, for which they are an indicator organism, as the absence of the index organisms then will ensure absence of the target pathogen in the sample. Several methods have been developed recently for rapid testing for the presence of *E. coli* (e.g. MicroSnapTM *E. coli*, Hygiena). In the future, these new methods could, after validation, potentially be used by farmers to enable them to monitor the hygiene status of different locations themselves. *Enterococcus* spp. could be an adequate hygiene-indicator organism for faecal contamination of surfaces (Gradel et al., 2004b; Luyckx et al., 2015). Gram-negative bacteria are intrinsically more resistant to disinfectants than enveloped viruses (see chapter 6 on cleaning and disinfection). Therefore it is assumed that if the Gram-negative bacterium *E. coli* is eliminated by disinfection, these viruses could probably also be eliminated if they are present in equal or lower numbers. In contrast, if *E. coli* survives the disinfection stage, then small non-enveloped viruses (intrinsically more resistant than Gram-negative bacteria) will probably also survive the disinfection stage.

3.1.1 Agar Contact Plates (ACP)

Agar contact plates (ACP) are agar plates that contain a convex agar surface that can be used for sampling by pressing it against a surface. ACPs taken before cleaning will often become overgrown or unreadable due to macroscopic particles. With the aid of ACP, you can quickly evaluate whether surfaces are 'clean'. The pressure plates measure and quantify the presence of bacterial contamination. In farms these samples are often taken routinely after production rounds (to evaluate the cleaning and disinfection procedure) or are implemented by the government when specific pathogens are found in samples on a farm (Vangroenweghe et al. 2009). At specific locations (e.g. floors, walls, feed hoppers, drinking water systems), samples are taken using ACPs and bacteriologically analysed. After counting bacterial colonies and scoring the plates between 0 and 5 (see below), a mean value for the plates is calculated. The results are expressed in colony-forming units (CFU) per plate, as is shown in the example of standards used for *Salmonella* in poultry houses below (Fig. 5.5). This procedure is often called the determination of a 'hygienogram'. Surfaces or zones that are less easy to sample using contact plates can in theory also be sampled using swabs or agar sausages.

Score	CFU per plate
0	0
1	1-40
2	41-120
3	121-400
4	> 400
5	countless

▲
Fig. 5.5: Scores used based on the number of colony forming units on an agar contact plate

3.1.2 Swab samples

Swab samples of a defined surface (625 cm²) can provide better insight into the initial bacterial load before cleaning. Different swab types and detection methods exist, the latter being direct streaking on agar versus elution followed by membrane filtration systems, and all have different sensitivities (Goverde et al., 2017). Differences in detection rates between cotton, rayon, flocked nylon swabs and foam swabs, when used on surfaces, have been described (Dalmaso et al., 2008; Hedin et al., 2010; Dolan et al., 2011).

3.2 Adenosine triphosphate (ATP) hygiene monitoring

Another quantitative method used for hygiene monitoring after cleaning is ATP analysis. This method has been widely adopted in the food industry (Betts and Chroleywood food research assocation, 2000) but until now has rarely been used in the primary animal production sector. ATP is a molecule involved in energy transfer for metabolic processes in cells, and is present in all eukaryotic and prokaryotic living cells. The principle of the analysis is based on the addition of a solution containing lysis reagent, the substrate luciferin and luciferase, to a swab sample. The lysis reagent allows the release of ATP from all living cells. Released ATP molecules are used by the enzyme luciferase to convert the substrate luciferin, resulting in a bioluminescent reaction. Measurements of the produced light can be immediately carried out using a specific piece of apparatus. ATP measurement is generally performed after cleaning. ATP analysis is capable of providing information about the level of biological residues (eukaryotic cells as part of soil and prokaryotic cells) and can be used therefore to identify badly cleaned or critical locations after cleaning animal houses. The study by Luyckx et al., (2015a) suggests a cut-off value of three log relative light units (RLU) as a warning level.

3.3 Visual inspection

In the past, the most frequently used criterion for assessing the efficacy of cleaning was the lack of visible organic material. There is no need to use agar contact plates, swabs or ATP measurements when visible organic material is still present on surfaces.

Table 5.2: Advantages and disadvantages given for each sampling method to assess the bacterial load. Examples of scientific studies carried out in chicken or pig facilities are given for each method.

Method	What monitored?	Advantages	Disadvantages	Studies
ACP[1]	Bacteria	– Ease of use – Fixed sampling area – No need for further processing after sampling – Pre-made available	– Limited sampling surface (25 cm²) – Only smooth, firm surfaces – Colony overgrowth – One ACP per specific organism – Need for standardised pressure	De Reu et al. (2006); Huneau-Salaün et al. (2010); Kim and Kim (2010)
Swab sampling	Bacteria	– Larger sampling surfaces[2] – Difficult to reach surfaces – ≥1 bacterial analyses/ swab – High upper enumeration limit	– Laboratory manipulation – No standardised protocol	Banhazi and Santhanam, (2013); Beloeil et al. (2007); Carrique-Mas et al. (2009); Davies and Breslin (2003a); Hancox et al. (2013); Mannion et al. (2007); Merialdi et al. (2013); Oliveira et al. (2006); Rathgeber et al. (2009); Rose et al. (2003); Schmidt et al. (2004); Ward et al. (2006)
ATP[3] analyses	Eukaryotic and prokaryotic cells	– Results within 1 minute	– Little scientific research in animal houses	Corrégé et al. (2003); Roelofs and Plagge (1998)
Visual inspection	Dirt	– Quick estimation of cleanliness	– Subjective	Huneau-Salaün et al. (2010)

[1] ACP, agar contact plates;
[2] Sponge swabs and environmental swabs may be used for surfaces that are at least 100 cm², however when using sponge swabs it is advisable to sample larger areas (Lahou and Uyttendaele, 2014);
[3] ATP, adenosine triphosphate.

3.4 Aspects to consider when monitoring the efficacy of C&D on farms

3.4.1 Locations

Inadequate cleaning and disinfection of animal houses or farm equipment can be an important source of infection for new incoming animals. To minimise the risk of round-to-round contamination, it is important to identify those locations in broiler and pig houses that are difficult to clean and disinfect in order to find a more efficient C&D protocol. It has been shown that drain holes as well as floor cracks are critical locations in broiler houses (Dewaele et al., 2012; Mueller-Doblies et al., 2010; Rajic et al., 2005; Luyckx et al., 2015). These locations may remain soiled because of the difficult access for cleaning and they are often still filled with water when disinfected. The residual organic material protects the bacteria from any contact with the disinfectants, affects the action of disinfectants and is a source of nutrients for the surviving bacteria. Therefore, floor cracks should be regularly repaired and filled in, whereas drain holes should be adequately rinsed after cleaning to flush out any residual organic material. Moreover, it is advisable to disinfect these locations twice as several studies showed that two disinfection rounds, rather than a single treatment, are more effective in eliminating pathogens such as *Salmonella* (Gradel and Rattenborg, 2003; Huneau-Salaün et al., 2010; Rose et al., 2000). Drinking cups were also identified as critical locations for C&D of broiler houses (Luyckx et al., 2015). Because of their fragile and angular construction, drinking cups are

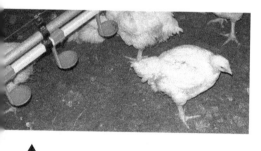

▲
Fig. 5.6: Soiled drinking cups in broiler houses after disinfection

difficult to clean (Fig. 5.6). Moreover, these cups are often filled with water after cleaning, which subsequently dilutes the applied disinfectant. Therefore, drinking cups should be emptied before disinfection.

In pig nursery units, slatted floors and drinking nipples were found to be critical locations as they are difficult to clean due to their specific design that features lots of edges (Luyckx et al., 2015).

Drinking cup and nipple contamination are considered to be critical because they can result in immediate oral inoculation of pathogens. In addition to the identified critical locations, many others also definitely exist because of the great variety in pig housing designs.

3.4.2 Composition and structure

It is also a known fact that the composition or structure of materials and the design of animal houses can be quite diverse. As a result, their ease of cleaning has an impact on the effectiveness of C&D. For example, there is a difference in the efficacy of C&D of battery-cage houses and on-floor houses, as battery-cage houses are more difficult to clean (Davies and Breslin, 2003b; Gradel and Ratteborg, 2003; Huneau-Salaün et al., 2010). Besides, wooden surfaces may be more difficult to clean than metal or plastic surfaces, probably because of the porous nature of wood (Rathgeber et al., 2009). Concrete is also often affected by numerous environmental factors, such as wear and tear caused by animals or vehicles and chemical degradation caused by feed or manure (Kymalainen et al., 2009). This all makes some elements difficult to clean and disinfect.

4 Conclusion

Measuring biosecurity is of utmost importance in benchmarking the disease prevention status of farms and identifying biosecurity shortcomings in order to improve biosecurity levels. Various questionnaire -based methods have been developed to describe and evaluate internal and external biosecurity. One of them, the Biocheck.UGent™, is a risk-based scoring system to quantify on-farm biosecurity and has been used worldwide to score biosecurity, identify biosecurity shortcomings and consequently provide advice on improving disease prevention. To evaluate the hygienic status on farms, most techniques use bacteriological detection methods to analyse surface contamination; agar contact plates and swab methods are the standard methods. ATP measurements yield information about the level of eukaryotic and prokaryotic cells present on surfaces, and are regarded as a measure of the cleanliness of a surface. When monitoring the hygienic status on farms, one should take into account the location to be sampled and the material structure and design of buildings.

References

American Association of Swine Veterinarians (AASV), 2007. PADRAP (Production Animal Disease Risk Assessment Program).

Australian Pork Industry, 2003. Australian pork industry Biosecurity program. Australia.

Australian Pork Industry, 2015. APIQ – Australian Pork Industry Quality Assurance Program. Barton, Australia.

Backhans A., Sjölund M., Lindberg A., Emanuelson U., 2015. Biosecurity level and health management practices in 60 Swedish farrow-to-finish herds. Acta Veterinaria Scandinavica 57, 14.

Backhans A., Sjölund M., Lindberg A., Emanuelson U., 2016. Antimicrobial use in Swedish farrow-to-finish pig herds is related to farmer characteristics. Porcine Health Management 2, 18.

Banhazi T. and Santhanam B., 2013. Practical evaluation of cleaning methods that could be implemented in livestock buildings in livestock housing: modern management to ensure optimal health and welfare of farm animals. Livestock housing: Modern management to ensure optimal health and welfare of farm animals. Wageningen Academic Publishers, 123-148.

Banhazi T.M., Currie E., Reed S., Lee I.B., Aarnik A.J.A., 2009. Controlling the concentration of airborne pollutants in piggery buildings in sustainable animal production. Wageningen Academic Publishers, Wageningen, the Netherlands.

Beloeil P.-A., Chauvin C., Proux K., Fablet C., Madec F., Alioum A., 2007. Risk factors for Salmonella seroconversion of fattening pigs in farrow-to-finish herds. Veterinary Research 38, 835-848.

Betts R.P., Chroleywood food research association, 2000. Conventional and rapid analytical microbiology in chilled foods, a comprehensive guide, 2nd edition, Woodhead Publishing Limited, Cambridge, England.

Carrique-Mas J.J., Marin C., Breslin M., McLaren I., Davies R., 2009. A comparison of the efficacy of cleaning and disinfection methods in eliminating Salmonella spp. from commercial egg laying houses. Avian Pathology 38, 419-424.

Corrégé I., De Azevedo Araujo C., Le Roux A., 2003. Mise au point d' un protocole de contrôle du nettoyage et de la désinfection en élevage porcin. Journées de la Recherche Porcine 26, 19-26.

Dalmaso G., Bini M., Paroni, R., Ferrari M., 2008. Qualification of high-recovery, flocked swabs as compared to traditional rayon swabs for microbiological environmental monitoring of surfaces. PDA Journal of Pharmaceutical Science and Technology 62, 191-199.

Davies R. and Breslin M., 2003a. Observations on Salmonella contamination of commercial laying farms before and after cleaning and disinfection. Veterinary Record 152, 283-287.

Davies R., Breslin M., 2003b. Investigation of Salmonella contamination and disinfection in farm egg-packing plants. Journal of Applied Microbiology 94, 191-196.

De Reu K., Grijspeerdt K., Herman, L., Heyndrickx M., Uyttendaele M., Debevere J., Putirulan F.F., Bolder N.M., 2006. The effect of a commercial UV disinfection system on the bacterial load of shell eggs. Letters in Applied Microbiology 42, 144-148.

Defra, 2007. Fact sheet 2: Biosecurity – Prevent the introduction and spread of classical swine fever – Advice for pig keepers. Department for environment, food and rural affairs (Defra), London, United Kingdom.

Dewaele I., Ducatelle R., Herman L., Heyndrickx M., De Reu K., 2011. Sensitivity to disinfection of bacterial indicator organisms for monitoring the Salmonella Enteritidis status of layer farms after cleaning and disinfection. Poultry Science 90, 1185-1190.

Dewaele I., Van Meirhaeghe H., Rasschaert G., Vanrobaeys M., De Graef E., Herman L., Ducatelle R., Heyndrickx M., De Reu K., 2012. Persistent Salmonella Enteritidis environmental contamination on layer farms in the context of an implemented national control program with obligatory vaccination. Poultry Science 91, 282-291.

Dolan A., Bartlett M., Mc Entee B., Creamer E., Humphreys H., 2011. Evaluation of different methods to recover meticillin-resistant Staphylococcus aureus from hospital environmental surfaces. Journal of Hospital Infection 79, 227-230.

Filippitzi M.E., Kruse A.B., Postma M., Sarrazin S., Maes D., Alban L., Nielsen L.R., Dewulf J., 2017. Review of transmission routes of 24 infectious diseases preventable by biosecurity measures and comparison of the implementation of these measures in pig herds in six European countries. Transboundary and Emerging Diseases. Http: "https://doi.org/10.1111/tbed.1275810.1111/tbed.12758.

Gelaude P., Schlepers M., Verlinden M., Laanen M., Dewulf J., 2014. Biocheck.UGent: A quantitative tool to measure biosecurity at broiler farms and the relationship with technical performances and antimicrobial use. Poultry Science 93, 2740-2751.

Ghent University, 2015. Biocheck.UGent. Ghent University – Faculty of Veterinary Medicine – Department of Reproduction, Obstetrics and Herd Health – Veterinary Epidemiology Unit, Merelbeke, Belgium.

Goverde M., Willrodt J., Staerk A, 2017. Evaluation of the Recovery Rate of Different Swabs for Microbial Environmental Monitoring. PDA Journal of Pharmaceutical Science and Technology 71, 33-42.

Gradel K.O., Jørgensen J.C., Andersen J.S., Corry J.E.L., 2004a. Monitoring the efficacy of steam and formaldehyde treatment of naturally Salmonella-infected layer houses. Journal of Applied microbiology 96, 613-622.

Gradel K.O. and Rattenborg E., 2003. A questionnaire-based, retrospective field study of persistence of Salmonella Enteritidis and Salmonella Typhimurium in Danish broiler houses. Preventive veterinary Medicine 56, 267-284.

Gradel K.O., Sayers A.R., Davies R.H., 2004b. Surface disinfection tests with Salmonella and a putative indicator bacterium, mimicking worst-case scenarios in poultry houses. Poultry Science 83, 1636-1643.

Hancox L.R., Le Bon M., Dodd C.E.R., Mellits K.H., 2013. Inclusion of detergent in a cleaning regime and effect on microbial load in livestock housing. Veterinary Record 173, 167-170.

Hedin G., Rynbäck J., Loré B., 2010. New technique to take samples from environmental surfaces using flocked nylon swabs. Journal of Hospital Infection, 75, 314-317.

Holtkamp D., Polson D., Wang C., Melody J., 2010. Quantifying risk and evaluating the relationship between external biosecurity factors and PPRS-negative herd survival. American Association of Swine Veterinarians, Omaha, Nebraska, USA.

Huneau-Salaün A., Michel V., Balaine L., Petetin I., Eono F., Ecobichon F., Bouquin S.L., 2010. Evaluation of common cleaning and disinfection programmes in battery cage and on-floor layer houses in France. British Poultry Science 51, 204-212.

Kim J.H. and Kim K.S., 2010. Hatchery hygiene evaluation by microbiological examination of hatchery samples. Poultry Science 89, 1389-1398.

Kymalainen H.R., Kuisma R., Maatta J., Sjoberg A.M., 2009. Assessment of cleanness of environmental surfaces of cattle barns and piggeries. Agricultural and Food Science 18, 268-282.

Laanen M., Bee, J., Ribbens S., Vangroenweghe F., Maes D., Dewulf J., 2010. Biosecurity in pig herds: development of an on-line scoring system and the results of the first 99 participating herds. Vlaams Diergeneeskundig Tijdschrift 79, 302-306.

Laanen M., Persoons D., Ribbens S., de Jong E., Callens B., Strubbe M., Maes D., Dewulf J., 2013. Relationship between biosecurity and production/antimicrobial treatment characteristics in pig herds. The Veterinary Journal 198, 508-512.

Lahou E. and Uyttendaele M., 2014. Evaluation of three swabbing devices for detection of Listeria monocytogenes on different types of food contact surfaces. International Journal of Environmental Research and Public Health 11, 804-814.

Luyckx K., Dewulf J., Van Weyenberg S., Herman L., Zoons J., Vervaet E., Heyndrickx M., De Reu K., 2015. Comparison of sampling procedures and microbiological and non-microbiological parameters to evaluate cleaning and disinfection in broiler houses. Poultry Science 94, 740-749.

Mannion C., Leonard F.C., Lynch P.B., Egan J., 2007. Efficacy of cleaning and disinfection on pig farms in Ireland. Veterinary Record 161, 371-375.

Merialdi G., Galletti E., Guazzetti S., Rosignoli C., Alborali G., Battisti A., Franco A., Bonilauri P., Rugna G., Martelli P., 2013. Environmental methicillin-resistant Staphylococcus aureus contamination in pig herds in relation to the productive phase and application of cleaning and disinfection. Research in Veterinary Science 94, 425-427.

Mueller-Doblies D., Carrique-Mas J.J., Sayers A. R., Davies R.H., 2010. A comparison of the efficacy of different disinfection methods in eliminating Salmonella contamination from turkey houses. Journal of Applied Microbiology 109, 471-479.

Oliveira C.J.B., Carvalho L.F.O.S., Garcia T.B., 2006. Experimental airborne transmission of Salmonella Agona and Salmonella Typhimurium in weaned pigs. Epidemiology & Infection 134, 199-209.

Pletinckx L.J., Dewulf J., De Bleecker Y., Rasschaert G., Goddeeris B.M., De Man I., 2013. Effect of a disinfection strategy on the methicillin-resistant Staphylococcus aureus CC398 prevalence of sows, their piglets and the barn environment. Journal of Applied Microbiology 114, 1634-1641.

Postma M., Backhans A., Collineau L., Loesken S., Sjölund M., Belloc C., Emanuelson U., Grosse Beilage E., Nielsen E.O., Stärk K.D.C., Dewulf J., 2016a. Evaluation of the relationship between the biosecurity status, production parameters, herd characteristics and antimicrobial usage in farrow-to finish pig production in four EU countries. Porcine Health Management 2, 1-11.

Postma M., Backhans A., Collineau L., Loesken S., Sjölund M., Belloc C., Emanuelson U., Grosse Beilage E., Stärk K.D.C., J., D., 2016b. The biosecurity status and its associations with production and management characteristics in farrow-to-finish pig herds. Animal 10, 478-489.

Postma M., Vanderhaeghen W., Sarrazin S., Maes D., Dewulf J., 2017. Reducing antimicrobial usage in pig production without jeopardizing production parameters. Zoonoses and Public Health 64, 63-74.

Rajic A., Keenliside J., McFall M.E., Deckert A.E., Muckle A.C., O'Connor B.P., Manninen K., Dewey C.E., McEwen S.A., 2005. Longitudinal study of Salmonella species in 90 Alberta swine finishing farms. Veterinary Microbiology 105, 47-56.

Ramvad C., Glavind A., Kruse A.B, Johansen C., Alban L., Nielsen L.R., 2017. Vurdering af smittebeskyttelse I 140 danske svinebesaetninger (Assessment of biosecurity in 140 Danish pig herds). Svin 8, 18-23.

Rathgeber B.M., Thompson K.L., Ronalds C.M., Budgell K.L., 2009. Microbiologic ion of poultry house wall materials and industrial cleaning agents. Journal of Applied Poultry Research 18, 579-582.

Roelofs P. and Plagge J., 1998. Cleaning of rooms for pigs after soaking with foam or water; costs and quality. F. Res. pig farming Report No. P 1.216, ISSN 0922-8586.

Rojo-Gimeno C., Postma M., Dewulf J., Hogeveen H., Lauwers L., Wauters E., 2016. Farm-economic analysis of reducing antimicrobial use whilst adopting improved management strategies on farrow-to-finish pig farms. Preventive Veterinary Medicine 129, 74-87.

Rose N., Beaudeau F., Drouin P., Toux J.Y., Rose V., Colin P., 2000. Risk factors for Salmonella persistence after cleansing and disinfection in French broiler-chicken houses. Preventive Veterinary Medicine 44, 9-20.

Rose N., Beaudeau F., Drouin P., Toux J.Y., Rose V., Colin P., 1999. Risk factors for Salmonella enterica subsp. enterica contamination in French broiler-chicken flocks at the end of the rearing period. Preventive Veterinary Medicine 39, 265-277.

Schmidt P.L., O'Connor A.M., McKean J.D., Hurd H.S., 2004. The association between cleaning and disinfection of lairage pens and the prevalence of Salmonella enterica in swine at harvest. Journal of Food Protection 67, 1384-1388.

Vangroenweghe F., Heylen P., Arijs D., Castryck F., 2009. Hygienograms for evaluation of cleaning and disinfection protocols in pig facilities. 8th International Symposium on the Epidemiology and Control of foodborne Pathogens in Pork, Safepork 30 September – 2 October 2009, Quebec, Canada 220-223.

Van Limbergen, T. Dewulf, J., Klinkenberg, M., Ducatelle, R., Gelaude, P., Méndez, J., Heinola, K., Papasolomontos, S., Szeleszczuk, P., Maes, D. on behalf of the PROHEALTH consortium. 2017, Scoring biosecurity in European conventional broiler production. Poultry Science, http://dx.doi.org/10.3382/ps/pex296.

Wageningen University, 2008. Checklist bestrijding Streptococcus suis door management-maatregelen. Wageningen University, Wageningen, the Netherlands.

Ward P.J., Fasenko G.M., Gibson S., McMullen L.M., 2006. A microbiological assessment of on-farm food safety cleaning methods in broiler barns. Journal of Applied Poultry Research 15, 326-332.

Winfield M.D. and Groisman E.A., 2003. Role of Non-host Environments in the Lifestyles of Salmonella and Escherichia coli. Applied and Environmental Microbiology 69, 3687-3694.

CHAPTER 6

CLEANING AND DISINFECTION

Filip Van Immerseel[1]

Kaat Luyckx[2]

Koen De Reu[2]

Jeroen Dewulf[3]

[1] Faculty of Veterinary Medicine, Department of Pathology, Bacteriology and Avian Diseases, University of Ghent, 9820 Merelbeke, Belgium

[2] Institute for Agricultural and Fisheries Research (ILVO), Technology and Science Unit, 9090 Melle, Belgium

[3] Faculty of Veterinary Medicine, Department of Obstetrics, Reproduction and Herd Health, Veterinary Epidemiology Unit, 9820 Merelbeke, Belgium

1 Introduction

In any infection control programme used in livestock production, animal breeding and animal shelters or veterinary practices/clinics, cleaning and disinfection is an essential component in preventing the persistence and spread of pathogens. The aim of cleaning and disinfection is to decrease microbial numbers on surfaces (and in the air) to a level that will ensure that most, if not all, animal pathogens and zoonotic agents are eliminated. Cleaning refers to the physical removal of organic matter and – where present – biofilms, so that the microorganisms and pathogens are optimally exposed to the disinfectant. Cleaning and disinfection of surfaces in stable environments will never yield full sterility, in contrast to disinfection of surfaces in clinical environments or sterilisation of medical instruments, where physical methods of disinfection (e.g. heat, radiation) are used. In the case of livestock production, cleaning and disinfection can be carried out between different rounds, so that young animals entering the facilities are placed in optimal conditions with an environment free, or at least with a low presence, of pathogenic micro-organisms. Cleaning and disinfection with animals present is more difficult. In such instances the corridors and animal-free spaces can be targeted, or partial and gradual cleaning and disinfection can be carried out in occupied stables or rooms, but this is less practical. Cleaning and disinfection may be carried out following a specific disease outbreak and in order to target specific pathogens, though in most cases it is a general prophylactic measure to reduce infection pressure and thus improve the overall health of the animals.

2 Practical aspects of cleaning and disinfection: a general protocol

2.1 Cleaning and disinfection procedure

In intensive animal production, cleaning and disinfection should be carried out each time when the stable is emptied. An important tool to facilitate hygiene and sanitation after cleaning and disinfection is the application of the 'all-in/all-out' principle, meaning that all animals are removed from a house or farm before cleaning and disinfecting, after which the animals can be let back in. This procedure can be performed simultaneously in all farm buildings. In many cases it is not possible to apply the 'all-in/all-out' principle, and if this is the case special measures should be taken to prevent cross-contamination.

A good cleaning and disinfection protocol consists of seven steps to ensure an optimal result. To start with a number of different cleaning procedures have to be taken aimed at the physical removal of dirt such as manure, litter, dust, feed and associated microorganisms and this before disinfecting the premises. This ensures effective disinfection of the remaining microorganisms as organic material hampers the activity of disinfectants; removing organic material also eliminates a source of nutrients for microorganisms present on floors and surfaces (Ruano et al., 2001; Moustafa Gehan et al., 2009). Biofilms also provide excellent protection for microorganisms (Akinbobola et al., 2017).

Contrary to popular belief, the cleaning stage is not only very important for ensuring the physical removal of organic matter but it also has a wider impact on the total reduction of microbial contamination than the disinfection stage. A recent study by Luyckx et al. (2015a), revealed that the mean total aerobic bacterial enumerations on swab samples taken in broiler houses, decreased by 2 log colony forming units (CFU)/625 cm^2 after cleaning and by 1.5 log CFU/625 cm^2 after disinfection. A good cleaning procedure therefore not only strongly reduces/removes microbiological contamination and organic material but also ensures that the subsequent disinfection stages have a greater impact on the remaining microbes. It is important to include the whole stable during the cleaning and disinfection process, including the ceiling, walls, the floor, pipelines, feeding troughs, drinking nipples and other equipment and material, to minimise potential contamination of previously cleaned areas. Some locations, such as dinking nipples, drain and floor cracks in broiler houses and grid floors and drinking nipples in pig nursery units also are more difficult to clean (Luyckx et al. 2015a; Luyckx et al. 2016a). A survey by Dewaele et al. (2012) discovered that hen houses were *Salmonella*-free after cleaning and disinfection but adjacent corridors and egg collecting areas were still contaminated and had not been cleaned sufficiently, which also underlines the importance of thorough cleaning and disinfection of all premises.

There are seven steps to ensure optimal cleaning and disinfection.

2.1.1 Dry cleaning

In general, stables need to be as empty as possible before cleaning and disinfection, without animals therefore; easy-to-dismantle equipment should also be removed and cleaned and disinfected outside the stable. Litter should then be removed and all visible dirt such as faecal matter, feed, crusts and dust should be removed including from pipes, window sills, and other materials. Appropriate equipment, such as shovels, scrapers and brushes (in some cases mounted on agricultural vehicles), are used during this step.

2.1.2 Soaking with water and a cleaning product

The next step is to soak all surfaces with water and a cleaning product. This step loosens and turns any organic material left after dry cleaning, into a solution. Foam is the preferred element for soaking as it has the advantage of a longer contact time with surfaces (including vertical surfaces) and makes it visually easier to differentiate treated and non-treated surfaces.

2.1.3 High-pressure cleaning

After a set contact time with the cleaning product (drying out needs to be avoided), the soaking liquid containing the loosened organic material needs to be removed by rinsing with high pressure (more than 50 atm but less than 120 atm) so that all organic debris and cleaning agents are removed; these may interfere later with the action of disinfectants. The more effective the soaking stage, the more efficient the high pressure cleaning will be. In practice cleaning products are not always used, although a study by Maertens et al. (2017) clearly shows lower counts using agar contact plate methods on surfaces when a cleaning product was applied in the cleaning and disinfection procedure.

The foaming-up rinsing-down principle must be used, meaning that during the soaking stage foam is applied floor to ceiling, and rinsing is done from ceiling to floor. It has been suggested that using hot water for cleaning would result in better results because of its ability to dissolve fat, although a study showed no significant difference in reducing the total aerobic bacterial counts and *Enterococcus* spp. contamination levels after cleaning broiler houses with hot or cold water (Luyckx et al., 2015b). An earlier study into animal houses also showed that the relevance of using hot water during cleaning of animal premises is negligible (Walters, 1967). One explanation could be that the action of cleaning products in combination with cold water is sufficient to dissolve fats and other organic material. There is a difference however in work comfort and required volume of water in favour of hot water (Luyckx et al., 2015a).

2.1.4 Drying

The next stage involves drying the stable before disinfection is carried out, as any remaining water will dilute the disinfectant concentration.

2.1.5 Disinfection

While cleaning will remove the residual organic material and the majority of the microbial population in a stable, disinfection will ideally kill most of the remaining microbes, although this depends on the type of disinfectant and the environmental conditions (see below). Surface disinfection or wet disinfection is often carried out with high pressure or an orchard sprinkler. In case of thermal fogging (i.e. dry disinfection), a highly concentrated disinfectant is heated and subsequently converted to a fog by a mobile or fixed fogger. Foam disinfection will improve the penetration into porous surfaces and increase the contact time. It also helps to visualise where the disinfection has already been applied and as such helps to avoid any forgotten areas.

To calculate the amount of solution needed to disinfect a stable one can use the following calculation methods:

1) First determine the floor surface of the stable (length of the stable * width of the stable).
2) Multiply the surface of the stable with a multiplication factor to account for the walls, ceiling, etc. As a rule of thumb this multiplication factor can be set to be 3.
3) Determine the volume of required water on the basis that one litre of water is required per 4 m^2.
4) Make a solution with the require dosing according to the manufacturer's guidelines.

As an example, in a pig stable of 10 m x 30 m (surface of 300m^2) an expected surface of 900m^2 (multiplication factor of 3) will need to be disinfected which requires 225 litres of water. If a disinfectant is used that requires application at 0.5% you will need 1.3 litres of disinfectant.

Disinfection can also be applied in a fumigation stage to ensure elimination of microbial agents in difficult-to-reach zones (ventilation, roof, air). When using fumigation, the volume of the stable needs to calculated first to determine the required amount of product. The volume can be calculated as:

Volume = (length of the stable * width of the stable * height of the stable) + ((length of the stable * width of the stable * highest point in the ceiling of the stable)/2)

Several products are registered for this form of application (see below), and a good ventilation after fumigation is needed.

Disinfectants must have sufficient contact time with surfaces in order to kill the bacteria concerned. Few disinfectants kill instantaneously. The amount of contact time needed will vary depending on the product used and the bacteria. 20-30 minutes is usually sufficient contact time for most disinfectants. The location of microorganisms should also be considered. Difficulties may arise in the penetration of a disinfectant in parts of equipment or infrastructure. Analysis of hygiene results in poultry farms showed better results if the disinfection stage was carried out by a specialised company rather than by farmers (Maertens et al., 2017). Analysis also showed that better results (lower agar contact plate counts) were obtained using two disinfectant products in one or two steps (Maertens et al., 2017).

2.1.6 Drying

After disinfection, the stable should be dried again to ensure that there are no remaining humid places where animals could come into contact with residues of the disinfectant products. Rinsing with water after disinfecting is not required. Only feeding troughs and drinking cups should be rinsed.

2.1.7 Testing efficacy

Verification of the efficacy of the cleaning and disinfection procedure is an essential step in the whole procedure to ensure that everything has been done appropriately. Different possibilities for measuring the hygiene are discussed in detail in chapter 5 of this book (how to measure biosecurity and hygiene).

If all the above steps are carried out appropriately, there will be no need for additional vacancy after cleaning and disinfection. In a recent study by Luyckx et al. (2016b), no additional reduction in the bacterial load of stable surfaces was observed with increased vacancy after thorough cleaning and disinfection. It also revealed that after a vacancy period of five days the bacterial load increased again, which could also be the result of recontaminated surfaces.

2.2 Cleaning products

The major compounds of cleaning products are detergents. Detergents have an amphipathic structure: a hydrophilic region and a hydrophobic region (hydrocarbon tail) (Field, 2014). Detergent monomers first reduce the surface and interfacial tension between air/water and soil/surface, which increases contact surface with detergent (mobilisation phase). When detergent monomer concentration exceeds the critical micelle concentration (CMC), molecules associate to form micelles (Fig. 6.1). This formation increases the solubility of hydrophobic compounds (solubilisation phase). The organic matter and/or bacteria are dispersed as micelle droplets in water (emulsification phase) and are washed away (Pacwa-Płociniczak et al., 2011).

Fig. 6.1: The relationship between surfactant concentration, surface tension and formation of micelles (adjusted Figure from Pacwa-Płociniczak et al., 2011)

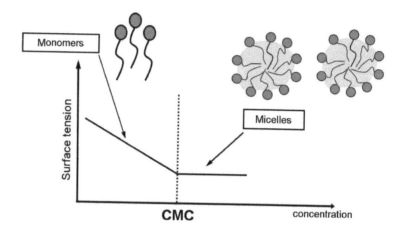

In addition to detergents, cleaning products include several other components such as chelating/sequestering agents, threshold agents, foam modifiers, corrosion inhibitors, pH modifiers, antimicrobials, emulsifiers, dyes, pigments, fragrances and water. Several of these compounds are discussed below.

2.2.1 Detergents

Four groups of detergents can be distinguished according to the head group (Porter, 1993; Salager, 2002).

1) Anionic detergents have a negatively charged head group. These detergents are the most commonly used detergents, are good emulsifiers when used at high temperatures and have strong foaming characteristics. They work in the same way as natural soaps except that they are less influenced by

hard-water ions. These detergents are the preferred choice for cleaning animal houses (Aceto, 2015).

2) Cationic detergents have a positively charged head group. These detergents are often used as fabric softeners in washing products. Quaternary ammonium compounds belong to this group and also have disinfecting properties.

3) Non-ionic detergents have an uncharged head and are the second most commonly used detergents. These detergents are good foam inhibitors and are therefore often used as industrial cleaning products, especially for cleaning on-site (CIP) applications. They are also less susceptible to pH changes and can be used in sour conditions.

4) Amphoteric detergents are negatively and positively charged. Depending on the pH, they can act as anionic and cationic detergents.

2.2.2 Other agents used in cleaning products

The content of dissolved minerals in tap water can vary from region. Because detergents have a higher binding affinity to these minerals than organic material, their activity is inhibited when used in hard water. To counteract this problem, chelating agents are added to cleaning products. These agents will bind the minerals and form soluble complexes, whereby free detergent monomers can actively bind organic material. Threshold agents are added to reduce the calcium deposit on the cleaned materials. Corrosion inhibitors inhibit corrosion formation on ferrous and non-ferrous metals. Alkaline substances or acids are added to influence the pH and application possibilities of the cleaning product. Alkaline cleaners are used to remove carbon-based organic compounds (e.g. fats, proteins, animal waste) and acidic cleaners for inorganic compounds (e.g. rust, corrosion, scale deposits). Depending on the degree of soiling, a weak or strong alkaline cleaner should be used for cleaning animal houses. In some cases, a solvent (e.g. glycol based compounds) is added to the cleaning product to remove tenacious soil (e.g. oily soils).

2.3 Disinfectants

Decontamination of surfaces can be carried out using physical inactivation of micro-organisms (e.g. heat, UV, ionizing radiation) or chemical compounds (disinfectants). Disinfectants are antimicrobial components that are used on inert surfaces. The term antiseptics is reserved for those antimicrobials that are sufficiently free from toxic effects so that they can be used on the body surface and wounds, but are still not safe enough to be administered systemically, in contrast to most antibiotics. Disinfectants can be used in a range of different ways and multiple classes of disinfectants exist, each containing many different molecules that can be used, depending on the actual aim of the application (surface, targeted microorganisms, environmental conditions, etc.). The ideal characteristics for a disinfectant would include the following:

1) fast action against a wide range of microorganisms;
2) limited inhibition of activity by environmental factors such as organic material or suboptimal temperature;
3) non-toxic for humans and animals;
4) stable in pure and diluted form;
5) water-soluble and not prone to inactivation in hard water;
6) homogenous in concentrated and diluted form;
7) easy-to-use;
8) penetrative;
9) non-corrosive.

2.3.1 Modes of action

Disinfectants have radical effects on the function of many different macromolecules (sugars, lipids, proteins, nucleic acids) and the respective microbial structures made up of combinations of these macromolecules. Structures on the outer microbial surface (such as bacterial cell wall, viral envelope) are particular targets, because these are the first that come into contact with the disinfectant molecules (McDonnell and Russell, 1999). After interaction with these outer surface structures of the microbial agents, other interactions (with cytoplasmic membrane, cytoplasm, DNA, cytoplasmic enzymes, etc.) may occur. This is in contrast to antibiotics, in which the modes of action are very specific. While physical methods of disinfection (i.e. sterilisation) transfer energy to the microbial agents that will cause death, the mode of action of disinfectants can be broadly broken down into three modes of action (McDonnell, 2008).

2.3.1.1 Coagulation or cross-linking of molecules

Cross-linking causes specific interactions between different macromolecules that lead to structure and function loss of these molecules. The most well-known types of disinfectants to cause cross-linking are aldehydes, alkylating agents, phenolic compounds and alcohols. Aldehydes for example cause strong covalent coupling of proteins (intra and inter) because of the cross-linking of free amine groups by the reactive aldehyde groups. The reactive groups in phenols and alcohols are the hydroxyl groups, while alkylating agents form alkyl or epoxide bounds between molecules.

2.3.1.2 Oxidation of molecules

The antimicrobial activity of oxidising agents is caused by the ability to remove electrons from proteins, fats and nucleic acids. This oxidation or loss of electrons is mainly caused by halogens and peroxides. Examples are oxidation of S-S bonds in proteins or unsaturated C-C bonds in lipids, and oxidation of nucleotide bases and the sugar-phosphate structure of DNA. Oxidised groups can initiate secondary reactions with other molecules.

2.3.1.3 Macromolecular structure disruption and membrane intercalation

Some types of disinfectants have rather specific primary action mechanisms, such as membrane intercalation. Examples are quaternary ammonium compounds and biguanidines (e.g. chlorhexidine) that penetrate the bacterial cell wall and interact with lipids and proteins in the cell membrane, resulting in leakage of cytoplasmic material and loss of membrane-associated functions, including transport of molecules and ATP production.

The choice of a disinfectant is often based on the targeted micro-organisms, the organic material load present on the surfaces, the environmental conditions (temperature for example) and the toxicity (risk for animals, human and environment). Quite a variety of product classes exist, and classification is mostly done by chemical structure. The characteristics of disinfectants (toxicity, spectrum, etc.) differ between product classes but variability can occur even within product class because of the chemical structure. A brief description is provided below of the most important product classes used in animal production and for veterinary purposes. The spectrum of activity is shown in Table 6.1. More detailed descriptions can be consulted in review papers by McDonnell and Russell (1999) and Suljagic (2008).

Table 6.1: The antimicrobial spectrum of disinfectants for most important chemical product classes and most important groups of micro-organisms. The table lists a general overview and within each class of disinfectants there are multiple compounds with different activities. Also within the groups of micro-organisms there is variability in characteristics in relation to resistance and sensitivity tio disinfectant molecules. (++ = in general very active; + = in general active; ± = limited activity; +/- : some molecules in this group are active). Adapted from http://www.cfsph.iastate.edu/pdf/antimicrobial-spectrum-of-disinfectants and *Linton* et al., 1987).

Group of micro-organisms	Acids	Alkalis	Alcohols	Aldehydes	Biguanides	QACs	Halogens	Peroxides	Phenols
Prions	-	-	-	-	-	-	-	-	-
Protozoal oocysts	-	+	-	-	-	-	-	-	+/-
Bacterial endospores	±	±	-	+	-	-	+	+	-
Mycobacteria	-	+	+	+	-	-	+	±	±
Non-enveloped viruses	-	±	-	+	-	-	+/±	±	-
Fungal spores	±	+	±	+	±	±	+	±	+
Gram negative bacteria	+	+	++	++	++	+	+	+	++
Enveloped viruses	+	+	+	++	±	±	+	+	±
Gram positive bacteria	+	+	++	++	++	+	+	+	++
Mycoplasmas	+	++	++	++	++	+	++	++	++

2.3.2.1 Acids and alkalis

Acids and alkalis are types of disinfectants, but most strong inorganic acids and alkalis are corrosive and hazardous to handle. Organic acids, for example, are used as feed additive in poultry and pig feed because of their antifungal (e.g. propionic acid) or antibacterial properties. Some are used in coated forms to control *Salmonella* or to enhance performance (e.g. butyrate). Alkalis contain sodium hydroxide and sodium carbonate for example but they are very corrosive, although they have been used to contain the foot-and-mouth virus. Ammonium sulphate combined with calcium carbonate and water yields calcium sulphate and ammonia, the latter having activity against *Eimeria* oocysts. Ammonium hydroxide also has been of value in killing *Eimeria* oocysts.

2.3.2.2 Aldehydes

Of the cross-linking agents, aldehydes are the most well-known. Aldehydes are broad-spectrum products (activity against bacteria, including spores, fungi and viruses) but some are very toxic and irritating and potentially carcinogenic, so precautions need to be taken when using these substances. The most widely used molecules are formaldehyde and glutaraldehyde. Formaldehyde is used as a fumigant and requires high humidity and temperatures above 15°C to be active. In several countries, formaldehyde is no longer authorised except in very low concentrations, due to its carcinogenic characteristics. Glutaraldehyde is known to be able to withstand rather high concentrations of organic matter and is therefore commonly used in preparations for stable disinfection.

2.3.2.3 Alcohols

Alcohols are compounds that are mostly used to disinfect hard material surfaces, or as hand or skin disinfectants. They exhibit a rapid and broad-spectrum antimicrobial activity against vegetative bacteria (not spores), viruses and fungi. The most commonly used compounds are ethanol, isopropanol and n-propanol. Because of its fast evaporation other active components are added to the disinfection in low concentrations to increase efficacy.

2.3.2.4 Phenolic compounds

Phenolic compounds are also cross-linking agents that cause denaturation of proteins. Originally obtained by distillation of coal, phenols are now synthesised chemically, and numerous products exist on the market with a wide range of toxicity and usage, from household products to disinfectants for surfaces. The basic structure is always a phenol ring, but side chains are present, ranging from simple methylations (cresols and xylenols (=dimethylphenols)) to complex structures (high molecular tar acids). Solubility in water also varies, and complex phenolic compounds (e.g. containing long aliphatic side chains) are often formulated in soap solutions or emulsions (to enhance solubility and penetration). In general, phenols are stable, non-corrosive, less prone to inactivation by organic material, but can cause irritation. As already indicated, there are exceptions to these general rules; chloroxylenol is a common household disinfectant (often in soap solution), and hexylresorcinol is used for non-toxic disinfection of air, and even as antiseptic.

2.3.2.5 Peroxides

The peroxides hydrogen peroxide and peracetic (peroxyacetic) acid are commonly used in peroxygen-based disinfectants. Oxidation is their main mode of action. Hydrogen peroxide is an environmentally-friendly product as it dissolves rapidly in water and oxygen. In addition, it exhibits a broad spectrum and rapid action against bacteria, yeast, viruses and bacterial spores. Peracetic acid, formed by a mixture of hydrogen peroxide and acetic acid in water, is considered bactericidal, viricidal and fungicidal in low concentrations. In addition, it remains more active in the presence of organic matter. A combination of both peroxygens is very effective as a farm disinfectant and is frequently used in animal husbandry (Maertens et al., 2017). However, a disadvantage is that these products are corrosive. Oxygen and hydroxyl radicals that oxidize molecules, including DNA, are the cause of the antimicrobial action of peroxides. A product with great promise is accelerated hydrogen peroxide (AHP), containing 0.5% hydrogen peroxide, combined with chelators, wetting agents and surfactants, so that the cleaning properties of the preparation is high (Holtkamp et al., 2017). Aerosolising peracetic acid is also carried out in order to disinfect whole rooms, Potassium peroxymonosulphate is a low-toxicity, broad-spectrum disinfectant that can cope with high organic loads and hard water environments. It is used for boot desinfection in stables, and is, in combination with a surfactant, sold as cleaning and disinfectant solution. Chlorine dioxide is a peroxygen compound that can be used for fumigation and is known for its ability to act on contaminations and biofilms in pipelines (Szabo et al., 2017). It is a small molecule that penetrates the biofilm better than peroxide and is more suitable therefore for biofilm removal (Rao et al., 2017). As a gas it can be used to sterilise rooms or buildings, without damaging electronic devices.

2.3.2.6 Halogens

Halogens are used as antiseptics and disinfectants, depending on the type of product and concentration. There are two types; the chlorine compounds and the iodine compounds or iodophors. The most well-known chlorine compound is household bleach (sodium hypochlorite), a broad-spectrum disinfectant easily inactivated by organic material. It is non-toxic but can be irritating, and is used for surface decontamination in low organic pollution environments (e.g. cleaned kennels). Organic chlorine compounds, for example, contain an N-Cl instead of an P-Cl bond as well as chloramine T, which can be used in boot disinfection baths since the inactivation by organic material is limited. Iodine products are broad-spectrum disinfectants and are mostly nowadays as iodophors – combinations of iodine and solubilising agents such as polyvinylpyrrolidine (povidone-iodine) – yielding an antiseptic product. Halogens are also prone to inactivation by organic material, hard water and surfactants. The mode of action of halogens has been attributed to oxidation, although cell wall penetration and protein and DNA structure disruption has also been proposed, depending on the compound. Their corrosive character is a minor point. A study by Maertens et al. (2017) also revealed poorer hygiene results compared to other disinfectant products in poultry stables.

2.3.2.7 Tenso-active compounds

Tensio-active compounds have been used as antiseptics, and are often used in disinfectant formulations to enhance penetration. Although multiple classes of tensio-active compounds exist, the *quaternary ammonium compounds* (QACs) are the main compounds used as antiseptics and surface detergents. Many different chemicals of this product class are used which means that they have a diverse range of specific action which is most frequently explained by cell membrane disruption. The spectrum is rather narrow and effective against Gram-positive vegetative bacteria, yeast, fungi and some viruses (especially enveloped). The QACs are easily inactivated by anionic detergents, hard water and organic material. Another class of positively charged compounds is the biguanides, containing chlorhexidine, an antiseptic chemical that is easily inactivated by anionic compounds and organic matter, and is often used as skin antiseptic. The spectrum is mainly antibacterial. As already mentioned, the list of disinfectant compounds discussed here is far from complete.

In practice, almost exclusively combination products containing multiple chemicals from different chemical classes are used for disinfecting surfaces in the animal production industry. They originate mostly from different product classes, combined with chelators (such as EDTA, to capture bivalent cations for activity in hard water), detergents (e.g. QACs for improving penetration) and stabilising agents. Mixtures of active compounds often aim at decreasing toxicity (lower dosage per compound), increasing action and broadening the antimicrobial spectrum.

Aerosols are used to disinfect surfaces or regions in stables or rooms that are not easily accessible via classical disinfection and for air disinfection. An aerosol consists of a very fine liquid phase in a gas phase and microbial killing occurs after condensation of the disinfectant product on the microorganisms. Nebulisation or aerosolising equipment is designed to generate the aerosols (foggers). Examples of compounds used are formadehyde, lactate, hexylresorcinol, and peroxides.

Few antibacterial agents are actively sporicidal. Disinfectants that are sporicidal, i.e. glutaraldehyde, formaldehyde, peracetic acid and hydrogen peroxide, often require higher concentrations and longer contact times for this effect than for bactericidal action. The mechanisms of sporicidal activity are poorly understood, probably due to the complex nature of bacterial spores and the fact that disinfectants may have more than one actual or potential target site.

2.4 Factors affecting efficacy of disinfectants

In addition to microorganisms and disinfectants, external factors also determine the outcome of disinfection. The impact of external factors differs according to the type of disinfectant. Factors such as concentration, contact time, temperature, relative humidity (RH), pH, extraneous materials (e.g. organic matter) and material cleanability, location and number of microorganisms, condition and susceptibility of the organism to the biocide, can influence the reaction between disinfectants and micro-organisms. This has been described in detail by Russell (1999).

2.4.1 Concentration of disinfectants

Using the appropriate concentration is a key element in the correct application of biocides. In addition to leading to reduced efficacy, over-dilution of biocides can lead to the survival of less-sensitive bacteria. Biocides which have to be applied in high concentrations, e.g., alcohols and phenolic compounds, are highly affected by changes in concentration, whereas those with a low recommended concentration, e.g., formaldehyde, are less influenced by this. Still, one has to keep in mind that dilution errors in disinfectant concentrations can occur.

2.4.2 **Contact time**

Disinfectants must have sufficient contact time with the surfaces in order to kill the microorganisms concerned. Few disinfectants kill instantaneously. The amount of contact time needed will vary depending on the product used and the targeted microorganisms. A quick splash of a dirty boot into a footbath will not accomplish anything except to give a false sense of security (cleaning before disinfection is crucial here). 20-30 minutes is usually sufficient contact time for most disinfectants.

2.4.3 **Temperature**

Disinfectant activity usually increases in line with an increase in temperature, although some disinfectants are more temperature-dependent than others. It has been reported that glutaraldehyde is effective at temperatures as low as 5°C, whereas formaldehyde requires a minimum around 16°C.

2.4.4 **Relative humidity**

In addition to temperature, the relative humidity in animal houses can also influence gaseous disinfectants, e.g. formaldehyde and chlorine dioxide. The relative humidity (RH) for disinfection with formaldehyde should be at least 70%.

2.4.5 **pH**

pH can influence the cell surface of bacteria as well as the action of the disinfectant. Firstly, when pH increases, the number of negatively charged groups on the cell surface of bacteria will increase. Therefore, positively charged or cationic disinfectants have an enhanced degree of binding. Secondly, if the disinfectant is an acid or a base, its degree of ionisation is dependent on the pH. For peracetic acid, the non-ionized molecule is the active form, and alkaline pH will decrease the action by forming ions. For QAC and glutaraldehyde, bactericidal action increases with pH and are best used under alkaline conditions therefore.

2.4.6 Extraneous material, cleanability and interactions with other molecules

Examples of extraneous materials include organic matter, surface active agents and cations. Organic matter may interfere with the microbiocidal activity of disinfectants. This reaction between the biocide and the organic matter (e.g., phospholipids in faeces), leaves a smaller antimicrobial concentration of the antimicrobial agent targeting microorganisms. This reduced activity is often noticed with highly reactive compounds, such as chlorine-based disinfectants and peroxides. As some surfaces in animal houses are difficult to clean and hence possibly still contain organic matter, these are likely sources of infectious agents. In addition, organic matter can protect organisms from disinfectant contact. The material to be disinfected is also of importance. Wood surfaces are more difficult to clean than plastic or metal, due to the porosity of wood (Rathgeber et al., 2009). It has been demonstrated that the performance of biocides on porous or rough surfaces such as wood and concrete is lower than on smooth surfaces such as metals and plastics (Harding et al., 2011). In addition to the type of material, the design of surfaces also has an impact on the cleanability. Animal houses are also often affected by numerous environmental factors such as wear and tear caused by animals and vehicles and chemical degradation caused by feeds and manure (Kymalainen et al., 2009), making them difficult to clean and disinfect. Surface active agents present in cleaning products can also reduce the action of QAC for example (Russell, 2004). Therefore it is important that animal houses are thoroughly rinsed with water after cleaning. Cations present in hard water (i.e. Ca^{2+} and Mg^{2+}) may reduce the action of disinfectants by interacting with them to form insoluble precipitates. Failure to make a fresh solution of disinfectant or a solution visibly contaminated by organic material like manure may result in a product that has lost its effectiveness. Even worse, it may generate a false sense of security. Sufficient concentration and contact time may overcome some of these problems with certain classes of disinfectants, but often increasing the concentration or contact time renders use of the product impractical, expensive, caustic, or dangerous to the users or to the animals. And finally, bacteriologically contaminated water used to dilute disinfectants may also be a problem because non-target bacteria also 'dilute' disinfectant activity. The location of microorganisms should also be considered. Difficulties may arise in ability of a disinfectant to penetrate parts of equipment or infrastructures (Fraise et al., 2004).

2.5 Resistance to disinfectants

Intrinsic and acquired resistance against disinfectants both exist, although it is believed that the latter is of little importance compared to the role it plays in antibiotic resistance. The reason is that many disinfectants are not used to target specific functions that may be modified using mutations, but to target general structural microbial components (e.g. amine groups in case of aldehydes). There are exceptions but the importance of acquired resistance in the field is believed to be limited. Different mechanisms of intrinsic resistance may be important.

The first form of intrinsic resistance is caused by the general microbial surface structure that can protect the microbes against disinfectant action. It is not within the scope of this chapter to cover the composition of microbial surface structures in detail. Because of differences in the bacterial cell wall, Gram-negative bacteria are considered to be less sensitive to the action of disinfectants as compared to Gram-positives and *Mycoplasma* spp. (without cell wall). Mycobacteria are even less sensitive than most Gram-negative bacteria (McDonnell and Russell, 1999; McDonnell, 2008). The envelope of viruses provides a target for disinfectants and as such viruses without envelope are less sensitive that viruses with an envelope (Maillard and Russell, 1997). These are general principles however and it is clear that there is a large variability within the different general classes of microorganisms. As an example, within the Gram-negative group, there is a huge variation in bacterial families, genera and species with differences in cell wall composition (e.g. LPS structure), causing potential variation in susceptibilities. However, the application of disinfectants in the correct doses and with sufficient contact time will, depending on the spectrum of activity, kill the microorganisms anyway. Dormant stages of microorganisms, such as spores, are the second form of intrinsic resistance against disinfectants. Some bacterial groups (e.g. Bacilli, Clostridia) may form endospores, which induce resistance to environmental factors such as heat and antimicrobial molecules, including disinfectants. It is not the aim of this chapter to describe the spore composition in detail, but the low water content, the presence of protective molecules and the high density of different layers that form the spore, mediate resistance. Exospores, such as those produced by *Actinomyces* and *Streptomyces* spp., and fungal spores are thought to be more sensitive than bacterial endospores. Coccidial oocysts are also resistant structures that require a special disinfection in poultry stables for example (often based on ammonia). Prions are the most resistant form of infectious compounds. The relative susceptibility of microorganisms to disinfectants, in general, is shown in Table 6.2.

Table 6.2: Relative susceptibility of groups of micro-organisms to disinfectants (adapted from *Fraise* et al., 2012)

Range	Group of micro-organisms
Resistant	Prions
	Bacterial endospores
	Protozoal oocysts
	Mycobacteria
	Small non-enveloped viruses
	Protozoal cysts
	Fungal spores
	Gram negative bacteria
	Moulds
	Yeasts
	Protozoa
	Large non-enveloped viruses
	Gram positive
Susceptible	Enveloped viruses

Growth phase responses can also cause intrinsic resistance, although these will not be able to fully confer resistance to well-executed disinfection rounds and are only relevant when doses and contact times are insufficient. These responses are typically induced in the stationary phase of bacterial growth and include motility (to zones with lower antimicrobial properties), oxidative stress (e.g. catalase) and heat shock responses (involved in the repair of molecular damage), slow metabolism, and efflux mechanisms (McDonnell, 2008). The latter means that bacteria can pump out antimicrobials through efflux pump systems and outer membrane channels (Poole, 2005). Here again, this system is not sufficient to withstand bacterial killing if disinfectants are used correctly. A very important form of intrinsic resistance is biofilm formation. These biofilms are three-dimensional structures of populations of microorganisms that develop on, or are associated with surfaces in a humid environment and may contain multiple microbial species (Branda et al., 2005; Jain et al., 2007). Biofilms produce an extracellular matrix that contains molecules such as cellulose or poly-ß-1.6-N-acetylglucosamine, and proteins. The composition of the matrix depends on the microbial composition, but may be involved in neutralisation of disinfectant molecules that, as a result, are unable to penetrate in the biofilm, while efflux pumps can also be activated (Tabak et al., 2007). Biofilms are well-known because they are important sources of contamination for medical equipment (catheters for example), drinking water lines as well as surfaces and floors. Oxidising agents are the most appropriate disinfectants for controlling biofilm, although prevention of biofilm formation on surfaces by preventing mineral deposition in water pipes for example (as material for adhesion of microorganisms) is also a possible solution (e.g. via electromagnetic water treatment, acidification, etc.). Enzymes can also potentially be used to break down the biofilm matrix.

3 Conclusion

Cleaning and disinfection is only effective if a full procedure made up of multiple stages is carefully followed. This includes dry and wet cleaning, rinsing and drying stages and thorough disinfection. Multiple cleaning and disinfectant products exist, and many different classes of products with different characteristics can be used so that the choice of product will depend on the application. The choice of disinfectant product also depends on whether specific pathogens are targeted, because different groups of microorganisms have different intrinsic resistance properties to disinfectant compounds. Environmental factors can also affect the cleaning and disinfection procedure and should be monitored.

6

References

Aceto, H. (2015). Biosecurity in hospitals; In: Robinson's current therapy in equine medicine, 7th ed. Elsevier Saunders, Missouri, USA.

Akinbobola, A., Sherry, L., McKay, W., Ramage, G., Williams, C. (2017). Tolerance of Pseudomonas aeruginosa in in-vitro biofilms to high-level peracetic acid disinfection. *Journal of Hospital Infection*, doi: 10.1016/j.jhin.2017.06.024.

Branda, S., Vik, A., Friedman, L., Kolter, R. (2005). Biofilms: the matrix revisited. *Trends in Microbiology* 13: 20-26.

Dewaele, I., Van Meirhaeghe, H., Rasschaert, G., Vanrobaeys, M., De Graef, E., Herman, L., Ducatelle, R., Heyndrickx, M., De Reu, K. (2012). Persistent *Salmonella* Enteritidis environmental contamination on layer farms in the context of an implemented national control programme with obligatory vaccination. *Poultry Science* 91, 282-291.

Field, C. (2014). Detergents. In: Encyclopaedia of lubricants and lubrication. Springer, Berlin Heidelberg, Germany.

Gradel, K.O., Sayers, A.R., Davies, R.H. (2004). Surface disinfection tests with *Salmonella* and a putative indicator bacterium, mimicking worst-case scenarios in poultry houses. *Poultry Science* 83, 1636-1643.

Harding, M., Howard, R., Daniels, G., Mobbs, S., Lisowski, S., Allan, N., Omar, A., Olson, M. (2011). A multi-well plate method for rapid growth, characterisation and biocide sensitivity testing of microbial biofilms on various surface materials. In: Science against microbial pathogens: communicating current research and technological advances A. Méndez-Vilas (Ed.).

Holtkamp, D., Myers, J., Thomas, P., Karriker, L., Ramirez, A., Zhang, J., Wang, C. (2017). Efficacy of an accelerated hydrogen peroxide disinfectant to inactivate porcine epidemic diarrhoea virus in swine faeces on metal surfaces. *Canadian Journal of Veterinary Research* 81: 100-107.

Gibson, H., Taylor, J.H., Hall, K.E., Holah, J.T. (1999). Effectiveness of cleaning techniques used in the food industry in terms of the removal of bacterial biofilms. *Journal of Applied Microbiology* 87, 41-48.

Jain, A., Gupta, Y., Agrawal, R., Khare, P., Jain, S.K. (2007). Biofilms: a microbial life perspective, a review. *Current reviews in therapeutic drug carrier systems* 24: 393-443.

Kymalainen, H., Kuisma, R., Maatta, J., SJoberg, A. (2009). Assessment of cleanness of environmental surfaces of cattle barns and piggeries. *Agricultural and Food Science* 18: 268-282.

Luyckx, K., Dewulf, J., Van Weyenberg, S., Herman, L., Zoons, J., Vervaet, E., Heyndrickx, M., De Reu, K. (2015a). Comparison of sampling procedures and microbiological and non-microbiological parameters to evaluate cleaning and disinfection in broiler houses. *Poultry Science* 94, 740-749.

Luyckx, K., VanWeyenberg, S., Dewulf, J., Herman, L., Zoons, J., Vervaet, E., Heyndrickx, M., De Reu, K. (2015b). On-farm comparisons of different cleaning protocols in broiler houses. *Poultry Science* 94, 1986-1993.

Luyckx K., Millet S., Van Weyenberg S., Herman L., Heyndrickx M., Dewulf J., De Reu K. (2016a). Comparison of competitive exclusion with classical cleaning and disinfection on bacterial load in pig nursery units. *BMC Veterinary Research* 12:189.

Luyckx K., Millet, S., Van Weyenberg, S., Herman, L., Heyndrickx, M., Dewulf, J., De Reu, K. (2016b). A 10-day vacancy period after cleaning and disinfection has no effect on the bacterial load in pig nursery units. *BMC Veterinary Research*. 12:236.

Maertens, H., De Reu, K., Van Weyenberg, S., Van Coillie, E., Meyer, E., Van Immerseel, F., Vandenbroucke, V., Vanrobaeys, M., Dewulf, J. (2017). Evaluation of the hygienogram scores and related data obtained after cleaning and disinfection of poultry houses in Flanders during the period 2007 to 2014. *Poultry Science*, 97, 620-627.

Maillard, J.-Y., Russell, A.D. (1997). Viricidal activity and mechanisms of action of biocides. *Science Progress* 80: 287-315.

McDonnell, G., Russell, A.D. (1999). Antiseptics and disinfectants: activity, action, and resistance. *Clinical Microbiology Reviews* 12, 147-179.

McDonnell, G. (2008). Biocides: modes of action and mechanisms of resistance. In: Disinfection and decontamination. Principles, applications and related issues. Gurusamy Manivannan (Ed.). CRC Press.

Moustafa Gehan, Z., Anwer, W., Amer, H, El-Sabagh, I., Rezk, I., Badawy, E. (2009). In-vitro efficacy comparisons of disinfectants used in commercial poultry farms. *International Journal of Poultry Production* 8, 237-241.

Pacwa-Płociniczak, M., Płaza, G.A., Piotrowska-Seget, Z., Cameotra, S.S. (2011). Environmental applications of biosurfactants: recent advances. *International Journal of Molecular Sciences* 12, 633-54.

Poole, K. (2005). Efflux-mediated antimicrobial resistance. *Journal of Antimicrobial Chemotherapy* 56: 20-51.

Porter, M.R. (1993). Handbook of surfactants. Springer Science Bussiness Media, New York.

Rathgeber, B., Thompson, K., Ronalds, C., Budgell, K., (2009). Microbiological evaluation of poultry house wall materials and industrial cleaning agents. *Journal of Applied Poultry Research* 18, 579-582.

Rao, T., Kumar, R., Balamurugan, P., Vithal, G. (2017). Microbial Fouling in a Water Treatment Plant and Its Control Using Biocides. *Biocontrol Science* 22: 105-119.

Ruano, M., El-Attrache, J., Villegas, P. (2001). Efficacy comparisons of disinfectants used by the commercial poultry industry. *Avian Diseases* 45, 972-977.

Russell, A.D. (1999). Factors influencing the efficacy of antimicrobial agents. In: Russell, A.D., Hugo, W.B., and Ayliffe, GA. J. Disinfection, preservation and sterilisation. Oxford, UK, Blackwell Science Ltd.

Salager, J.-L. (2002). Surfactants; types and uses. http://nanoparticles.org/pdf/Salager-E300A.pdf

Suljagic, V. (2008). A pragmatic approach to judicious selection and proper use of disinfectant and antiseptic agents in healthcare settings. In: Disinfection and decontamination. Principles, applications and related issues. Gurusamy Manivannan (Ed.). CRC Press.

Szabo, J., Meiners, G., Heckman, L., Rice, E., Hall, J. (2017). Decontamination of *Bacillus* spores adhered to iron and cement-mortar drinking water infrastructure in a model system using disinfectants. *Journal of Environmental Management* 187: 1-7.

Tabak, M., Scher, K., Hartog, E., Romling, U., Matthews, K., Chikindas, M., Yaron, M. (2007). Effect of triclosan on *Salmonella* Typhimurium at different growth stages and in biofilms. *FEMS Microbiology Letters* 267: 200-206.

Walters, A. (1967). Hard surface disinfection and its evaluation. *Journal of Applied Bacteriology* 30: 56-65.

CHAPTER 7

HYGIENIC ASPECTS OF AIR AND DECONTAMINATION OF AIR

Steven J. Hoff

Department of Agricultural and Biosystems Engineering, Iowa State University, 4331 Elings Hall, Ames, Iowa USA

1 Introduction

Biosecurity measures in animal housing systems have been in place for many years. Protocols for at-the-gate and pre-entry to a facility are well developed throughout the world. The majority of these measures aim to secure physical entry through some tangible vector such as clothes, shoes, truck traffic, and rendering. Less developed, but equally important, is the fact that measures for air transmission of disease into and from animal housing systems are gaining in popularity. Measures aimed at mitigating air vector transmission are in many cases very costly relative to other physical vectors and failure to abide by some basic principles can negatively affect other aspects of production systems, such as fresh-air exchange rates, and overall air quality for employees and animals. This chapter will focus on air as a vector of disease transmission, especially viruses associated with pigs and poultry, and the measures being taken to address this disease vector.

2 Air as a disease transmission vector

Tests regarding aerosol transmission of livestock viruses have been conducted in both lab and field settings to test the viability of specific viruses after aerosol transmission, the distance a virus can travel, and the particles that carry the virus.

Lab and field work conducted in an attempt to confirm the transfer of viruses via aerosols yield different results. A 2002 study attempted to transmit PRRSV by aerosols in field conditions where 210 pigs housed in a swine finishing facility were broken down into 10 uninfected indirect contact pigs in one pen, no pigs in another pen, and 15 to 16 infected and 6 to 7 uninfected direct contact pigs in nine remaining pens. In addition, two trailers, each with 10 pigs, were parked on either side of the facility, one 30 metres from the exhaust fans and the other 1 metre away. The sentinel pigs in the trailers were exposed to the air from the infected barn for three days before being moved to the buildings 30 and 80 metres from the infected barn. After a 21-day monitoring period, the direct and indirect contact pigs became infected, while the sentinel pigs did not (Otake S. , Dee, Jacobsen, Torremorrell, & Pijoan, 2002). A similar study conducted in 2004 at the same disinfected, virus free site was set up in the same manner, except that the sentinel pigs in one trailer were positioned 15 metres from the exhaust fans with a longer exposure time period of 7 days. The results were the same; the direct and indirect contact pigs became infected while the sentinel pigs tested negative. Researchers speculated that the air supply from the infected barn could have been too low; the pigs too young to excrete the virus, or the virus had attached itself to the walls of the tube connecting the airspaces of the barn and trailer (Trincado, et al., 2004).

A laboratory model was followed a year later in 2005 by some of the same researchers. In this model, seven pigs were placed in a chamber at the end of a 150-metre long tunnel through which an aerosolised PRRS virus travelled. After exposure for 3 hours, 3 of the 6 pigs exposed to the virus contracted PRRS. However, this experiment was conducted under ideal conditions while high amounts of the virus were present for an extended length of time. This experiment only confirms the potential of the virus to transfer over extended distances and still be viable. It does not provide any proof of the virus's viability in the field and suggests that the transmission of PRRSV in the field over this distance is rare (Dee S. , et al., 2005). Another lab test focused on the rate of infection based on varying rates of air transfer between two chambers. Exposed to a rate of 70% air transfer from an infected chamber to an uninfected chamber, 94% of the pigs in the second chamber tested positive for PRRSV. At 10% transfer, 100% of the pigs in the second chamber tested positive for PRRSV, and a transfer rate of 1% yielded the same result (Kristensen, Botner, Takai, Nielsen, & Jorsal, 2004). Although the rate of transfer varied in this experiment, the actual amount of air transferred between neighboring barns is estimated at approximately 2% (Bjerg, 2000).

Across these studies, a trend emerges showing that results from lab tests were much more successful in having a viable virus after transporting it some distance than tests in a field setting. Although tests conducted in labs may not be accurate in the field, they do provide valuable information on the range of a virus in ideal conditions and their viability (Dee S. , et al., 2005). Laboratory tests may not be as accurate as field tests because of the amount of dust (Spekreijse D. , Bouma, Koch, & Stegeman, 2011). In true field settings, a much higher volume of dust is present, providing more opportunities for the virus to attach to these particles, and larger particles in turn have an increased probability of carrying a virus. In addition, the viability of IAV and PRRSV depends on the size of the particles. Size also affects the distance viruses can travel as well as their ability to survive. Finally, relative humidity, temperature, and airspeed have a strong impact on the settling time of the dust particles. A table in the report entitled 'Concentration, Size Distribution, and Infectivity of Airborne Particles Carrying Swine Viruses' summarises particle size distribution for airborne viruses PRRS, PEDV, and IAV-S (Alonso, Raynor, Davies, & Torremorell, 2015). In one reported incidence, an outbreak of PRRSV occurred in 6 farms that had no direct contact with each other. Each strain was identical, every case was from the same source; the only connection was the relative location of the farms to each other. After studying the pattern and time that these outbreaks occurred, researchers concluded that as a virus disperses, it fans out from the original source (Lager, Mengeling, & Wesley, 2001).

Another prominent area of testing is the range of a virus and its viability at that point. Foot-and-mouth disease is known to travel 60 km over land and 100 to 280 km over sea (Donaldson, Gloster, Harvey, & Deans, 1982). A virus with a much shorter range, Aujeszky's Disease, has been confirmed to travel 1.3-1.8 km (Grant, Scheidt, & Rueff, 1994). Two studies in 2009 and 2010 confirmed that PRRSV can travel up to 9.2 km and still be infectious to pigs. However, 9.2 km was the outer range of the testing field around the infectious site so there is still the possibility that PRRSV can travel greater distances, although it may not remain viable (Otake S. , Dee, Corzo, Oliveira, & Deen, 2010); (Dee, Otake, Oliveira, & Deen, 2009). A study into the transmission of PEDV in 2014 in Oklahoma USA detected genetic material of PEDV 16 km downwind from the infected site. However, the virus was only viable in areas within 1,6 km of the site. Research-ers suggested that solar light, temperature, or UV radiation could have deactivated the virus beyond 1,6 km (Alonso, et al., 2014). A study on IAV-S returned results showing that 75% of the infected barns were expelling the virus from their exhaust fans and 50% of the sites showed that the virus was still present 2.1 km downwind (Corzo, Culhane, Dee, Morrison, & Torremorell, 2013).

A 2008 study attempted to evaluate the infectivity of pathogens expired by infected pigs. Pigs were infected with PRRSV, Porcine circovirus 2, swine influenza, porcine respiratory coronavirus, Mycoplasma hyopneumoniae, and Bordatella bronchiseptica. Expired air samples were collected for 5 minutes from pigs whose snouts were placed in a large canine surgical mask connected to an impinger with sterile collection fluid. Nasal or oral (PRRSV) swabs were also collected for all pathogens. The first day of detection and frequency varied according to pathogen. Swabs for all pathogens in the upper respiratory tract tested positive. In the expired air however, only pigs infected with Mycoplasma hyopneumoniae and Bordatella bronchiseptica were positive. This could be attrib-uted to the fact that only small quantities of the pathogen were aerosolised from individual pigs or that the pathogen was present in quantities smaller than the detection device could recognise (Hermann, Brockmeier, Yoon, & Zimmermann, 2008).

One final area of testing attempted to quantify the rate at which a virus will spread. A 2011 study on Avian Influenza in the Neth-erlands focused on short-range transmission and attempted to quantify the rate at which the virus spread. The researchers used HPAI H5N1 in an experiment with a total of 160 chickens, some infected and some not. Across their experiments, they varied the number of chickens in a room, the number of chickens in each pen in the room, and the spacing of the pens. Air and dust samples were also collected for each test. Infected chickens were placed at 0 metres, and two other pens were placed at varying distances from the inoculated pen. The tests in the rooms with more chickens resulted in a greater rate of infection than the tests in the rooms with a lower total number of chickens. The varying distances of the pens from each other made it possible to quantify the rate at which H5N1 spread. For example, a non-infected pen at 0.2 metres from the infected pen was estimated to have an infection rate of 0.13 new infections/day. Similarly, a 0.4 metre spacing was estimated at 0.21 infections/day and direct exposure was estimated at 1.43 infections/day. This study concluded that airborne transmission was possible over short distances, although not likely. However, the researchers suggested that if the same experiment was conducted in a true field setting with more dust present, infection rates would increase (Spekreijse D. , Bouma, Koch, & Stegeman, 2011). The rate of infection by low pathogenic avian influenza H9N2, via aerosol inoculation in chickens, was tested finding that 41.7% of the chickens that inhaled a dose of 57 EID_{50} were infected, while the chickens that inhaled a dose of 3.7 x 10^3 EID_{50} were 91.7% susceptible. This study effectively demonstrated the possible transmission of LPAI H9N2 or similar viruses via aerosols over short distances (Guan, Fu, Chan, & Spencer, 2013).

3 Aerosol size and physical capture and non-contact virus destruction considerations

Because aerosol transmission of viruses such as PEDV, IAV-S, and PRRSV among others has been identified as a possible route of infection between farms (Alonso, et al., 2014) (Corzo, Culhane, Dee, Morrison, & Torremorell, 2013) (Dee, Otake, Oliveira, & Deen, 2009) (Otake S. , Dee, Corzo, Oliveira, & Deen, 2010), the latest challenge has become how to best combat this issue. Physical capture methods include the use of High-Efficiency Particulate Arrestance (HEPA) filters, antimicrobial filters, low-cost and bag filters, and a filtration system integrated into evaporative coolers. Several studies comparing these physical capture methods, in addition to non-contact ultraviolet light (UV) destruction have been carried out, some of which are summarised below.

Filters have been given a rating scale to classify the particle removal capability of the filters. Typically, filters rank between 1 and 16 Minimum Efficiency Reporting Value (MERV), but the scale sometimes extends to 20. Particulate concentration, measured before and after passing through the filter, determines the MERV rating, based on the worst result. A MERV 16 filter, commonly used in swine facilities, removes particles ranging from 0.3 to 1.0 μm at >95% capture efficiency (What are MERV Ratings and How Do They Work?, 2010). Typically, IAV-S, PRRSV, and PEDV range from 0.5-10.0 μm in size (Alonso, Raynor, Davies, & Torremorell, 2015), making MERV 16 filters an effective choice. However, MERV 16 filters restrict airflow more than a MERV 14 filter thus reducing the effective airflow delivery to a barn with typical agricultural fan systems (Dee, Pitkin, & Deen, 2009). Engineered ventilation systems are needed to properly size any added filtration system to ensure adequate ventilation needs for the employees and housed animals.

With regards to non-contact UV virus destruction applied to animal housing, and typically swine housing, the majority of implementations have taken place within the last 15 years. However, extensive work has already been carried out in the past using UV radiation as early as 1892 with studies on its effects on microorganisms (Ward, 1892). Work has been carried out on its 'germicidal' effects (Barnard & Morgan, 1903), in hospital operating rooms (Wells & Wells, 1938), controlling rubella virus in army and navy barracks (Wheeler, et al., 1945), slowing measles spread in classrooms (Perkins, Bahlke, & Silverman, 1947), and controlling tuberculosis in hospital wards (Riley, 1961). UV radiation is able to deactivate viruses because the photons induce molecular transformation in the DNA and RNA of the virus. Typically, UV radiation in wavelengths between 210 nm and 260 nm has the best effect (Jagger, 1967) and has been shown to reduce the concentration of airborne microorganisms (Berg, Bergman, & Hoborn, 1991). UV radiation of 254 nm has been adopted as a standard for inactivation of infectious agents. Ultraviolet C (UVC), or also referred to as Ultraviolet Germicidal Irradiation (UVGI), which ranges between 200nm and 280 nm is known as the 'germicidal spectrum' because it has the ability to reduce concentrations of microorganisms. Although UV light has been proven successful in reducing microorganism concentrations, it may only be practically applied in conjunction with another technology, such as photocatalysis or filtration, in order to completely deactivate any bioaerosols. This can be explained by the Lambert-Beer Law and Grotthus-Draper Law, which states that some of the UV_{254} energy will be absorbed by the surroundings and that not all the energy striking the object is absorbed (Cutler & Zimmerman, 2011).

In one study, UV radiation was applied to 12 different materials commonly found in swine facilities in order to deactivate PRRSV. One sample of each material was exposed to UV light and another to incandescent light for 24 hours. After 10 minutes under the UV light, all sample materials tested negative for PRRSV, whereas 5 of the 12 samples were still positive after one hour under the incandescent light, and 1 of the 12 remained positive after 24 hours of exposure (Dee, Otake, & Deen, 2011). Although this study returned positive results for the use of UV radiation to inactivate viruses, more studies should be conducted to determine how long the bioaerosols should be exposed, because 10 minutes was the minimum length of time tested in this study. A 2012 study determined how the UV inactivation constants changed in response to temperature and relative humidity. As temperature increased, inactivation constants lowered. The constant was highest in ranges of 25%-79% relative humidity and lowest above 80% (Cutler, Chong, Hoff, & Zimmerman, 2012). The lamp design and performance are the most critical elements in inactivation of viruses. The design of the bulb should match environmental conditions. In addition, the use of a medium- or high-pressure polychromatic bulb will contribute to the efficiency of inactivation, although it is an additional expense (Cutler & Zimmerman, 2011).

Although UV radiation has the ability to reduce airborne viruses, it may not be the best means of bioaerosol removal, as was revealed in a 2006 study when it was compared to a HEPA system and a low-cost filter. The low-cost filter was made out of a mosquito netting pre-filter, a fiberglass furnace filter, and an electrostatic furnace filter. The UV radiation emitted a wavelength of 253.7 nm. All three of these filters, along with a control set, were tested 10 times by passing PRRSV at a concentration 1×10^8 $TCID_{50}$ through each treatment. Particles ranged from 0.3 to 3.0 μm. After passing through the filters, 9 of 10 control (no filter) trials tested positive for PRRSV, 8 of 10 UV, 4 of 10 low-cost, and none of the HEPA filter tests were positive for PRRSV (Dee, Batista, Deen, & Pijoan, 2006). A second study in 2006 compared a HEPA filter, low-cost filter, a bag filter (made up of an EU8 filter and a MERV 14 filter), and a dioctylphthalate (DOP) filter with a similar rating to a MERV 15 filter. This study returned 0 of 10 positive results for PRRSV through the HEPA filter, 2 of 10 positive through the bag filter, 4 of 10 positive from the low-cost filter, and 0 of 10 positive from the DOP filter. Upon further evaluation of the HEPA and DOP filters, 0 of 76 tests from the HEPA filter were positive, while 2 of 76 tests on DOP filters were positive (Dee S. A., Deen, Cano, Batista, & Pijoan, 2006).

One final comparison study in 2009 compared four MERV 16 filters from four different manufacturers, one MERV 14 filter, three antimicrobial filters, and a disinfectant integrated into an evaporative cooler pad system (EVAP). The antimicrobial filters control growth and colonisation of viruses on the surface of the filter, although they may not possess the ability to totally inactivation a virus such as PRRSV (Price, Simmons, Crow, & Ahearn, 2005). The disinfectant integrated into the EVAP system was known to deactivate PRRSV on contaminated surfaces (Dee S. , Deen, Burns, Douthit, & Pijoan, 2005), but its effectiveness on bioaerosols was not previously known. Seven concentrations of the virus were passed ten times through all the filtration systems, and results were recorded for detection of the virus. All MERV filters were tested at an air velocity of 1.1 m/s and pressure of 0.3-0.8 Pa. For brand A MERV 16, there were no positive results for PRRSV through all 7 concentrations. For brands B and C MERV 16, as well as brand A MERV 14, all 10 samples resulted positively for PRRSV in the highest concentration (1×10^7) with no positive results in the lowest six concentrations. Brand D MERV 16 was the least successful. All 10 samples were positive in the highest concentration, 3 of 10 in the second highest, and no samples were positive in the lowest five concentrations. Antimicrobial filters were tested at an airspeed of 1.1 m/s and pressure of 1.2-1.8 Pa. The 20- and 15-layer filters successfully filtered all seven concentrations of the virus. For the 10-layer filter, 4 of 10 samples in the highest concentration of the virus were positive for PRRSV. Finally, for the disinfectant in the EVAP system, all 7 concentrations tested positive to some degree for PRRSV. However, when analysed with a bioassay, all samples were negative, which suggests some success in the disinfectant. Although the EVAP with disinfectant method was somewhat successful, it is not the most practical solution because EVAP coolers are used in warmer months, and viruses tend to spread in cooler weather (Dee, Pitkin, & Deen, 2009).

Two studies using a production region model were conducted in 2008 and 2010. The first used three barns over the course of 1 year; one infected with PRRSV and the other two 120 m downwind (potentially) from the infected barn. One of the downwind barns was unfiltered and the other used MERV 16 filtration. In the filtered barn, none of the samples returned positive for PRRSV, while the unfiltered barn returned 31% positive samples for PRRSV (Pitkin, Deen, & Dee, 2009). In the 2010 study, four barns were used in the 2-year study; one infected with PRRSV and 3 placed 120 m downwind. One of the downwind barns was unfiltered, one used MERV 16 filtration, and the last used antimicrobial filters. None of the samples taken from the filtered barns were positive, while 54% of the samples from the non-filtered barn were positive for PRRSV (Dee, Otake, & Deen, 2010). More proof of the effectiveness of filters can also be seen in reports published between 2010 and 2013. These reports identified barns in high-density swine regions and analysed infection rate data in filtered versus non-filtered barns. All of the studies revealed that filtered barns were much more effective in remaining infection-free (Alonso, Murtaugh, Dee, & Davies, 2013) (Spronk, Otake, & Dee, 2010) (Dee, Spronk, Reicks, Ruen, & Deen, 2010). One 2012 report revealed that filtered barns have an infection rate that is eight times lower than non-filtered barns and that the time between infections for filtered barns is 30 months compared to 11 months for non-filtered barns (Dee, et al., 2012).

4 Methods and system design for aerosol capture

Because it has been confirmed that viruses like PRRSV and PEDV have the ability to transmit via bioaerosols, there is a need to identify methods to mitigate these viruses. Filter barn designs in the USA have evolved from two basic platforms, based on the operating pressure of the barns relative to outside ambient conditions. The negative pressure system (figure 7.1) was the first type of filtered barn system to be designed; used primarily as a retrofit for existing negative pressure ventilation systems. In this system, normal agricultural-use exhaust fans, combined with existing fresh-air inlets, are retrofitted with MERV 8 rating pre-filters combined with a MERV 14 or 16 primary filter. Integrating virus filtration into negative pressure barns is challenging. In negatively pressurised systems, any opening in the building will act as an inlet for outside air, allowing non-filtered and potentially contaminated air into the barn. These leaks could arise from poor building design, improper craftsmanship or installation, poor management, or wear and tear of building materials (Jadhav, Hoff, Harmon, Jacobson, & Hetchler, 2015). Other points of entry for non-filtered air could be backdrafted air through idle fans (Alonso, Otake, Davies, & Dee, 2012).

In 2012, a group of researchers recognised the need for further analysis of backdrafted air movement through idle fans. They believed that that the backdraft through idle fans posed a significant risk to biosecurity because of bioaerosols. An experiment was set up in a 25 m^2 facility with 6 polypropylene MERV 14 filters, 6 inlets, and 2 exhaust fans, one of which was idle for this experiment. Both exhaust fans were equipped with a standard 6-slat plastic shutter and an external hood. PRRSV in concentrations of 1 x 10^1 TCID$_{50}$/L, 1 x 10^3 TCID$_{50}$/L, 1 x 10^5 TCID$_{50}$/L, and 1 x 10^7 TCID$_{50}$/L were misted at 100 mL/minute 45 cm from the idle fan. A cyclonic collector inside the chamber detected PRRSV. In addition, an anemometer collected airspeed data. After testing, results indicated that the minimum velocity of air required for backdraft through the idle fan with only the standard shutters applied was 0.76 m/s. No positive results of PRRSV were recorded for the methods of double shutters, air chutes, and canvas covers. Researchers suggest that swine facilities apply double shutters, or remove the hood from the outside of the fan and install an air chute to effectively deter viruses from entering barns (Alonso, Otake, Davies, & Dee, 2012).

Fig. 7.1: Negative pressure filtration systems for swine housing.
Red arrows indicate unfiltered air entry through unplanned openings.

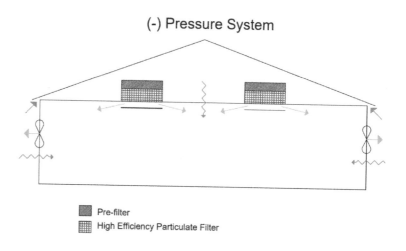

An additional location of infiltration in negative pressure filtered barns is through ventilation curtains. This could occur through the curtain itself, through the top seam, or at the end pocket closures. Through a series of tests with various wind velocities and curtain types, a guideline was established for essential overlaps of the curtains at the top seam. For agricultural use curtains, a two-inch overlap is required (Hoff, Assessing Air Infiltration Rates of Agricultural Use Ventilatoin Curtains, 2001). By identifying the proper placement of curtains, infiltration rates can be significantly reduced, thereby reducing the risk of airborne viruses entering barns in negative pressure systems.

In order to combat infiltration in negative pressure animal housing, it is important to understand how much air enters through unplanned leakage points. Measurements can be achieved through pressurisation tests, tracer gas, acoustics tests, or thermographic surveys (Masse, Munroe, & Jackson, 1994). Quantified tests have been conducted to show how much air is able to move through these unplanned leakage areas. In a 2015 study, results were recorded for 18 swine finishing barns in four different styles ranging in size from 1124 m^3 to 3032 m^3. The average leakage rates across all 18 finishing barns (air exchange per hour, ACH) at a 20 Pa pressure differential was 6.43±1.68 ACH in total with 1.47±0.71 ACH entering through curtains (23% of total), 1.63±0.77 ACH entering through idle fan shutter and pump-outs (25% of total), and 3.33±1.23 ACH entering through other unidentified locations such as ceiling panels and wall/ceiling joints (Jadhav, Hoff, Harmon, Jacobson, & Hetchler, 2015). A 1994 study attempted to determine the level of air leakage, quantify the variation between farm buildings (style, builder), and make recommendations. Conditions for the inclusion of the 13 barns in the study were that they had to be of recent construction, completely enclosed, mechanically ventilated, and empty at the time of testing. At a pressure difference of 50 Pa and average barn size of 1529 m^3, the average recorded leakage rate across all 13 barns was 14.7 ACH. After analysing the data, no evidence was found to support the fact that style of the building had effect on leakage. Also, no clear difference between buildings by different builders was observed (Masse, Munroe, & Jackson, 1994). Finally, when the results from these tests were compared to the ASHRAE prediction for leakage rates, the actual result with a pressure difference of 15 Pa was 7.6 ACH, compared to the 1.8 ACH predicted by ASHRAE (ASHRAE, 1985).

Due to the extreme variability in leakage rates during negative pressure barn operation, a movement in the USA towards positive pressure filtered barns has become more prominent. In positive pressure barns (figure 7.2), high pressure fans force air through HEPA filters and any auxiliary components such as evaporative coolers. The barns come under higher pressure relative to outside ambient conditions, and thus any leakage in the barn is forced out through the barn shell, preserving complete use of filtered air for the ventilation process. A myriad of positive pressure barn designs exist, but the general objective is that shown in figure 7.2. The major drawback for positive pressure barn ventilation is that in cold climates, warm moisture-laden air will be forced out through leakage points, resulting in interior wall condensation and structural rotting, which can significantly reduce barn life. Therefore, positive pressure filtered barn designs need attention to detail during the construction phase in order to limit leakage.

Fig. 7.2: Positive pressure filtration systems for swine housing.

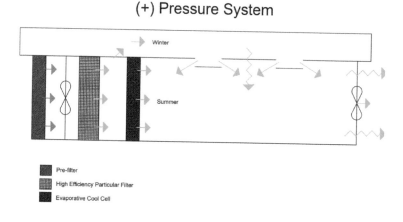

(+) Pressure System

Pre-filter

High Efficiency Particular Filter

Evaporative Cool Cell

5 Summary

Transmission of livestock and poultry diseases via aerosolised transport has become a focal point for many researchers, with mitigation methods being implemented at field level. Filtration systems add complications to overall ventilation processes, and caution is needed when retrofitting existing non-filtered barns to filtered systems. Whether they are positive or negative ventilated filtered designs, the overall structural integrity of the barns needs to be improved in order to significantly reduce outside unfiltered air from entering the barn (negative pressure systems) or to reduce internal moisture-laden air from exiting the barn (positive pressure systems).

Acknowledgements

The author would like to thank Sara Weyer, Undergraduate Research Assistant, Department of Agricultural and Biosystems Engineering, Iowa State University for her help with the extensive literature review.

7

References

Alonso, C., Goede, D. P., Morrison, R. B., Davies, P. R., Rovira, A., Marthaler, D. G., & Torremorrel, M. (2014). Evidence of infectivity of airborne porcine epidemic diarrhea virus and detection of airborne viral RNA at long distances from infected herds. *Veterinary Research, 45*(73). doi:10.1186/s13567-014-0073-z

Alonso, C., Murtaugh, M. P., Dee, S. A., & Davies, P. R. (2013). Epidemiological study of air filtration systems for preventing PRRSV infection in large sow herds. *Preventative Veterinary Medicine*, 109-117. doi:10.1016/j.prevetmed.2013.06.001.

Alonso, C., Otake, S., Davies, P., & Dee, S. (2012). An evaluation of interventions for reducing the risk of PRRSV introduction to filtered farms via retrograde air movement through idle fans. *Veterinary Microbiology*, 304-310. doi:10.1016/j.vetmic.2012.01.010

Alonso, C., Raynor, P. C., Davies, P. R., & Torremorell, M. (2015). Concentration, Size Distribution, and Infectivity of Airborne Particles Carrying Swine Viruses. *PLoS One*. doi:10.1371/journal.pone.0135675

ASHRAE. (1985). Handbook of Fundamentals. Atlanta, GA: American Society of Heating, Refrigeration, and Air Conditioning Engineers.

Barnard, J., & Morgan, H. (1903). The physical factors in phototherapy. *British Medical Journal*, 1269-1271.

Berg, M., Bergman, B., & Hoborn, J. (1991). Ultraviolet Radiation compared to an ultra-clean air enclosure. *Journal of Bone and Joint Surgery*, 811-815.

Bjerg, B. (2000). Use of tracer gas and numerical simulations to simulate airborne transmission of pathogens in a pig unit. *Research Gate*, 364-369.

Corzo, C. A., Culhane, M., Dee, S., Morrison, R. B., & Torremorell, M. (2013). Airborne Detection and Quantification of Swine Influenza A Virus in Air Samples Collected Inside, Outside and Downwind from Swine Barns. *PLoS ONE, 8*(8). doi:10.1371/journal.pone.0071444

Cutler, T. D., Chong, W. C., Hoff, S. J., & Zimmerman, J. J. (2012). Effect of temperature and relative humidity on ultraviolet (UV254) inactivation of airborne porcine respiratory and reproductive syndrom virus. *Veterinary Microbiology, 159*(1-2), 47-52. doi:10.1016/j.vetmic.2012.03.044

Cutler, T., & Zimmerman, J. J. (2011). Ultraviolet irradiation and the mechanisms underlying its inactivation of infectious agents. *Animal Health Research Reviews*, 15-23. doi:10.1017/S1466252311000016

Dee, S. A., Batista, L., Deen, J., & Pijoan, C. (2006). Evaluation of systems for reducing the transmission of Porcine reproductive and respiratory syndrome virus by aerosol. *The Canadian Journal of Veterinary Research, 70*(1), 28-33.

Dee, S. A., Deen, J., Cano, J. P., Batista, L., & Pijoan, C. (2006). Further Evaluation of alternative air-filtration systems for reducing the transmission of Porcine reproduce and respiratory sydrome virus by aersol. *The Canadian Journal of Veterinary Research*, 168-175.

Dee, S., Cano, J. P., Spronk, G., Reicks, D., Ruen, P., Pitkin, A., & Polson, D. (2012). Evaluation of the Long-Term Effect of Air Filtration on the Occurrence of New PRRSV Infections in Large Breeding Herds in Swine-Dense Regions. *Viruses, 70*(3), 654-662.

Dee, S., Deen, J., Burns, D., Douthit, G., & Pijoan, C. (2005). An evaluationn of disinfectants for the sanitation of porcine reproductive and respiratory syndrome virus-contaminated transport vehicles at cold temperatures. *The Canadian Journal of Veterinary Research, 69*(1), 64-70.

Dee, S., Deen, J., Jacobson, L., Rossow, K., Mahlum, C., & Pijoan, C. (2005). Laboratory model to evaluate the role of aerosols in the transport of porcine reproductive and respiratory syndrome virus. *Veterinary Record*, 501-504.

Dee, S., Otake, S., & Deen, J. (2010). Use of a production region model to assess the efficacy of various air filtration systems for preventing airborne transmission of porcine reproductive and respiratory syndrome virus and Mycoplasma hypneumoniae: Results from a 2-year study. *Virus Research, 154*(1-2), 177-184. doi:10.1016/j.virusres.2010.07.022

Dee, S., Otake, S., & Deen, J. (2011). An evaluation of ultraviolet light (UV254) as a means to inactivate porcine reproductive and respiratory syndrome virus on common farm surfaces and materials. *Veterinary Microbiology, 150*(1-2), 96-99. doi:10.1016/j.vetmic.2011.01.014

Dee, S., Otake, S., Oliveira, S., & Deen, J. (2009). Evidence of long distance airborne transport of porcine reproductive and respiratory syndrome virus and mycoplasma hyopneumoniae. *Veterinary Research*. doi: 10.1051/vetres/2009022

Dee, S., Pitkin, A., & Deen, J. (2009). Evaluation of alternative strategies to MERV 16-based air filtration systems for reduction of the risk of airborne spread of porcine reproductive and respiratory syndrome virus. *Veterinary Microbiology, 138*(1-2), 106-113. doi:10.1016/j.vetmic.2009.03.019

Dee, S., Spronk, G., Reicks, D., Ruen, P., & Deen, J. (2010). Further assessment of air filtration for preventing PRRSV infection in large breeding pig herds. *Veterinary Record, 167*(25), 976-977. doi:10.1136/vr.c6788

Donaldson, A., Gloster, J., Harvey, L., & Deans, D. (1982). Use of prediction model to forecast and analyze airborne spread during the foot-and-mouth disease outbreaks in Brittany, Jersey and the Isle of Wight in 1981. *Vet. Rec., 110*(3), 53-57.

Grant, R. H., Scheidt, A. B., & Rueff, L. R. (1994). Aerosol transmission of a viable virus affecting swine: Explanation of an epizootic pseudorabies. *International Journal of Biometerorology, 38*(33), 33-39. doi:10.1007/BF01241802

Guan, J., Fu, Q., Chan, M., & Spencer, J. L. (2013). *Aerosol Trasmission of an Avian Influenza H9N2 Virus with a Tropism For the Respiratory Tract of Chickens*. American Association of Avian Pathologists. doi:10.1637/10486-010913-Reg.1

Hermann, J. R., Brockmeier, S. L., Yoon, K.-J., & Zimmermann, J. J. (2008). Detection of repiratory pathogens in air samples from acutely infected pigs. *The Canadian Journal of Veterinary Research, 72*(4), 367-370.

Hoff, S. (2001). Assessing Air Infiltration Rates of Agricultural Use Ventilatoin Curtains. *Applied Engineering in Agriculture, 17*(4), 527-531. doi:10.13031/2013.6469

Jagger, J. (1967). *Introduction to Research in Ultraviolet Photobiology*. Englewood Cliffs, NJ: Prentice-Hall, Inc.

Jadhav, H., Hoff, S., Harmon, J., Jacobson, L., & Hetchler, B. (2015). *Infiltration Characteristics of Swine Finishing and Gestation Buildings: Review and Quantification*. ASABE Annual International Meeting: ASABE. doi:10.13031/aim.20152190046

Kristensen, C., Botner, A., Takai, H., Nielsen, J., & Jorsal, S. (2004). Experimental airborne transmission of PRRS virus. *Veterinary Microbiology, 99*(3-4), 197-202. doi:10.1016/j.vetmic.2004.01.005

Lager, K. M., Mengeling, W. L., & Wesley, R. D. (2001). Evidence for local spread of porcine reproductive and respiratory syndrome virus. *Journal of Swine Health and Production, 10*(4), 167-170.

Masse, D., Munroe, J., & Jackson, H. (1994). Air leakage through farm building envelopes in Eastern Ontario. *Canadian Agricultural Engineering, 36*(3), 159-163.

Otake, S., Dee, S., Corzo, C., Oliveira, S., & Deen, J. (2010). Long-distance airborne transport of infectious PRRSV and mycoplasma hyopneumoniae from a swine population incected with multiple viral variants. *Veterinary Microbiology, 145*(3-4), 198-208. doi:10.1016/j.vetmic.2010.03.028

Otake, S., Dee, S., Jacobsen, L., Torremorrell, M., & Pijoan, C. (2002). Evaluation of aerosol transmission of porcine reproductive and respiratory syndrome virus under controlled field conditions. *The Veterinary Record, 150*(26), 804-808. doi:10.1136/vr.150.26.804

Perkins, J., Bahlke, A., & Silverman, H. (1947). Effect of ultraviolet irradiation of classroom on the spread of measles in large rural central schools. *American Journal of Public Health, 37*(5), 529-537. doi:10.2105/AJPH.37.5.529

Pitkin, A., Deen, J., & Dee, S. (2009). Use of a production region model to assess the airborne spread of porcine reproductive and respiratory syndrome virus. *Veterinary Microbiology, 136*(1-2), 1-7. doi:10.1016/j.vetmic.2008.10.013

Price, D. L., Simmons, R. B., Crow, S. A., & Ahearn, D. G. (2005). Mold colonization during use of preservative-treated and untreated air filters, including HEPA filters from hospitals and commerical locations over an 8-year period (1996-2003). *J Ind Microbial Biotechnol, 32*(7), 319-321. doi:10.1007/s10295-005-0226-1

Riley, R. (1961). Airborne pulmonary tuberculosis. *Bacteriol*, 243-248.

Sergeev, A. A., Demina, O., Pyankov, O., Pyankova, O., Agafonov, A., Kiselev, S., . . . Sergeev, A. (2012). Infection of Chickens Caused by Avian Influenza Virus A/H5N1 Delivered by Aerosol and Other Routes. *Transboundary and Emerging Diseases*, 159-165. doi:10.1111/j.1865-1682.2012.01329.x

Spekreijse, D., Bouma, A., Koch, G., & Stegeman, J. (2011, August). Airborne transmission of a highly pathogenic avian influenza virus strain H5N1 between groups of chickens quantified in an experimental setting. *Veterinary Microbiology, 152*(1-2), 88-95. doi:10.1016/j.vetmic.2011.04.024

Spronk, G., Otake, S., & Dee, S. (2010). Prevention of PRRSV infection in large breeding herds using air filtration. *Veterinary Record*, 758-759. doi: 10.1136/vr.b4848

Trincado, C., Dee, S., Jacobsen, L., Otake, S., Rossow, K., & Pijoan, C. (2004). Attempts to transmit porcine reproductive and respiratory syndrome virus by aerosols under controlled field conditions. *Veterinary Record, 154*(10), 294-297. doi:10.1136/vr.154.10.294

Ward, M. (1892). Experiments of the action of light on Bacillus anthracis. *Proceedings of the Royal Society of London, 52*, 393-403.

Wells, W., & Wells, M. (1938). Measurement of sanitary ventilation. *American Journal of Public Health*, 343-350.

What are MERV Ratings and How Do They Work? (2010). Retrieved from Air Purifier Guide: http://www.airpurifierguide.org/faq/merv-ratings

Wheeler, S. M., Ingraham, H., Hollaneder, A., Lill, N., Gershon-Cohon, J., & Brown, E. (1945). Ultraviolet light control of airborne infections in a naval training center. *American Journal of Medicine*, 457-468.

CHAPTER 8

FEED HYGIENE

Steven C. Ricke

Center for Food Safety, Department of Food Science, University of Arkansas, Fayetteville, AR 72704

1 Introduction

Animal feed continues to be a major economic component in live-stock production. Depending on the animal species and the corresponding nutritional requirements both the minor and major ingredients that make up the complete feed ration may vary considerably. As a general rule ruminants are fed high fibre forage diets depending on the production cycle and final animal product; pasture grazing cow-calf operations for instance versus grain-fed finishing beef cattle in feedlots. Dairy cattle during peak milk production in particular, may be fed forage in the form of silage supplemented by silage inoculants such as lactic acid bacteria (Weinberg and Muck, 1996). Non-ruminants rely on cereal grain-based diets usually consisting primarily of a combination of corn and soybean in order to meet the energy and protein demands of the animal complemented by a range of micronutrients such as minerals and vitamins to provide for the specific dietary requirements of individual animal species. In some cases, such as poultry, crystalline forms of amino acids (usually lysine and methionine) are added as supplements to achieve a more ideal protein quality balance to maximize growth performance. This is particularly important when non-corn/soybean diets are substituted with more economical protein sources which may be deficient in some of the essential amino acids. Regardless of the diet composition or animal species, feed contains a diverse range of microorganisms most of which are relatively harmless but some of which are pathogenic to the animal being fed and/or to humans consuming the animal-based products. In this chapter we will discuss the ecology of these organisms, means of identification, control measures, and future strategies for understanding feed hygiene.

2 Feed microbial ecology

Given the diverse nature of feed sources and the environments associated with their production, milling and processing, storage, and feeding facilities it comes as no surprise that the microbiota associated with feed are also fairly diverse (Sauer et al., 1992;

Maciorowski et al., 2007). In addition to the bacteria, bacterio-phage, fungi, and yeast have also been identified in feeds as commonly occurring biological contaminants (Maciorowski et al., 2001, 2007; Oguz, 2011). Feed fungi and the production of mycotoxins are issues associated with feed storage and can have a detrimental impact on animal nutrition (Ricke, 2005; Maciorowski et al., 2007). Several environmental factors can influence the microbial and fungal composition and the corresponding biological activities of feed. These include water activity and exposure to vectors such as mice, wild birds, and insects that can carry and cross-contaminate batches of feed (Fenlon, 1985; Pelhate, 1998; Pedersen, 1992; Maciorowski et al., 2007). In addition, use of thermal processes such as pelleting can also influence the final microbial composition of the feed product.

3 Feed Contamination

3.1 Overview

As discussed earlier, given the great many sources and environments in which feed ingredients originate, it is no surprise that biological contamination can be traced to a very wide range of diverse points of origin some of which are shown in figure 8.1. The microorganisms found in soils where cereal grain crops are grown would certainly appear to be contributors but other sources, some more obvious than others, also contribute to this ecosystem. In the fresh produce industry, obvious sources such as irrigation water have been well documented as a potential source of foodborne pathogens such as *Salmonella* (Hanning et al., 2009) and would certainly be anticipated as contributors via row crop production when irrigation is used. Likewise, airborne routes for transmission of numerous bacterial contaminants have considerable potential for extensive dissemination not only on the row crops that are being produced for feed but at the feed mill as well as the animal housing where feed in dispensed (Pillai and Ricke, 2002). Biological vectors such as insects, mice, rats, cats, and wild birds among others have all been identified as potential carriers of various foodborne pathogens and could certainly contaminate feed (Park et al., 2008). Less obvious sources might include trucks and other means of transporting cereal grains to be milled for feed production and for delivering mixed feeds to livestock farms; feed mill and livestock workers who carry biological contaminants on clothing and shoes, and the animal housing environment itself via ventilation fans and flooring for instance. The following sections take a look at the different biological contaminants that present the most probable concern with regards to animal feeds.

Fig. 8.1: Potential Environmental Sources of Microbial Contamination in Feed Manufacturing

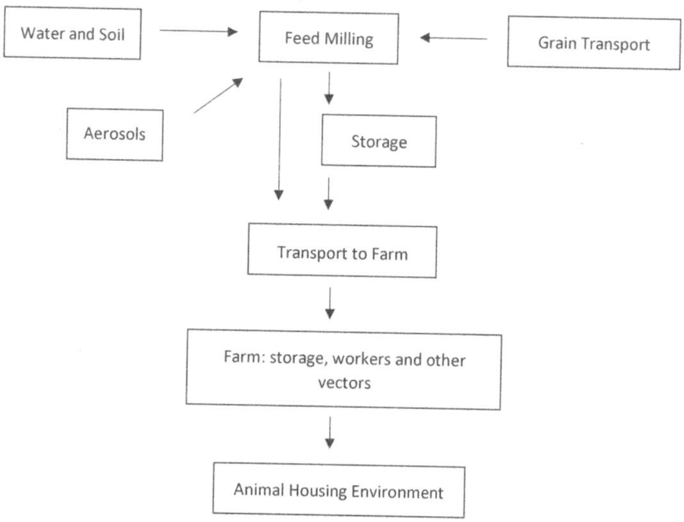

3.2 Bacteriophage

Bacteriophages are essentially viruses that target bacteria and in turn, are able to either immediately propagate in the host bacteria and cause eventual lysis of the bacterial cell or insert into the chromosome and enter a somewhat dormant lysogenic or prophage physiological state which can then enter a lytic state at some point in the future (Ricke et al., 2012). While not documented extensively there is no reason to imagine that bacterial viruses would not be found in feed materials given the diverse bacterial background. Maciorowski et al. (2001) screened both fresh and stored feeds and feed ingredients along with poultry diets suspected of containing *Salmonella* spp. Using enrichment for isolation and detection, they detected both male-specific and somatic coliphages in all of the feed sources and most of the feeds contained RNA somatic phages. There is also a potential for lactic acid bacteria bacteriophage when starter cultures are used in silage fermentations (Weinburg and Muck, 1996).

More recently, Vongkamjan et al. (2012) found that nearly half of the silage samples from two dairy farms contained listeriaphages. Greater interest in bacteriophage ecology in animal feeds will no doubt receive increased attention in the future as the use of bacteriophages against bacterial pathogens are being promoted as an alternative to antibiotics in animal diets. It is assumed that future research would not only focus on feeds as a potential source of bacteriophage candidates with properties to ensure their survival in dry feeds, but that efforts would also be made to screen bacteriophage additives for determining the best means of delivering them in a dry feed matrix to be effectively consumed by the target animal.

3.3 Fungi

Toxigenic fungi have continued to be of considerable concern in the animal feed industry. Not only do they impact on feed quality but they can be the source of secondary metabolites collectively known as mycotoxins that are produced by *Aspergillus*, *Penicillium*, and *Fusarium* (Hesseltine, et al., 1976; Wilson and Abramson, 1992; Dänicke, 2002; Ricke, 2005). These toxins include aflatoxins, ochratoxins, trichothecens, zearlenone and fumonisins which can lead to a series of pharmacological effects on the consuming animal that in turn cause physiological responses that are detrimental to the victim (Miller, 1995; Dänicke, 2002; Ricke, 2005). Control measures have generally focused on either detoxification of mycotoxins via the removal of the respective toxin or preventing fungal growth and therefore initial production of the fungal metabolite (Ricke, 2005; Maciorowski et al., 2007; Oguz, 2011). Given the stability of mycotoxin compounds, detoxification has proven to be a challenge whether the approach has been to destroy the toxin outright or to attempt to remove it from the contaminated animal feed. More emphasis has been placed therefore on means of preventing fungal contamination or retarding growth of fungi already present in the animal feed by complementary physical treatments such as addition of heat or incorporating chemicals such as organic acids that are inhibitory to fungal growth into the feed matrix.

3.4 Bacteria

3.4.1 Indigenous feed microbiota

Indigenous feed microbiota could be defined as commonly occurring microorganisms, in this case bacteria, that could be considered part of the characteristic or 'native' feed microbial community. As such they would be expected to possess at least some of the phenotypic and physiological traits that fit with the environmental conditions typically associated with feed-based ecosystems. Consequently one would expect bacteria that can tolerate and survive in the presence of low water activity, exist under limited nutrient availability conditions, survive variable amounts of aeration and cope with highly complex surfaces for attachment to form the bulk of the microbial community. Certainly, the capacity for producing a spore under adverse conditions and mounting various stress responses would be considered advantageous for adapting to feed matrices and the corresponding environmental conditions. The following sections delineate some of these groups of bacteria, their ecology, and means for persisting as members of feed ecosystems.

3.4.2 Spore formers

Bacterial spore formers present a unique challenge to feed manufacturing since these bacteria in the spore form are able to survive some of the thermal processes associated with feed milling such as *Clostridium perfringens* in pelleted feed (Greenham et al, 1987). Certainly, microorganisms in the spore state might also be expected to survive non-thermal stresses such as the introduction of acids or other chemicals. Consequently, preventing spore formation in the first place and keeping numbers of the spore formers low remains a viable strategy and is probably where interventions would be best employed (Ricke, 2005). Other *Clostridium* isolates from feed include *Clostridium botulinum* which has been associated with non-acidified and plastic wrapped silage (Lindström et al., 2010).

A more recent introduction of a spore former to feeds and which represents a deliberate contamination of feeds is the administration of *Bacillus* spores into feeds as a source of probiotics, particularly for chickens (Ricke and Saengkerdsub, 2015). The perceived advantage of adding *Bacillus* spores is that they are capable of resisting thermal processing that occurs during feed processing and once ingested can subsequently germinate into vegetative bacterial cells thus providing benefit to the host as a probiotic in the gastro-intestinal tract (Ricke and Saengkerdsub, 2015). As more genetic modifications and developments are made with these strains, it is anticipated that such organisms will receive widespread commercial adaptation as feed amendments for a variety of feeds and animal diets.

3.4.3 *Listeria*

Listeria spp. are often associated with cattle farms and *Listeria monocytogenes* that causes disease in humans and mammals and *L. ivanovii* that causes disease in ruminants are considered as the primary *Listeria* species pathogens (Milillo et al., 2012a). In a survey of seven dairy farms where some cows were diagnosed with *Listeria* mastitis, Skovgaard and Morgen (1988) found that 82 % of the feed samples contained *Listeria* spp. and 62% were contaminated specifically with *L. monocytogenes*. *Listeria* has also been identified in silage (Fenlon, 1985, 1986; Caro et al., 1990; Ryser et al., 1997; Vongkamjan et al., 2012). Silage conditions and resulting quality of the final product may be a factor. For example, Ryser et al. (1997) screened corn, hay and grass silages and observed differences in isolation frequencies related to the silage-fermented source. Nearly all (92%) of the hay silage which was classified as low quality (pH equal or above 4) samples yielded recoverable *Listeria* spp. but even the silages where the pH level was below 4 contained *Listeria* spp. This led Ryser et al. (1997) to conclude that even silages that would be considered high-quality represented a risk for *Listeria*.

The consistent prevalence of *Listeria* spp. in silage is still somewhat unclear but Vongkamjan et al., (2012) isolated *L. monocytogenes* and listeriaphages from two dairy farms and noted that only 4.5 % of the silage samples were positive for *L. monocytogenes* but 47.8 % were positive for listeriaphages. They concluded that based on the wide host range and genomic diversity of the characterised silage listeriaphages phages were an important component in *L. monocytogenes* ecology on dairy farms. This would also seem to suggest that *Listeria* may be present in silage on a fairly consistent basis. Finding *Listeria* in silage is not completely surprising given its ability to grow in reduced oxygen atmospheres (Lungu et al., 2009). The listeriaphage presence in silage may also suggest that bacteriophage could be an effective control approach for reducing *Listeria* levels in silage.

While ruminants have perhaps received greater attention from the view of farms, other farm animal species have also been associated with *Listeria*. Milillo et al., (2012b) isolated *Listeria* from pasture flock poultry ceca and pasture environments suggesting that poultry could pick up and harbour *Listeria*. *Listeria* spp. have been identified in poultry feeds even after post-heat processing (Blank et al., 1996; Whyte et al., 2003). It was reported by Whyte et al. (2003) that much of the feed mill equipment was contaminated with *Listeria* including the pellet cooler air inlet. The environmental dissemination of *Listeria* is conceptually consistent with the environmental persistence of *Listeria* observed in food processing environments (Milillo et al., 2012a).

3.4.4 *Campylobacter*

Campylobacter are Gram-negative spiral shapes that grow under microaerophillic atmospheric conditions (Humphrey et al., 2007; Silva et al. 2011). They are found in most food animals and some species such as *C. jejuni* and *C. coli* are considered to be the major foodborne disease-causing species and campylobacteriosis is considered one of the major foodborne diseases worldwide (Humphrey et al., 2007; Horrocks et al., 2009; Silva et al., 2011). While transmission routes for various food animals have been suggested and debated, we know that for chickens at least the primary ecological niche for *Campylobacter* is the gastrointestinal tract where its survival and protection from the host intestinal immune system is believed to be supported by other intestinal tract bacteria (Silva et al., 2011; Indikova et al., 2015). Survival outside the gastrointestinal tract has also been proposed by Indikova et al. (2015) due to its association with other microorganisms in mixed culture matrices such as biofilms.

Animal feed as a potential transmission vehicle for *Campylobacter* spp. has not been established (Silva et al., 2011). Over the years several published poultry feed surveys have looked for campylobacters but the results revealed either infrequent and/or undetectable levels of the organism thus supporting the concept that *Campylobacter* spp. were sensitive to the dry form of most poultry feeds (referenced in a review by Ricke, 2005). More recently, Ge et al. (2013) screened 201 feed ingredient samples, that were either animal or plant byproducts, for several microorganisms including *Campylobacter*. They used Bolton broth for enrichment of potential *Campylobacter* from the feed ingredients followed by plating on *Campylobacter* selective agar plates and culture identification testing of presumptive colonies. However, they were unable to recover *Campylobacter* from any of the feed ingredient samples via this approach and concluded that feed was a relatively unimportant source of *Campylobacter*. However, as Ricke (2005) has pointed out, since it is known that *Campylobacter* is able to convert to a viable non-culturable physiological form this could cause culture-based recovery approaches to be less conclusive.

3.4.5 *Salmonella*

Foodborne *Salmonella* spp. have a long history with food animals and are considered as one of the primary agents for causing human cases of foodborne illnesses. While identified with most food animals and pets as well, poultry remains one of the more identifiable farm animals associated with *Salmonella* (Foley et al., 2011, 2013). The dissemination routes for *Salmonella* spp. in poultry are diverse and can occur both vertically as well as horizontally during poultry production (Park et al., 2008). Consequently, control measures have been implemented and/or suggested for all facets of poultry production from the hatchery through the broiler grower houses and processing facilities (Park et al., 2008; Finstad et al., 2012). This also holds true for layer hen flocks and egg production (Howard et al., 2012). Certainly, poultry feeds for breeder flocks, broilers and layers have all been identified as potential sources of concern and several studies over the years have recovered a variety of *Salmonella* serovars from poultry feeds (Williams, 1981a; Maciorowski et al., 2004, 2006b; Jarquin et al., 2009).

Given that foodborne *Salmonella* spp. have clearly been identified with a broad spectrum of feeds, it stands to reason that *Salmonella* occurrence and control in feeds and feed ingredients has received the bulk of attention both from a research and a perception standpoint (Williams, 1981a; Maciorowski et al., 2004, 2006b; Jones, 2011). There are several reasons for this. First of all, *Salmonella* serovars are relatively ubiquitous in environments and are likely to come in contact with feed at various stages of production as illustrated in figure 8.2 (Maciorowski et al., 2004, 2006b; Park et al., 2008). In addition, numerous vectors such as rodents, wild birds, insects, pets among others may serve as conduits for *Salmonella* transmission routes (Park et al, 2008). This presents a challenging time component for controlling *Salmonella* as it also appears to possess considerable survival capabilities in feed matrices ensuring that once *Salmonella* has become a contaminant, it can persist through the lifecycle of a feed or feed ingredient (Ha et al., 1998a,b). However, survival in feed may also be *Salmonella* strain-dependent as indicated by the comparison of multiple serovars inoculated into poultry feeds by Andino et al., (2014). While this study was only carried out with one feed type if such results hold true among multiple feed types and ingredients this could further complicate the assessment of appropriate control measures for *Salmonella* in feeds. Feed type and source may be critical as well. For example, Ge et al. (2013) reported that animal byproducts exhibited a substantially higher recovery of over 30 % positive samples compared to plant by-product samples which were approximately 5% positive.

Fig. 8.2: *Salmonella* Potential Feed Transmission Routes

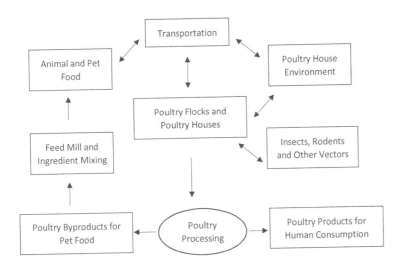

4 Feed Hygiene Practices – Physical

4.1 Overview

Physical control measures typically involve some form of external change of environmental conditions in the target matrix such as animal feed. With feed processing, this is mostly associated with the application of heat during feed milling to produce specific types of feed such as processes associated with pelleting feed. Other physical processes such as irradiation that have been examined and/or have potential but are not necessarily extensively used in routine feed manufacturing have been discussed in detail elsewhere (Williams, 1981c; Ricke, 2005; Maciorowski et al., 2007) and will not be discussed in the current review.

4.2 Thermal

The pelleting process in feed manufacturing has been described in detail previously by Jones (2011) and only will be discussed briefly here. Jones (2011) lists three primary steps in commercial pelleting, namely steam introduction to the mash form of the feed; pressing (pelleting) the feed through the corresponding metal die form; and finally, air cooling. While spores of spore formers would be able to withstand such temperatures the level of reduction of *Salmonella* during the addition of steam to start the pelleting process depends on several factors, in particular, the length of application time, the temperature used for heating, and the moisture level (Ricke, 2005; Jones, 2011). Further reduction of *Salmonella* can be achieved either by applying expanders and extruders to administer combinations of temperature and pressure and/or including antimicrobials which are activated during the steam process (Jones, 2011). Such combinations may lead to synergistic reduction of *Salmonella*. For example, Milillo and Ricke (2010) and Milillo et al. (2011) demonstrated that the combination of organic acids and sublethal heat led to a synergistic reduction of *S*. Typhimurium in the presence of a chicken meat broth.

While thermal application may be considered as an effective lethal step in *Salmonella* reduction, several factors may counteract this lethality. Some *Salmonella* serovars vary in their thermo-tolerance and if the level of heat is sublethal for some reason, this may in turn lead to resistance through thermal shock resistant systems such as the formation of heat shock proteins (Jarvis et al., 2016; Dawoud et al., 2017). In terms of management the other problem is the potential recontamination by *Salmonella* after the feed has been pelleted and is being air-cooled (Ricke, 2005; Jones, 2011). Jones and Richardson (2004) observed that sources of *Salmonella* recontamination included dust in the feed mill and therefore they emphasised that mill design should be reviewed in order to avoid potential cross-contamination between areas of the mill operation. Isolation of *Salmonella* from meat rendering plants supports this concept of cross-contamination during thermal processing as the same serovars were found in both the initial raw materials as well as the finished meat meal (Gong and Jiang, 2017). Jones (2011) suggested that the addition of chemical disinfectants should alleviate some of the potential for recontamination. The chemicals currently being used in the feed industry will be discussed in the next section.

5 Feed Hygiene Practices – Chemical and Biological Additives

5.1 Overview

Historically there has been an extensive effort to identify chemicals and biological compounds that can potentially be added to animal feeds to serve a variety of purposes but their use as fungistats and to retard pathogenic bacterial proliferation have been among the more well-documented applications. While properties may vary among the chemicals and biological compounds, several criteria need to be considered when it comes to routine commercial use in feed manufacturing. It is true that efficacy that is consistent across a broad spectrum of organic loads characteristic of the complex feed matrices would be a priority but other factors such as cost would also be important given the large volumes of feeds milled and subsequently mixed for food animal operations. In addition, governmental regulatory approval for use in animal diets would be critical. Other factors such as ease and safety of use for the feed mill workers and minimal negative impact on feed mill equipment would be important considerations as well. The following subsections provide a brief overview of some of the compounds being considered or being used in feeds but it does not represent a comprehensive list of all the potential additives that have been or are being considered. For more comprehensive descriptions please refer to several previously published reviews (Williams, 1981c; Maciorowski et al., 2004, 2007; Ricke, 2005, Wales et al., 2010).

5.2 Essential Oils and Related Botanicals

Essential oils (EOs) and related botanicals are extracted aromatic and volatile secondary plant metabolites which can be derived from a wide range of plant materials and have historically been used in medical, culinary, and cosmetic applications (O'Bryan et al., 2015). More recently they have received attention as potential antimicrobial compounds in order to combat foodborne pathogens in foods (Calo et al., 2015). Mechanistically, their antimicrobial activity and growth inhibition probably derives from a combination of these compounds being lipophilic and easily able to cross the bacterial cell membrane causing disruption of internal cell metabolism and resulting in leakage of cell contents among other related cell responses (Calo et al., 2015; O'Bryan et al., 2015). Given the complexity and varied chemical structure a more precise description of antimicrobial mechanisms remains elusive. Extensive feeding trials have been conducted with EOs as feed additives in attempts to decrease pathogen colonisation and improve animal health and performance and will not be discussed here (see reviews by Calo et al., 2015; O'Bryan et al., 2015). However, experiments to examine the potential of EOs to prevent recontamination of animal feeds are limited. When Cochrane et al. (2016) compared an EO blend (garlic oleoresin., turmeric oleoresin, capsicum oleoresin, rosemary extract, and wild oregano) with a control without chemical treatment and various commercial chemical blends on the survival of S. Typhimurium over 42 days in four rendered protein meals (feather, blood, meat and bone, and poultry by-product meals) S. Typhimurium populations were reduced but not to the extent of some of the other feed additives.

5.3 Acids

Acids cover a broad group of compounds but essentially consist of organic (carbon based) and inorganic (non-carbon based) with organic acids further categorised by carbon chain length. Much of the research relating to food production has focused on short-chain fatty acids (SCFA) due to their use as preservatives and in production during food fermentation as well in the gastrointestinal tract (Ricke, 2003). Antimicrobial mechanisms essentially involve bacterial cell pH gradients and disruption of intracellular regulation of pH, but other toxic impacts on bacterial cells have also been suggested (Cherrington et al., 1991; Russell, 1992; Ricke, 2003; Van Immerseel et al., 2006; Wales et al., 2010). Much of the research efforts into organic acids and commercial application in feeds have involved propionic and formic acids either singly or as mixtures and have been discussed in detail elsewhere (Van Immerseel et al., 2006; Wales et al., 2010). However, some general observations can be made. The ability of these compounds to directly reduce *Salmonella* levels in feeds appears to be a function of both concentration and final pH of the feed as buffered versions tend to be less effective even when added in higher concentrations (Ha et al., 1998a; Wales et al., 2010). Consequently, Wales et al., (2010) has suggested that higher concentrations should only be used in individual feed ingredients prior to feed mixing to avoid animal palatability issues and feed mill equipment deterioration. In addition, Van Immerseel et al. (2006) has pointed out that antibacterial activity in feeds depends on temperature and moisture content of the feed.

Inorganic acids and medium-chain fatty acids (MCFA) have also been considered as antimicrobial feed amendments but only limited studies involving feed matrices have been conducted with these types of compounds. Cochrane et al., (2016) compared an MCFA blend (caproic, caprylic, and capric acids) with an organic acid blend (lactic, formic, propionic and benzoic acids), an EO blend, sodium bisulfate, and a commercial formaldehyde product on rendered protein feed ingredients by treating the rendered protein matrix initially with the corresponding chemical followed by inoculation with a S. Typhimurium strain. They concluded that the MCFA blend and formaldehyde commercial product were equal in their responses and the most effective in reducing S. Typhimurium compared to the control treatment with no chemical added over a 42 day post-inoculation time period. However, they also noted that the efficacy depended on the time of exposure and the type of rendered protein which supported their initial hypothesis that a specific chemical may interact differently with a particular feed matrix. In addition to these contributions to efficacy variability, *Salmonella* strain and serovar differences in tolerance response to stressors such as acids should also be considered (González-Gil et al., 2012; Lianou and Koutsoumanis, 2013). Therefore, multiple *Salmonella* isolates should probably be examined in screening experiments when more comprehensive conclusions need to be drawn.

5.4 Aldehydes

Formaldehyde is the aldehyde used primarily in commercial feed treatments and has been shown to exhibit antibacterial efficacy by irreversible cross-linking proteins (Carrique-Mas et al., 2007; Wales et al., 2010). When used as a feed additive it has been shown to be one of the more effective compounds for reducing *Salmonella* levels in feeds (Carrique-Mas et al., 2007; Cochrane et al., 2016). However, Carrique-Mas et al., (2007) pointed out that concerns have been raised regarding safety to humans (Arts et al., 2006). More recent risk assessments (EFSA, 2014) have concluded that formaldehyde used for animal nutrition purposes would not be expected to present a risk for the environment, but anyone handling the product should avoid exposure to the respiratory tract, skin, and eyes. The other consideration when using formaldehyde is the potential to reduce feed protein availability for digestion. Tamminga et al. (1979) concluded from studies conducted with ruminants that formaldehyde was effective in treating feed proteins so that they became resistant to proteolytic rumen microorganisms in the rumen and thus escape relatively unscathed to the lower part of the digestive tract where they can be used by the ruminant animal. However, Tamminga (1979) also noted that excessively high concentrations resulted in over-protection where not only were proteins protected from rumen microbial proteolysis but they were also now resistant to ruminant animal proteolytic enzymes resulting in a negative ruminant animal nutritional response. Formaldehyde as an antimicrobial feed additive has not been generally observed to cause adverse responses in animals

(Wales et al., 2010). However, the impact on protein availability for the concentrations of formaldehyde used as a feed antimicrobial treatment may need to also be considered.

6 Detection and Analyses

6.1 Overview and the Issue of Sampling

Detection of microorganisms in feed matrices continues to be a challenge. There are several reasons for this. First of all, the sheer size of batches of feed that need to be screened and thus appropriately sampled remains a daunting challenge. Unlike liquid bulk sources which are relatively homogenous and therefore somewhat amendable to samples being taken, which should be representative of the entire lot, feed is a solid that is of a potentially fairly heterogeneous composition. Thus single samples suffer from the question of just how representative they are of the entire lot especially when several tons of feed are being produced on an hourly basis (Ricke, 2005). While suggestions for a set number of feed samples have been recommended over the years, Jones (2011) concluded – based on previous work by Davies and Wales (2010) – that dust and other materials around feed mill equipment represented a more sensitive sampling protocol than direct feed sampling. Coupled with the fact that important pathogens such as *Salmonella* may only be associated with a few feed particles within that ton of feed (Jones and Ricke, 1994) one begins to appreciate the magnitude of the issue of retrieving a representative sample that comes even close to detecting highly random appearances of such organisms. Hence the need for identification and characterisation of more commonly occurring indicator microorganisms and that are therefore more likely to be detected in quantifiable numbers. This will be discussed in more detail in a later section. The other primary challenge is the choice of detection methods to ensure consistent identification of the target microorganisms depending upon the goal-accurate enumeration of a particular microbial population. The following sections describe some of the approaches that have been or are currently being used for detection and quantification of microorganisms associated with animal feeds.

6.2 Cultural Growth-Based Methods

Classic microbiological characterisation has generally consisted of collecting representative samples, removing a portion for inoculating serial dilution tubes, followed by plating of either general media or media that is more selective for the specific bacteria of interest as outlined in figure 8.3. Depending on the goal, further efforts can be made to not only identify the organisms present but to enumerate the levels of bacterial contamination. Over the years, efforts to improve on general methodology for specific microorganisms have been made. For example, development of selective media to exclude potential fungal overgrowth, incorporation of minimal media to improve representative general bacterial numeration, and screening sample extraction procedures in order to dislodge bacteria attached to feed particles more effectively have all been reported (Ha et al., 1995a,b; Maciorowski et al., 2002a,b).

Fig. 8.3: Feed Bacterial Detection by Growth Culture

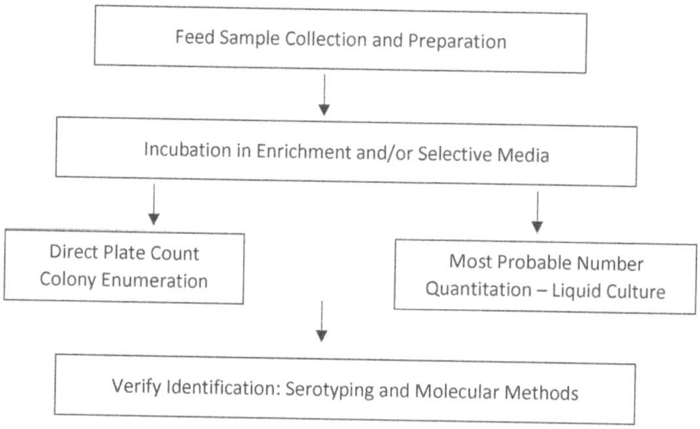

Certainly an extensive amount of research has been devoted to methods for isolating, cultivating and enumerating *Salmonella* spp. from feeds and these will not be discussed in detail here (see reviews by Williams, 1981b; Ricke et al., 1998; Maciorowski et al., (2004, 2005, 2006a,b; Jarquin et al., 2009). In short, most of the strategies for culturing *Salmonella* from other biological sources such as food substances also apply to culturing *Salmonella* from feeds as well. However, some problems with cultural-based methods for feeds have been encountered. Soria et al., (2011) compared two culture methods for recovery of motile and non-motile *Salmonella* strains and concluded that that the detection levels of cultural methods were different for the two *Salmonella* groups with the nonmotile isolates being more difficult to detect. In addition, general caution when culturing *Salmonella* from feeds is also warranted particularly when feed amendments such as acids or other chemicals are introduced. Carrique-Mas et al. (2007) demonstrated that organic acids and formaldehyde could mask the recovery of *Salmonella* from the respective treated feeds unless some sort of counter-compound to neutralise the inhibition of the chemical present in the pre-enrichment broth was included. Consequently, without considering the potential impact of antimicrobial chemical carryover into the culture media there is a viable risk of either underestimating the levels of *Salmonella* present in the feed sample or even failure to detect *Salmonella* altogether.

6.3 Molecular-Based Methods

Given some of the difficulties associated with cultural approaches such as inconsistent recovery, problems with identification and the need for further characterisation such as serotyping for *Salmonella*, interest in alternative non-cultural-based methods began to receive more interest when carrying out feed analyses. In addition, a further driver towards non-cultural methods is the desire to speed up completion of bacterial analyses of feeds and reduce costs (Maciorowoski et al., 2005, 2006b; Malorny et al., 2008). As expected, much of the focus in feed microbial analyses has centered on *Salmonella*. Options that have been considered over the years have included both immunological and molecular methods but early on molecular approaches received more developmental input (Ricke et al., 1998; Maciorowski et al., 2005, 2006a) Much of the progress made in molecular approaches for *Salmonella* detection and identification in feeds as well as related matrices have been well documented elsewhere and will only be covered briefly in the current review (Maciorowski et al., 2005, 2006b; Malorny et al., 2008; Jarquin et al, 2009; Ricke et al., 2013; Park et al., 2014).

Polymerase chain reaction (PCR) approaches both for detection (see figure 8.4 for an overview) and in some cases quantification have been developed over the years with animal feeds (Maciorowski et al., 2005; Malorny et al., 2008). As these methods have been improved and optimised, opportunities to glean more information from a specific feed sample have emerged. For example, Park et al., (2011) used the primers that are specific to the virulence *hilA* regulatory gene in *S*. Typhimurium to demonstrate the impact of thermal stress on survival and virulence response at gene expression level. In the future, identification of additional potential indicator genes found in specific pathogens such as *Salmonella* as well as more commonplace indicator organisms in order to evaluate feed processing effectiveness may have considerable utility for a more rapid means to evaluating processing steps before and after critical control steps. Simultaneous detection of multiple *Salmonella* serovars and even unrelated pathogens would also be attractive from a sampling and cost standpoint. While not used directly on feed, Park and Ricke (2015) developed multiplex and quantitative PCR assays that allow for the simultaneous detection of not only the *Salmonella* genus, but *Salmonella* subspecies I, *S*. Enteritidis, *S*. Heidelberg, and *S*. Typhimurium. Having a broad *Salmonella* detection capability with genera-based *Salmonella* PCR assay offers the opportunity to gain 'a first look' to determine if any *Salmonella* spp. are present regardless of serovar and as more serovar-specific PCR assays become available the opportunity to either simultaneously or at least rapidly elucidate which serovars present will be of value for trouble-shooting potential issues with feed contamination or recontamination and sources of cross-contamination.

Being able to quantify *Salmonella* present in feeds will be useful to not only evaluate effectiveness of control methods but potentially in quantitative risk assessment of feeds. To achieve more accurate quantification Schelin et al. (2013) compared pre-PCR processing methods to enumerate *S. enterica* in naturally contaminated feeds using a combined most probable number-PCR approach to recover low numbers of *Salmonella* from feeds. The initial introduction of DNA microarrays and the more recent application of whole genome sequencing (WGS) will further improve on the ability to track and identify sources of contamination both within the feed mill as well in outside sources including transportation, farm sites, and associated environments in a similar fashion as occurs in the food industry (Alvarez et al., 2003; Koynucu et al., 2011; Ricke et al., 2013; Park et al., 2014).

Fig. 8.4: Molecular Detection of Feed Microorganisms

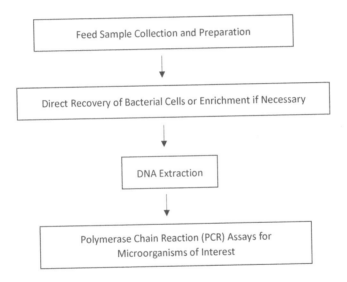

6.4 Indicator Organisms

Given the inconsistencies and infrequent occurrence of most pathogenic microorganisms in the typical feed matrix, even the best combinations of sampling and detection methodologies will struggle to assess the level of contamination and just as importantly the effectiveness of hygienic practices. This is a common dilemma in many food production systems. Consequently, identification of suitable indicator organisms which approximate the target pathogen behaviour and responses to exposure to various stresses are continually sought after and appraised. Ideally, such microorganisms should not only approximate the tendencies of the pathogen but be present in sufficiently high numbers that they are always detectable and consistently prevalent so that they can be guaranteed as being present in the feed at all locations and in all environmental conditions. There are several potential candidates. For example, Jones and Richardson (2004) collected over 800 samples from feed ingredients, dust samples and feed from feed mills to enumerate *Salmonella* and *Enterobacteriaceae* and found that sources contaminated with *Salmonella* also contained significantly higher *Enterobacteriaceae* counts. Based on this they suggested that *Enterobacteriaceae* might be indicative of *Salmonella* contamination. Depending on the microorganism to be monitored, such qualities as thermal tolerance may also be a desired characteristic particularly for spore formers. For example, Okelo et al (2008) concluded that the addition of *Bacillus stearothermophilus* spores served as a suitable surrogate organism to evaluate efficiency of feed sterilisation during extrusion.

6.5 Future Detection Approaches – Feed Microbiome

During the characterisation of the microbiota of animal feed materials, most of the information was generated by classic microbiological techniques that relied on recovery of organisms from complex feed matrices, growth on some sort of culture or solid plate type media and presumptive visual, biochemical and physiological profiling (Sauer et al., 1992). As molecular methods became more advanced and therefore more routine, more precise identification and taxonomical assignments became possible. Approaches such as denaturing gradient gel electrophoresis (DGGE) allowed for a composite microbial population comparison to be made based on banding patterns on gels followed by band excision and DNA sequencing of visually prominent or otherwise selected bands to identify an individual organism. In the case of feeds, Maciorowski et al., (2002c,d) demonstrated the utility of using bacterial ribosomal gene detection for assessing the microbial quality of poultry and animal feed. When next generation sequencing (NGS) technologies emerged and became commercially viable for more routine laboratory use, 16S rRNA gene sequencing for profiling entire microbial populations on a genetic basis became a reality. This sequencing capacity to generate large volumes of raw data coupled with the development of computer software pipelines that could transform the data into biologically interpretable taxonomic information revolutionised the study of microbial ecosystems, particularly of gastrointestinal tract microbial communities.

While NGS 16S rRNA gene sequencing has been extensively applied in gastrointestinal tract ecosystems and other environments, minimal effort has been made to survey animal feeds. It is not entirely clear why this is so. There would certainly be several reasons to conduct such studies more routinely (see figure 8.5 for an outline of a general approach). First of all, since feed is a source of a variety of microorganisms it would seem that at least some contribution from such sources could influence the makeup of the animal gastrointestinal tract microbiota at least in very young animals with a minimally developed gastrointestinal tract microbial ecology. How this impacts on the host animal immune system and later establishment of the microbial population more characteristic of a mature animal could be a revealing answer and possible consideration for feed formulation as well as feed hygienic management in ways that have not been previously considered.

8

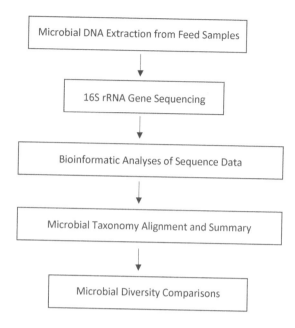

Secondly, microbiome profiles offer a more comprehensive means of assessing the effectiveness of feed hygiene in terms of the impact on the feed microbial contaminants. For example, does the before and after microbial population change and if so how does the chemical and/or physical treatment select microbial populations and in turn impact the quality of the feed? Likewise, the microbiome profiling offers a new tool for better defining and identifying potentially optimal indicator microorganisms that approximate pathogen patterns in the respective feed or feed ingredient better. Finally, comprehensive profiling offers the opportunity to improve tracking of potential sources of cross-contamination as well as recontamination during feed mill processing.

7 Feed Hygiene Management

Even with the advances made in feed intervention development and improving analytical capabilities with more sensitive and sophisticated detection technologies, feed hygiene management is still paramount to achieving overall improvement in feed mill and feed hygiene quality. This in turn requires systematic appraisal of all potential issues associated with either ongoing feed hygiene problems or anticipation of those that are most likely to occur. However, fundamental problems such as designing optimal representative sampling protocols and the frequency needed for sampling time intervals remain unresolved. While any attempt to arbitrarily increase sampling sites or frequency in taking samples would seemingly offer optimistic progress on precision and by default accuracy, the logistical practicality of such approaches is elusive. Therefore, an attempt must be made to prioritise where the greatest vulnerabilities occur and focus on them for in-depth analytics. There is a precedent for this in the food industry with the introduction of Hazard Analysis Critical Control Point (HAACP). Essentially such approaches identify critical control points within a food system to identify sites and locations in the process where contamination of a pathogen is more likely to occur. Jones and Ricke (1994) proposed a HACCP planning approach for feed manufacturing that encompassed most of the areas that could be considered as vulnerable and therefore a potential critical control point (CCP). An extensive list of such CCPs, starting with receiving and unloading with the initial CCP being the pre-unloading inspection, are described in detail by Jones and Ricke (1994) and will only be discussed briefly in the current review. Typically, inspection for visible signs of contamination such as animal faecal material including wild birds along with anything else out of the ordinary concerning the appearance of the feed would be considered a viable issue. Certainly, the means used to transport feed ingredients such as trucks and other equipment could also be a CCP. When it comes to transportation equipment, record keeping is an important component. For example, the history of the haulage of trucks carrying material(s) and whether they have been satisfactorily cleaned prior to the delivery of the feed ingredient could be critical in determining if a contamination problem is likely (Jones and Ricke, 1994). In short, this type of systematic assessment and identification of CCPs along with the appropriate corrective measures could be developed for every step in the feed milling process as described in detail by Jones and Ricke (1994).

Obviously, individual CCPs may vary among feed mill operations depending on mill design and other factors, but the general implementation of good manufacturing practices (GMPs) to reduce overall feed contamination in problematic areas such as feed bins, feed augers and other potential contamination areas should lead to an improvement (Maciorowski et al., 2004). The ability to control contamination at various stages of feed manufacturing will no doubt improve as technology for the application of disinfectant, sampling feeds and ingredients, and detection systems evolve. In addition, over the years, there has been some talk of developing a more risk-based approach to feed contamination with the idea of achieving risk minimisation rather than no contamination at all (Maciorowski et al., 2004). The precedent for risk modelling of heterogeneous matrices such as ground poultry meat (Rajan et al., 2017) would suggest that similar approaches could be taken with complex feed matrices as well. While numerous feed sources and ingredients would result in a more complex product than ground meat the concept is essentially the same. One would expect that each ingredient and feed source could be developed and assigned a level of risk in terms of potential exposure to the target animal consuming the final feed product. Recently, van der Fels-Klerx et al., (2017) published a model for risk-based monitoring of feed ingredient contaminants using dioxin and dl-PCBs with the potential to contaminate feeds which could in turn lead to these chemicals being introduced to susceptible animals. Development of the model allowed them to rank individual feed ingredients according to the potential for exceeding acceptable limits for these chemicals and thus assign risk accordingly. As the ability to quantify *Salmonella* in feeds improves, quantitative risk modelling should become possible (Malorny et al., 2008; Schelin et al., 2013). Such approaches depending on the database available for *Salmonella* contamination in feeds and feed ingredients could certainly be quite useful for accomplishing similar models for feed ingredients.

8 Conclusions

Feed hygiene has evolved over the years as more knowledge has become available about sources of contamination and in turn how contaminated feed affects susceptible animals that consume the contaminated feed. Part of this is due to a better understanding of how and when animals are most likely to become colonised by a specific foodborne pathogen. Along with this, more research has also been conducted into the mechanisms that pathogens such as *Salmonella* use to respond to exposure to stresses such as those encountered during feed processing. Parallel to these developments, considerable effort has been put into developing technologies to prevent or limit contamination of animal feeds. The success of any specific treatment remains somewhat difficult to appraise given the complex nature of feed matrices and the corresponding problems with sampling and detection of foodborne pathogens in large batches of feed. Certainly, pathogen detection methods have improved over the years and have in turn become more economical, but representative sampling is still a problem. Resolving this may require a combination of identifying suitable non-pathogenic indicator organisms that could be more easily and predictably recovered. Introduction of techniques such as microbiome sequencing to profile microbial feed populations offers a potentially comprehensive approach to accomplishing this. A different approach that might be complementary or at least supportive is the development of HACCP plans for feed processing to identify CCPs for the strategic application of control measures along with risk modelling to better predict which feed ingredients are most likely to represent unacceptable contamination.

References

Alvarez, J., Porwollik, S., Laconcha, I., Gisakis, V., Vivanco, A.B., Gonzalez, I., Echenagusia, S., Zabala, N., Blackmer, F., McClelland, M., Rementaria, A., and Garaizar, J. (2003) Detection of *Salmonella enterica* serovar California strain spreading in Spanish feed mills and genetic characterization with DNA microarrays *Applied and Environmental Microbiology* 69, 7531-7534.

Andino, A., Pendleton, S., Zhang, N., Chen, W., Critzer, F., and Hanning, I. (2014) Survival of *Salmonella enterica* in poultry feed is strain-dependent. *Poultry Science* 93, 441-447.

Arts, J.H., Rennen, M.A., and Mr, C. (2006) Inhaled formaldehyde: Evaluation of sensory irritation in relation to carcinogenicity. *Regulatory Toxicology and Pharmacology* 44, 144-160.

Blank, G. Savoie, S., and Campbell, L.D. (1996). Microbiological decontamination of poultry feed – evaluation of steam conditioners. *Journal of the Science of Food and Agriculture*, 72, 299-305.

Calo, J.R., Crandall, P.G., O'Bryan, C.A., and Ricke, S.C. (2015) Essential oils as antimicrobials in food systems – A review. *Food Control*. 54, 111-119.

Caro, M.R., Zamora, E., León, L., Cuello, F., Salinas, J., Megias, D., Cubero, M.J., and Contreras, A. (1990) Isolation and identification of *Listeria monocytogenes* in vegetable by-product silages containing preservative additives and destined for animal feeding. *Animal Feed Science and Technology* 31, 285-291.

Carrique-Mas, J.J., Bedford, S., and Davies, R.H. (2007) Organic acid and formaldehyde treatment of animal feeds to control *Salmonella*: Efficacy and masking during culture. *Journal of Applied Microbiology* 103, 88-96.

Cherrington, C.A., Hinto, M., Mead, G.C., and Chopra, I. (1991) Organic acids: Chemistry: antimicrobial activity and practical applications. *Advances in Microbial Physiology* 32, 87-108.

Cochrane, R.A., Huss, A.R., Aldrich, G.C., Stark, C.R., and Jones, C.A. (2016) Evaluating chemical mitigation of *Salmonella* Typhimurium ATCC 14028 in animal feed ingredients. *Journal of Food Protection* 79, 672-676.

Dänicke, S. (2002). Prevention and control of mycotoxins in the poultry production chain: A European view. *World's Poultry Science Journal* 58, 451-474.

Davies, R.H. And Wales, A.D. (2010) Investigation into *Salmonella* contamination in poultry feed mills in the United Kingdom. *Journal of Applied Microbiology* 109, 1430-1440.

Dawoud, T.M., Davis, M.L., Park, S,H. Kim, S.A, Kwon, Y.M., Jarvis, N., O'Bryan, C., Shi, Z., Crandall, P.G., and Ricke, S.C. (2017) *Salmonella* thermal resistance – Molecular responses. *Frontiers in Veterinary Sciences* 4: (Article 93) doi: 10.33889/fvets.2017.00093.

EFSA FEEDAP Panel (EFSA Panel on Additives and Products or Substances used in Animal Feed), 2014. Scientific Opinion on the safety and efficacy of formaldehyde for all animal species based on a dossier submitted by Regal BV. *EFSA Journal* 2014;12(2):3561, 24 pp. doi:10.2903/j.efsa.2014.3561

Fenlon, D.R. (1985). Wild birds and silage as reservoirs of *Listeria* in the agricultural environment. *Journal of Applied Bacteriology* 59, 537-543.

Fenlon, D.R. (1986). Rapid quantitative assessment of the distribution of listeria in silage implicated in a suspected outbreak of listeriosis in calves. *The Veterinary Record* 118, 240-242.

Finstad, S., O'Bryan, C.A., Marcy, J.A., Crandall, P.G., and Ricke, S.C. (2012) *Salmonella* and broiler production in the United States: relationship to foodborne salmonellosis. Food Res. Int. 45: 789-794.

Foley, S.L., Johnson, T.J., Ricke, S.C., Nayak, R. and Danzeisen, J. (2013) *Salmonella* pathogenicity and host adaptation in chicken-associated serovars. *Microbiology and Molecular Biology Reviews* 77, 582-607.

Foley, S., Nayak, R., Hanning, I.B., Johnson, T.J., Han, J. and Ricke, S.C. (2011) Population dynamics of *Salmonella enterica* serotypes in commercial egg and poultry production. *Applied and Environmental Microbiology* 77, 4273-4279.

Ge, B., LaFon, P.C., Carter, P.J., McDermott, S.D., Abbott, J., Glenn, A., Ayers, S.L., Friedman, S.L., Paige, J.C., Wagner, D.D., Zhao, S., McDermott, P.F., and Rasmussen, M.A. (2013) Retrospective analysis of *Salmonella*, *Campylobacter*, *Escherichia coli*, and *Enterococcus* in animal feed ingredients. *Foodborne Pathogens and Disease*. 10, 684-691.

Gong, C. and Jiang, X. (2017) Characterizing *Salmonella* contamination in two rendering processing plants. *Journal of Food Protection* 80, 263-270.

González-Gil, F., Le Bolloch, A., Pendleton, S., Zhang, N., Wallis, A. and Hanning, I. (2012) Expression of *hilA* in response to mild acid stress in *Salmonella enterica* is serovar- and strain-dependent. Journal of Food Science 77, M292-M297.

Greenham, L.W., Harber, C., Lewis, E., and Scullion, F.T. (1987). *Clostridium perfringens* in pelleted feed. *The Veterinary Record* 120, 557.

Ha, S.D., Maciorowski, K.G., Jones, F.T., Kwon, Y.M., and Ricke, S.C. (1998a). Survivability of indigenous feed microflora and a *Salmonella typhimurium* marker strain in poultry feed treated with buffered propionic acid. *Animal Feed Science and Technology* 75, 145-155.

Ha, S.D., Maciorowski, K.G., Kwon, Y.M., Jones, F.T. and Ricke, S.C. (1998b). Indigenous feed microflora and *Salmonella typhimurium* marker strain survival in poultry feed with varying levels of protein. *Animal Feed Science and Technology* 76, 23-33.

Ha, S.D., Pillai, S.D., and Ricke, S.C. (1995a) Growth response of *Salmonella* spp. to cycloheximide amendment in media. *Journal of Rapid Methods in Automation and Microbiology* 4, 77-85.

Ha, S.D., Pillai, S.D., Maciorowski, K.G., and Ricke, S.C. (1995b) Cycloheximide as a media amendment for enumerating bacterial populations in animal feeds. *Journal of Rapid Methods in Automation and Microbiology* 4, 95-105.

Hanning, I., Nutt, J.D., and Ricke, S.C. (2009). Salmonellosis outbreaks due to fresh produce: Sources and potential intervention measures. *Foodborne Pathogens and Disease* 6, 635-648.

Hesseltine, C.W., Shotwell, O.L., Kwolek, W.F., Lillehof, E.B., Jackson, W.K., and Bothast, R.J. (1976). Aflatoxin occurrence in 1973 corn at harvest. II. Mycological studies. *Mycologia* 68, 341-353.

Horrocks, S.M., Anderson, R.C., Nisbet, D.J., and Ricke, S.C. (2009) Incidence and ecology of *Campylobacter* in animals. *Anaerobe* 15, 18-25.

Howard, Z.R., O'Bryan, C.A., Crandall, P.G., and Ricke, S.C. (2012) *Salmonella* Enteritidis in shell eggs: Current issues and prospects for control. *Food Research International* 45, 755-764.

Humphrey, T., O'Brien, S., and Madsen, M. (2007) Campylobacters as zoonotic pathogens: A food production perspective. *International Journal of Food Microbiology* 117, 237-257.

Indikova, I., Humphrey, T.J., and Hilbert, F. (2015) Survival with a helping hand: *Campylobacter* and microbiota. *Frontiers in Microbiology* 6 (Article 1266): 1-6. doi: 10.3389/fmmicb.01266.

Jarquin, R., Hanning, I., Ahn, S., and Ricke, S.C. (2009). Development of rapid detection and genetic characterization of *Salmonella* in poultry breeder feeds. *Sensors* 9, 5308-5323.

Jarvis, N.A., O'Bryan, C.A., Dawoud, T.M., Park, S.H., Kwon, Y.M., Crandall, P.G., and Ricke, S.C. (2016) An overview of *Salmonella* thermal destruction during food processing and preparation. *Food Control* 68, 280-290.

Jones, F.T. (2011) A review of practical *Salmonella* control measures in animal feed. *Journal of Applied Poultry Research* 20, 102-113.

Jones, F.T., and Richardson, K.E. (2004) *Salmonella* in commercially manufactured feeds. *Poultry Science* 83, 384-391.

Jones, F.T. and Ricke, S.C. 1994. Researchers propose tentative HACCP plan for feed manufacturers. *Feedstuffs* 66 (18), 32, 36-38, 40-42.

Koyuncu, S., Andersson, G., Vos, P., and Häggblom, P. (2011) DNA microarray for tracing *Salmonella* in the feed chain. *International Journal of Food Microbiology* 145, 518-522.

Lianou, A. and Koutsoumanis, K.P. (2013) Strain variability of the behaviour of foodborne bacterial pathogens: A review. *International Journal of Food Microbiology* 167, 310-321.

Lindström Department of Food and Environmental Hygiene, Faculty of Veterinary Medicine, University of Helsinki , Finland , M., Myllykoski, J., Department of Food and Environmental Hygiene, Faculty of Veterinary Medicine , University of Helsinki , Finland Sivelä, S. Department of Food and Environmental Hygiene, Faculty of Veterinary Medicine, University of Helsinki, Finland and Korkeala, H. (2010) Clostridium botulinum in cattle and dairy products. *Critical Reviews in Food and Nutrition* 50, 281-304.

Lungu, B., Ricke, S.C., and Johnson, M.G. (2009). Growth, survival, proliferation and pathogenesis of *Listeria monocytogenes* under low oxygen or anaerobic conditions: A review. *Anaerobe* 15, 7-17.

Maciorowski, K.G., Herrera, P., Jones, F.T., Pillai, S.D., and Ricke, S.C. (2007). Effects on poultry and livestock of feed contamination with bacteria and fungi. *Animal Feed Science and Technology* 133, 109-136.

Maciorowski, K.G., Hererra, P., Jones, F.T., Pillai, S.D., Ricke, S.C. (2006a) Cultural and immunological detection methods for *Salmonella* spp. in animal feeds – A review. *Veterinary Research Communication* 30, 127-137.

Maciorowski, K.G., Herrera, P., Kundinger, M.M., and Ricke, S.C. (2006b) Animal feed production and contamination by foodborne *Salmonella*. *Journal of Consumer Protection and Food Safety* 1, 197-209.

Maciorowski, K.G., Pillai, S.D. Jones, F.T., and Ricke, S.C. (2005) Polymerase chain reaction detection of foodborne *Salmonella* spp. in animal feeds. *Critical Reviews in Microbiology* 31, 45-53.

Maciorowski, K.G., Jones, F.T., Pillai, S.D., and Ricke, S.C. (2004). Incidence, sources, and control of food-borne *Salmonella* spp. in poultry feed. *World's Poultry Science Journal* 60, 446-457.

Maciorowski, K.G., Pillai, S.D., Jones, F.T., and Ricke, S.C. (2002a) Low nutrient R2A culture medium for bacterial enumeration from poultry feeds. *Journal of Rapid Methods in Automation and Microbiology* 10, 59-68.

Maciorowski, K.G., Pillai, S.D., and Ricke, S.C. (2002b) Comparison of media and a liquid detergent extraction step on bacterial recovery from animal feeds. *Journal of Environmental Science and Health Part B* 37, 255-264.

Maciorowski, K.G., Pillai, S.D., and Ricke, S.C. (2002c) Rapid assessment of poultry feed microbial quality using polymerase chain reaction detection of microbial ribosomal gene sequences. *Journal of Rapid Methods in Automation and Microbiology* 10, 9-18.

Maciorowski, K.G., Pillai, S.D., and Ricke, S.C. (2002d) Polymerase chain reaction detection of bacterial ribosomal genes from fresh and stored animal feeds. *Journal of the Science of Food and Agriculture* 82, 1398-1404.

Maciorowski, K.G., Pillai, S.D., and Ricke, S.C. (2001). Presence of bacteriophages in animal feed as indicators of faecal contamination. *Journal of Environmental Science and Health Part B* 36, 699-708.

Malorny, B., Löfström, C., Wagner, M., Krämer, N., and Hoorfar, J. (2008). Enumeration of *Salmonella* in food and feed samples by real-time PCR for quantitative microbial risk assessment. *Applied and Environmental Microbiology* 74, 1299-1304.

Mililllo, S.R., Friedly, E.C., Saldivar, J.C., Muthaiyan, A., O'Bryan, C.A., Crandall, P.G. Johnson, M.G., and Ricke, S.C. (2012a). A review of the ecology, genomics and stress response of *Listeria innocua* and *Listeria monocytogenes. Critical Reviews in Food Science and Nutrition* 52, 712-725.

Mililllo, S.R., Stout, J.C., Hanning, I.B., Clement, A., Fortes, E.D., den Bakker, H.C., Wiedemann, M., and Ricke, S.C. (2012b). Characteristics of *Listeria* from pasture-reared poultry reveals *L. monocytogenes* and hemolytic *L. innocua* in poultry ceca and the pasture environment. *Poultry Science* 91, 2158-2163.

Mililllo, S.R., Martin, E., Muthaiyan, A., and Ricke, S.C. (2011) Immediate reduction of *Salmonella enterica* serotype Typhimurium following exposure to multiple-hurdle treatments with heated, acidified organic acid salt solutions. *Applied and Environmental Microbiology* 77, 3765-3772.

Mililllo, S.R. and Ricke, S.C. (2010) Synergistic reduction of *Salmonella* in a model raw chicken media using a combined thermal and organic acid salt intervention treatment. *Journal of Food Science* 75, M121-M125.

Miller, J.D. (1995) Fungi and mycotoxins in grain: Implications for stored product research. *Journal of Stored Product Research* 31, 1-16.

O'Bryan, C.A., Pendleton, S.J., Crandall, P.G., and Ricke, S.C. (2015) Potential of plant essential oils and their components in animal agriculture – *in vitro* studies on antibacterial mode of action. *Frontiers in Veterinary Science* 2 (Article 35): 1-8. doi: 10.3389/fvets.2015.00035

Oguz, H. (2011). A review of experimental trials on detoxification of aflatoxin in poultry feed. *Eurasian Journal of Veterinary Sciences* 27, 1-12.

Okelo, P.O., Joseph, S.W., Wagner, D.D., Wheaton, F.W., Douglass, L.W., and Carr, L.E. (2008) Improvements in reduction of feed contamination: An alternative monitor of bacterial killing during feed extrusion. *Journal of Applied Poultry Research* 17, 219-228.

Park, S.H. and Ricke, S.C. (2015) Development of multiplex and quantitative PCR assays for simultaneous detection of *Salmonella* genus, *Salmonella* subspecies I, *S.* Enteritidis, *S.* Heidelberg, and *S.* Typhimurium. *Journal of Applied Microbiology* 118, 152-160.

8

Park, S.H., Aydin, M., Khatiwara, A., Dolan, M.C., Gilmore, D.F., Bouldin, J.L, Ahn, S., and Ricke, S.C. (2014) Current and emerging technologies for rapid detection and characterization of *Salmonella* in poultry and poultry products. *Food Microbiology* 38, 250-262.

Park, S.H., Jarquin, R., Hanning, I., Almeida, G., and Ricke, S.C. (2011) Detection of *Salmonella* spp. survival and virulence in poultry feed by targeting the *hilA* gene. *Journal of Applied Microbiology* 111, 426-432.

Park, S.Y., Woodward, C.L., Kubena, L.F., Nisbet, D.J., Birkhold, S.G., and Ricke, S.C. (2008). Environmental dissemination of foodborne *Salmonella* in pre-harvest poultry production: Reservoirs, critical factors and research strategies. *Critical Reviews in Environmental Science and Technology* 38, 73-111.

Pedersen, J. (1992). Insects – identification, damage, and detection. In: Sauer, D.B. (ed.) *Storage of Cereal Grains and Their Products, 4th edition*, pp. 435-489, American Association of Cereal Chemists, St. Paul, MN.

Pelhate, J. (1988). Microbiology of moist grains. In: Multon, J.L. (ed.). *Preservation and Storage of Grains, Seeds, and Their By-Products*, pp. 328-346, Lavoisier Publishing, Inc., New York, NY.

Pillai, S.D. and Ricke, S.C. (2002). Aerosols from municipal and animal wastes: Background and contemporary issues. *Canadian Journal of Microbiology* 48, 681-696.

Rajan, K, Shi, Z., and Ricke, S.C. (2017) Potential application of risk strategies for understanding *Salmonella* contamination in ground poultry products. *Critical Reviews. In Microbiology* 43, 370-392.

Ricke, S.C. (2005). Chapter 7. Ensuring the Safety of Poultry Feed. In: Mead, G.C. (ed.) *Food Safety Control in Poultry Industry*, pp. 174-194, Woodhead Publishing Limited, Cambridge, UK..

Ricke, S.C. (2003) Perspectives on the use of organic acids and short-chain fatty acids as antimicrobials. *Poultry Science* 82, 632-639.

Ricke, S.C., and Saengkerdsub, S. 2015. Chapter 19. *Bacillus* probiotics and biologicals for improving animal and human health: Current applications and future prospects *In:* V. Ravishankar Rai and A Jamuna Bai (eds.) *Beneficial Microbes in Fermented and Functional Foods*, pp. 341-360, CRC Press/Taylor & Francis Group, Boca Raton, FL.

Ricke, S.C. , Khatiwara, A., and Kwon, Y.M. (2013) Application of microarray analysis of foodborne *Salmonella* in poultry production: A review. *Poultry Science* 92, 2243-2250.

Ricke, S.C., Hererra, P., and Biswas, D. (2012) Chapter 23. Bacteriophages for potential food safety applications in organic meat production. In: S.C. Ricke, E.J. Van Loo, M.G. Johnson and C.A. O'Bryan (Eds.), *Organic Meat Production and Processing*. pp. 407-424, Wiley Scientific/IFT, New York, NY.

Ricke, S.C., Pillai, S.D., Norton, R.A., Maciorowski, K.G., and Jones, F.T. (1998) Applicability of rapid methods for detection of *Salmonella* spp. in poultry feeds: A review. *Journal of Rapid Methods and Automation in Microbiology* 6, 239-258.

Russell, J.B. (1992) Another explanation for the toxicity of fermentation acids at low pH: Anion accumulation versus uncoupling. *Journal of Applied Bacteriology* 73, 363-370.

Ryser, E.T., Arimi, S.M., and Donnelly, C.W. (1997) Effects of pH on distribution of *Listeria* ribotypes in corn, hay, and grass silage. *Applied and Environmental Microbiology* 63, 3695-3697.

Sauer, D.B., Meronick, R.A., Christenesen, C.M. (1992). Microflora. In: Sauer, D.B. (ed.) *Storage of Cereal Grains and Their Products, 4th edition*, pp. 313-340, American Association of Cereal Chemists, St. Paul, MN.

Schelin, J., Andersson, G., Vigre, H., Norling, B., Häggblom, P. Hoorfar, J., Rädström, P., and Löfström, C. (2013) Evaluation of pre-PCR processing approaches for enumeration of *Salmonella enterica* in naturally contaminated feed. *Journal of Applied Microbiology* 116, 167-178.

Silva, J., Leite, D., Fernandez, M., Mena, C., Gibbs, P.A., and Teixeira, P. (2011) *Campylobacter* spp. as a foodborne pathogen: A review. *Frontiers in Microbiology* 2 (Article 200): 1-12 doi:10.3389/fmicb.2011.00200.

Skovgaard, N. and Morgen, C.-A. (1988). Detection of *Listeria* spp. in faeces from animals, in feeds, and in raw foods of animal origin. *International Journal of Food Microbiology* 6, 229-242.

Soria, M.C., Soria, M.A., Bueno, D.J., and Colazo, J.L. (2011) A comparative study of culture methods and polymerase chain reaction assay for *Salmonella* detection in poultry feed. *Poultry Science* 90, 2606-2618.

Tamminga, S. (1979) Protein degradation in the forestomachs of ruminants. *Journal of Animal Science* 49, 1615-1630.

Van der Fels-Klerrx, H.J., Adamse, P., de Jong, J., Hoogenboom, R., and de Nijs, M. (2017) A model for risk-based monitoring of contaminants in feed ingredients. Food Control 72, 211-218.

Van Immerseel, F., Russell, J.B., Flythe, M.D., Gantois, I., Timbermont, L., Pasmans, F., Haesebrouck, F. And Ducatelle, R. (2006) The use of organic acids to combat *Salmonella* in poultry: A mechanistic explanation of the efficacy. *Avian Pathology* 35, 182-188

Vongkamjan, K., Switt, A.M., den Bakker, H.C., Fortes, E.D., and Wiedmann, M. (2012) Silage collected from dairy farms harbours an abundance of listeriaphages with considerable host range and genome size diversity. *Applied and Environmental Microbiology* 78, 8666-8675.

Wales, A.D., Allen, V.M., and Davies, R.H. (2010) Chemical treatment of animal feed and water for the control of *Salmonella. Foodborne Pathogens and Disease* 7, 1-15.

Weinberg, Z.G. and Muck, R.E. (1996). New trends and opportunities in the development and use of inoculants for silage. *FEMS Microbiological Reviews* 19, 53-68.

Williams, J.E. (1981a) Salmonellas in poultry feeds – A worldwide review. Part I. Introduction. *World's Poultry Science Journal* 37, 6-19.

Williams, J.E. (1981b) Salmonellas in poultry feeds – A worldwide review. Part II. Methods in isolation and identification. *World's Poultry Science Journal* 37, 19-25.

Williams, J.E. (1981c) Salmonellas in poultry feeds – A worldwide review. Part III. Methods in control and elimination. *World's Poultry Science Journal* 37, 97-105.

Wilson, D.M. and Abramson, D. (1992). Mycotoxins In: Sauer, D.B. (ed.) *Storage of Cereal Grains and Their Products, 4th edition*, pp. 341-391, American Association of Cereal Chemists, St. Paul, MN.

Whyte, P., McGill, K., and Collins, J.D. (2003). A survey of the prevalence of *Salmonella* and other enteric pathogens in a commercial poultry feed mill. *Journal of Food Safety* 23, 13-24.

CHAPTER 9

DRINKING WATER HYGIENE AND BIOSECURITY

Andrew Olkowski

University of Saskatchewan, Saskatoon Canada

1 Introduction

Contemporary, constantly expanding, global agriculture is facing ever increasing water security challenges. One of the most critical factors that limit water security in agriculture is water availability, but when it comes to the animal production sector, water security is delineated not only by quantity but also by quality and biosecurity of drinking water.

The most significant threats to drinking water security for the animal industry include industrial, municipal and agricultural pollution, which cumulatively contribute to contamination of global drinking water sources at an alarming rate. Biological contaminants of drinking water sources are of increasing concern, presenting real and present threats to water biosecurity in both developing and developed countries.

The increasing risk of biological contamination in water sources is strongly linked to human population growth, followed by the expansion of the animal industry, both of which, in turn, produce large quantities of biological waste. This waste is discharged into the environment and directly or indirectly into surface and ground water bodies, frequently untreated and uncontrolled. Therefore, the animal industry itself has become a major threat to the biosecurity of drinking water.

Biosecurity of drinking water is inadvertently linked to food biosecurity. Therefore, the availability of good-quality drinking water for farm animals is also the critical element in the strategy safeguarding against hazards associated with waterborne contaminants for both humans and animals. However, sustainable biosecurity of drinking water for farm animals is not a trivial task and requires proper technical resources as well as extensive understanding of water hygiene principles along with solid practical knowledge of water chemistry, basic water physiology and the nature of contaminants that impact on animals.

2 Drinking Water Hygiene

Drinking water hygiene is an essential concept that focuses on mitigating potential hazards associated with natural and/or anthropogenic contaminants present in water. Fundamental principles of hygiene involve promotion and safeguarding health based on procedures designed to endorse and maintain cleanliness.

One of the most important goals pertinent to drinking water hygiene is to provide a strategic platform for biosecurity, which is in essence a comprehensive set of preventive measures designed to protect animals and humans from non-infectious contaminants such as toxins or from infectious agents such as viruses, bacteria, fungi, and parasites.

One very specific aspect of biosecurity of drinking water as it relates to the animal industry sector is reducing the risk of disease transmission between animals, between animals and humans and between humans and animals.

This integrated approach is described by the US Center for Disease Control and Prevention as the One Health concept (https://www.cdc.gov/onehealth/), which recognizes that the health of humans is inadvertently linked to the health of animals and the environment. Therefore, the biosecurity strategy for food-producing animals must be all-inclusive, encompassing the biosecurity not only of animals, but of animal products and consumers.

Biosecurity of drinking water for animals is an important element in any comprehensive biosecurity strategy. Hygiene protocol to ensure drinking water biosecurity therefore should be based on thorough analysis and solid understanding of water contaminants. Key strategic points should include continuous and diligent identification of potential hazards, exposure assessment, risk characterization, and risk management.

9

3 Significance of Water Hygiene in the Contemporary Animal Industry

Water sources used by the animal industry vary according to different regions, but in practice farm drinking water is obtained mostly from central municipal supplies or local sources (underground or surface water). In each instance the water hygiene strategy will require different considerations.

Farms that are located around urban centres are most likely to benefit from centrally supplied municipal water which is generally treated. Since the municipal water quality is routinely monitored, the risk of any adverse effects is generally very low and water hygiene strategy in such situations should focus on points where water is distributed to animals on the farm.

On the other hand, the approach to water hygiene on farms located in rural areas that rely on local water sources may be variable, and frequently have to be considered on a case by case basis.

In the majority of cases, drinking water from surface water sources runs a higher risk of biological and chemical contamination of agricultural or industrial origin, whereas underground water generally presents a low to moderate risk of biological or industrial contamination, but may contain high levels of naturally occurring chemical contaminants, some with high toxicity potential.

Nevertheless, regardless of the water source, it is important to realise that source water quality can change abruptly, and the safety of drinking water offered to animals therefore should be monitored on a regular basis.

Inadequate attention to drinking water hygiene may impact on the health and performance of animals in many different ways. In more extreme situations, poor quality drinking water and poor hygiene may have an immediate and dramatic effect on the health of animals, including morbidity and mortality. However, in practice, clinically affected animals only represent the proverbial tip of the iceberg and the most likely scenario from an on-farm perspective is that in the vast majority cases, many animals exposed to poor quality, contaminated, water are affected at a subclinical level, which usually manifests itself as subtle metabolic changes affecting performance rather than health.

Subclinical effects of drinking water contaminants deserve thorough consideration. Given that the commercial success of the modern food animal industry is largely measured in terms of animal performance parameters (growth rate, feed conversion ratio, reproductive success, and product quality), taken together at a herd or flock level, even small changes in any of these performance parameters may have far-reaching economic consequences.

Diligent monitoring of water quality on a regular basis would be a highly desirable strategy from an economic impact perspective. However, in practice, water-related problems are most probably underestimated, and drinking water analyses are often performed on a crisis management basis only. Consequently, subtle effects of poor quality water on animal performance remain obscured for a long time.

Because water contaminants can cause a wide range of non-specific metabolic changes, detecting the problems may present a considerable challenge. For that reason, an effective approach to the management of putative problems associated with water quality and hygiene would require a thorough understanding of drinking water chemistry and the possible effects on water physiology and metabolism.

4 Chemistry of Drinking Water

In chemical terms, water is a simple molecule made up of one atom of oxygen and two atoms of hydrogen. However, in natural environments, water does not occur in its chemically pure form and it is important to understand that the water we drink or offer to animals as "drinking water" is not just water, but rather a complex mixture of various substances, where water is merely a solvent. Thus, from the perspective of water hygiene, anything in drinking water that is not water should be regarded as a contaminant.

In practical terms, the chemistry of drinking water is broadly characterised by the makeup of its contaminants, whereas chemical, physical, and biological characteristics of specific contaminants are determining factors of drinking water quality and safety for human or animal consumption. Drinking water chemistry is a key factor in determining water palatability and thus may have a great impact on voluntary water intake and physiology.

5 Impact of Contaminants on Water Intake and Physiology

A continuous supply of drinking water is an unconditional requirement for sustaining life. Animals must have unrestricted access to good quality drinking water in order to be productive. Physiological requirements for water are regulated at the central nervous system level, with the thirst centre being located in the hypothalamus.

An important aspect of water physiology is that drinking water chemistry may affect voluntary water intake by animals in several different ways. Some chemical contaminants present in drinking water may induce excessive thirst and cause increased water intake, whereas some water contaminants limit water intake by animals. In some situations, water contaminants may even cause animals to refuse water.

Increased water intake may have a detrimental effect on animal physiology, but water rejection can be an outright danger to health. At any rate, prolonged water deficiency will rapidly affect all metabolic functions, and in more extreme cases may lead to serious health problems or even death. However, even mild water insufficiency will eventually depress metabolism and ultimately impact animal performance, particularly in highly productive genotypes. Given that the animal industry depends to a large degree on genotypes selected for high performance characteristics, adequate intake of drinking water is critically important in fulfilling the requisite metabolic and physiological demand of highly producing animals, as water is an essential nutrient.

Water physiology is subject to tight homeostatic control and even small changes in water homeostasis may have significant systemic effects. In these terms it is important to understand that in its biological role, water serves as a solvent and metabolic medium unreservedly required for all basic physiological and metabolic body functions and is a critically vital solvent and medium for excretion of harmful metabolic by-products.

The bulk of body water for physiological and metabolic functions in particular, is obtained from drinking water absorbed from the alimentary tract where water acts as a solvent and medium for transporting not only nutrients, but also contaminants. Therefore, a good understanding of drinking water chemistry in the context of water physiology is critically important in order to appreciate the potential adverse effects of water contaminants.

6 Biosecurity Aspect of Drinking Water Contaminants

Drinking water contaminants with the potential to cause adverse health effects in humans or animals are of particular concern, and many contaminants commonly found in various water sources may present a real concern for drinking water biosecurity.

Contaminants in water may represent extremely diverse structures and forms in which they occur. However, from the perspective of biosecurity, commonly occurring water contaminants are best broken down into two general categories; 1) chemical contaminants (organic and inorganic) and 2) biological (biotic) contaminants (bacteria, viruses, fungi, and parasites). Each of these categories characterises agents of different origins and modes of action, and thus present different challenges to water hygiene issues.

6.1 Mineral Chemical Contaminants

Drinking water problems attributed to chemical contaminants are associated with naturally occurring mineral contaminants or contaminants of industrial origin. Some minerals commonly present in various water sources have high toxicity potential and may present a significant risk of chronic or even acute toxicity to animals. Furthermore, some water contaminants may be transferred to animal products (milk, meat, eggs) and present a biosecurity risk to consumers.

A large number of the problems associated with drinking water quality for animals can be attributed to minerals inherently present in many natural water sources or that are of anthropogenic origin. Of particular importance in terms of biosecurity are those mineral contaminants with a high inherent toxicity potential (e.g. fluorine, nitrites, selenium, mercury, arsenic, cadmium, lead). The presence of these toxic compounds in drinking water should always trigger hazard evaluation. Of the toxic mineral contaminants, heavy metals such as mercury, cadmium, and lead present an especially high threat to biosecurity because of their strong potential to accumulate in edible animal products such as liver, kidney, meat or milk. Many mineral contaminants commonly found in water sources, e.g. calcium, magnesium, manganese, sodium, potassium, copper, carbonate, or phosphorus have a low (if any) potential to cause harm, but these minerals may have an indirect impact on water hygiene and biosecurity. The mere presence of otherwise harmless metals such as calcium, magnesium, sodium or potassium in water may alter the physicochemical characteristics of water such as hardness, salinity, and shift the pH of water into the alkaline range. These kinds of physicochemical changes may have an indirect impact on biosecurity, for instance by affecting the effectiveness of water sanitation or the efficacy of medicines and vaccines delivered with drinking water.

Another practical concern linking drinking water mineral contaminants and biosecurity stems from the fact that some water minerals readily precipitate on water delivery equipment, providing scaffolding for biofilm formation (Figure 9.1).

By providing a medium for the formation of biofilm, as clearly evidenced in Fig. 1a, 1b, and 1c, mineral precipitation presents a real threat to drinking water biosecurity by furnishing a breeding ground for pathogenic micro-organisms.

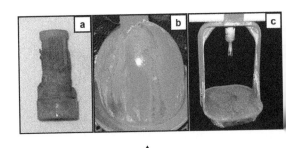

▲

Fig. 9.1: Typical examples of poultry water delivery equipment: in-line filter (a), bell drinker (b), and nipple drinker (c) surfaces, showing mineral deposits and biofilm formation associated with mineral contaminants present in drinking water (Olkowski, unpublished observations).

In addition, mineral precipitation in water delivery systems can result in a plethora of plumbing problems which may affect biosecurity. For instance, as Fig. 1b and 1c illustrate, mineral precipitation may prevent proper sealing of drinkers' valves and cause water leakages. Leaky valves increase the risk of cross-contamination in the water distribution system by facilitating access of pathogens to low-pressure water lines. Furthermore, spills of water on the floor resulting in wet litter may have a significant impact of biosecurity by providing an environment that is conducive for the proliferation of pathogens and the development of parasites eggs. Wet litter in particular, is a major threat to overall hygiene in poultry facilities with far-reaching consequences for biosecurity and animal welfare.

6.2 Biologically Active Chemical Contaminants

Over the last few decades, considerable risks of drinking water source contamination have been tied to intensification of agriculture, and specifically the exponential growth of the animal industry. In recent years, contamination of water sources by biologically active industrial contaminants, and especially by pharmaceuticals and biologically active metabolites present in human and animal waste, has become an increasingly recognized problem.

A variety of human and veterinary pharmaceuticals have been detected for some time in surface waters (Zuccato et al., 2000; Iglesias et al., 2012; Hughes et al., 2013) and in groundwater (Bartelt-Hunt et al., 2011; Fram and Belitz, 2011). Although concerns about the potential impact of pharmaceuticals on humans and animals have been raised, these compounds are found in drinking water at very low levels, and so far there has been no evidence that waterborne drugs pose an imminent threat to human or animal health (Bruce et al., 2010; WHO, 2012).

Nevertheless, the occurrence of pharmaceuticals in water sources should be closely monitored, as some drugs may have a strong potential to cause adverse effects at very low concentrations, and may be potentially problematic in susceptible individuals.

Recently, a good deal of attention has been devoted to the contamination of water sources with pharmaceuticals and industrial chemicals which remain biologically active in drinking water. Those with immune-suppressive properties, hormonally active compounds, and antimicrobial agents demand particularly closer scrutiny.

6.3 Immunomodulatory Compounds

No data currently exist on the immune modulatory effect of contaminants in drinking water on farm animals. However, based on several studies in laboratory animals (Yang and Healey, 1993; Jadhav et al., 2007; Kozul et al., 2009), water contaminants with the potential to suppress immune functions in farm animals should be closely monitored.

Immunosuppressive contaminants should be considered as a real threat to biosecurity, because compromised immune systems always carry a considerable risk of increased susceptibility of animals to infectious agents.

Hormonally Active Compounds

Chemical contaminants found in drinking water sources that are known to act on the endocrine system are collectively called endocrine disruptors. These include pharmaceuticals, natural hormones excreted by humans and animals, and a wide range of industrial agents such as organochlorine pesticides, various phenolic compounds, dioxins and furans. A number of hormonally active agents have been detected in various water sources (Kolpin et al., 2002; Bartelt-Hunt et al., 2011), and the detrimental effects thereof on aquatic wildlife have been demonstrated, but at present, the physiologically measurable effects of hormonally active water contaminants on farm animals or humans remain unclear. One case study from the Netherlands (Meijer et al., 1999) reported that dairy cattle exposed to drinking water contaminated with sewage overflows showed a reduction in reproductive performance, but in a recent review Magnusson and Persson (2015) concluded that the clinical evidence of endocrine disruption caused by hormonally active compounds in water is weak.

Nevertheless, even if clinical evidence is weak, the concerns associated with hormonally active contaminants in drinking water for livestock should not be ignored. Many of these compounds have a strong potential to affect reproductive performance at a sub-clinical level (e.g. poor sperm motility, silent estrus, poor conception etc.). We cannot exclude the possibility therefore that some fertility problems experienced at a herd level are associated with waterborne hormonally active contaminants.

6.4 Antimicrobial Agents

For many years, antimicrobial agents used in human and veterinary medicine for therapeutic purposes, and in the food animal industry for prophylactic purposes have been shown to occur in the aquatic environment (Cabello, 2006; Baquero et al., 2008; Fram and Belitz, 2011; Iglesias et al., 2012; Burke et al., 2016; Carvalho and Santos, 2016). Also, rapidly expanding commercial aquaculture has become a major contributor to global water contamination with antimicrobial agents due to the widespread application of antimicrobial agents in prophylaxis and therapy (Cabello, 2006; Done et al., 2015; Liu et al., 2017).

One of the major concerns arising from the contamination of drinking water with antimicrobial agents is that persistent exposure of bacteria to low levels of antibiotics will inevitably lead to the development of antimicrobial resistant bacteria strains (You and Silbergeld, 2014). Bacteria from aquatic ecosystems have been found to carry resistance genes, which can act as a reservoir of resistance for human and animal pathogens (Lupo et al., 2012).

Taken together, it is apparent that water has become an important reservoir of antimicrobial agents, resistant bacteria, and resistance genes (Baquero et al., 2008; Carvalho and Santos, 2016), and the occurrence of drug-resistant bacteria (including pathogens) in water sources has been well documented (Sapkota et al., 2007; Xi et al., 2009; Li et al., 2014; Bergeron et al., 2015; Khan et al., 2016; Yao et al., 2017). Therefore, the mere presence of antimicrobial drug residues in water sources should be recognized as a major threat to biosecurity (FAO 2016).

6.5 Biological Contaminants

Water is an important reservoir of bacteria, fungi, viruses and parasites of human and animal origin (Puschner et al., 1998; Cabral, 2010; Kotila et al., 2013; Gall et al., 2015; Oliveira et al., 2016). Pathogenic biotic contaminants present a real challenge to drinking water hygiene and remain a significant threat to biosecurity.

The health hazards associated with bacteria, viruses and parasites in both humans and livestock have been well documented, but in practical terms, the most significant threat to on-farm biosecurity is mostly limited to certain specific bacteria, protozoal parasites and viruses. Although fungi are common in many water sources, their potential impact on biosecurity is not clear at present, but should not be ignored.

6.5.1 Fungi

Historically, water sources have not been routinely screened for fungal contamination. However, recently, the putative role of fungi as a threat to drinking water biosecurity has been deliberated (DEFRA Report, 2011). The potential threat of waterborne fungi to biosecurity is highly relevant because drinking water sources can be readily colonized by fungi. Although the risk of infection to humans or animals by waterborne fungi is relatively low, the issue of water biosecurity ought to be considered as many fungi species have a strong potential to produce toxic metabolites (mycotoxins), which are known to cause severe health hazards to humans and animals when ingested.

The potential threat comes from biofilms which have been shown to be an important habitat for fungi in drinking water systems (Doggett, 2000; Paterson and Lima, 2005; Siqueira, et al., 2013). Fungi species producing mycotoxins, including *Penicillium* spp., *Aspergillus* spp., *Fusarium* spp. and *Claviceps* spp., have been identified in underground water sources (Oliveira et al., 2016). It is worth noting that mycotoxins have been detected in bottled drinking water (Mata et al., 2015).

6.5.2 Viruses

Several viruses of significance to public health can be transmitted by drinking water (Gall et al., 2015). However, the role of drinking water in the epidemiology of viral diseases of importance in the livestock industry is not clear. Poultry operations dependent on surface water as a source of drinking water may be at risk of exposure to a waterborne viral agent of high epidemiological significance, because the surface water provides a habitat for waterfowl species, which are known to be a reservoir for several very important viral poultry diseases such as Newcastle Disease, Infectious Bronchitis, Marek's Disease, and Avian Influenza (Amaral, 2004; Brown et al., 2007; Domanska-Blicharz et al., 2010).

9

6.5.3 **Parasites**

The major threat to on-farm water biosecurity relevant to livestock concerns two protozoal parasites; *Giardia spp.*, and *Cryptosporidium spp.*, as infections associated with these organisms may cause serious health problems and spread rapidly, particularly in young animals.

Cryptosporidiosis is an important gastrointestinal disease in humans and animals. Contaminated water is the most common and epidemiologically significant source of the parasite. C. *parvum* is a common cause of enteric infection in livestock, with a high rate of morbidity and mortality. C. *parvum* can survive outside of mammalian hosts for several months depending upon water temperature.

Giardiasis is a chronic, intestinal protozoal infection seen worldwide in humans and animals. Infection is common in dogs, cats, ruminants, and pigs. *Giardia* infection is recognized as a common cause of waterborne disease in humans and animals worldwide.
It is important to stress that Giardia cysts, and Cryptosporidial oocytes more particularly, are resistant to chlorine, and may thus present a significant challenge to maintaining proper water hygiene when chlorine-based disinfectants are used. Widespread presence of these parasitic agents in some waters is of major epidemiological concern for humans.

6.5.4 **Bacteria**

Water contaminated with faecal matter may contain a wide diversity of bacteria, including all known human pathogens (Cabral 2010). However, some bacteria that occur naturally in surface water may present a significant health hazard and challenge to biosecurity.

One specific health hazard among livestock is associated with cyanobacteria Microcystis spp., a phylum of bacteria that obtain their energy through photosynthesis, commonly known as Blue-

Green Algae. Many cyanobacteria can produce potent toxins causing serious illness or even death in animals (Puschner et al., 1998), but the risk of exposure is mostly limited to hot summer months, and predominantly among animals watered directly from surface water reservoirs (lakes, dugouts, dams, ponds).

On-farm drinking water contamination with faeces is a common way for bacterial pathogens to spread from animal to animal. At a herd or flock level, a very discrete and insidious threat to biosecurity stems from the fact that farm animals are commonly asymptomatic carriers of the most significant zoonotic bacterial pathogens such as *E. coli*, *Salmonella*, or *Campylobacter*.

Although drinking water can be a direct source of infection among humans, animal products (meat, milk, eggs) from infected animals are more likely to present a significant threat to public health. Therefore, controlling the spread of bacterial pathogens via drinking water among animals is pertinent to both animal and human biosecurity.

It is estimated that nearly two-thirds of human infections arise from pathogens shared with wild or domestic animals, with about a billion cases of illness in people and millions of deaths every year being attributed to zoonotic pathogens (Karesh et al., 2012). The majority of foodborne diseases in humans are associated with food products obtained from infected animals, and contamination of drinking water is a major cause of animal infections.

6.6 Significant Zoonotic Pathogens Associated with Drinking Water

Drinking water is a major contributor to the dissemination of zoonotic pathogens in the food animal industry. Several pathogens commonly occurring in water sources are of particular concern to on-farm biosecurity because of their high public health significance in very low infective doses (Table 1).

Table 9.1. Biotic drinking water contaminants with public health significance, their zoonotic hosts, and infective doses.

Pathogen	Zoonotic Host	Infective Dose
Salmonella sp; S. enterica, the Typhimurium serotype is the most common cause of gastroenteritis in humans.	Poultry, cattle, swine are natural, non-symptomatic reservoirs of *Salmonella spp.*; under suitable environmental conditions, *Salmonella* can survive several weeks in water.	100-1,000 cells
Escherichia coli; of concern are highly pathogenic strains known as enterohaemorrhagic *E. coli*, especially those belonging to the serogroups O157.	Ruminants and swine are natural reservoirs *of E. coli*; mostly prevalent in the gastrointestinal tract of young calves, lambs, and piglets. *E. coli* can multiply in water.	5-10 cells
Campylobacter spp.; *C. jejuni* is recognized as being the most common cause of infections.	Poultry, cattle, and swine are natural reservoirs of *Campylobacter*; majority of infections in humans are linked to chickens.	< 500 cells
Cryptosporidium spp.; only a few species are of epidemiological significance in humans; *C. parvum* is the most common.	Young ruminants (calves, lambs, goats) are natural reservoirs of *C. parvum* with a high rate of morbidity and mortality; sporadic infections in pigs documented;	10-1,000 oocysts
Giardia spp.; many identified but *G. lamblia* is the most common cause of mammalian infection.	Wildlife and domestic animals; most common in dogs, cats, ruminants, and pigs.	10-25 cysts

Source: EPA Reports 2009 and 2013

The widespread occurrence of zoonotic pathogens listed in Table 1 presents a significant biosecurity problem to the animal industry worldwide, and cross-contamination of drinking water is a major contributor (LeJeune et al., 2001; Ogden et al., 2007; Levantesi et al., 2012; Pitkänen, 2013; Galanis et al., 2014). Therefore, a diligent approach to monitoring on-farm water safety is absolutely essential.

7 Evaluating Drinking Water Safety

Quality of water from any source must be carefully monitored to ensure drinking water safety. Knowing how to recognize the potential hazards associated with water contaminants is essential for the rapid detection of problems and timely recognition of potential threats to water biosecurity is critically important for effective prevention of potential adverse effects.

In considering drinking water safety, the evaluation protocol should include key strategic points outlined in Figure 9.2.

Figure 9.2. Flow chart illustrating a logistical approach to ensuring on-farm drinking water safety.

BASIC STRATEGY FOR DRINKING WATER SAFETY EVALUATION AND RISK MANAGEMENT

Hazard Identification
The identification of biological, chemical, and physical agents capable of causing adverse health effects which may be present in water source considered to be used as drinking water for animals

Hazard Characterization
Analysis of the potential to cause harm and evaluation of the nature of the adverse health effects associated with contaminants present in water

Exposure Assessment
Evaluation of the intake of biolocial, chemical, and physical agents via water as well as exposures from other sources

Risk Characterization
The qualitative and quantitative analyses of the probability of occurrence and severity of known or potential adverse effects in a given population based on hazard characterization and exposure assessment

Risk Management
The process of selecting appropriate prevention and control options, based on risk benefit analysis taking into account the economic consequences and the feasibility

The identification of biological, chemical and physical agents, which may be present in water sources, is an important step of the hazard identification process. Drinking water contaminants that have a potential to cause adverse health effects in humans or animals must always be classified as hazardous contaminants.

Detection of potentially hazardous contaminants in drinking water should trigger the process of hazard characterisation, which should include a qualitative and quantitative evaluation of the nature of the adverse effects associated each hazardous agent. An exposure assessment and risk analysis should be carried out for each factor, but it is important to stress that the adverse effects of individual contaminants should not be examined as a "stand alone" problem. When carrying out risk analyses thorough consideration must also be given to possible additive, cumulative or synergistic effects, along with specific pathophysiological responses of the host. Frequently, the interaction between contaminants may have a more significant impact on biosecurity than the simple fact of their presence.

Risk characterisation should always be based on all available data (basic research, epidemiological surveillance, quantitative and qualitative information). A thorough qualitative and quantitative assessment, including uncertainties, centred on the probability of occurrence and severity of known or potential adverse health effects based on hazard identification, hazard characterisation and exposure assessment should be conducted. The presence of hazardous contaminants in drinking water should always be considered as a risk factor, not only from the perspective of animal health and animal performance, but also from the perspective of quality and safety of products derived from food producing animals, as well as safety of consumers.

7.1 Water Analyses

At the very least, routine drinking water analyses should provide basic information about water chemistry and sanitary status. It is advisable to test water at the source, at the point of entry to the animal facility, and at the point of watering devices. To allow for an accurate evaluation of the water quality it is important that water samples are collected with due care to avoid contamination. To ensure this, the following steps should be respected:

a) Before the sample is taken, the area at the point of entry of the water on the transfer or discharge device should be cleaned using a suitable disinfectant (e.g. 70% Alcohol or 3% hydrogen peroxide).

b) Prior to sample collection, water should be allowed to run for about 10 min, and then, a representative sample should be collected in a sterile container while avoiding contact between container and the source.

c) The water sample can be stored in a refrigerator overnight if necessary, but should be transferred to the lab as soon as possible.

Routine tests should be carried out annually in order to avoid potential problems that may arise from waterborne hazards. However, it is important to stress that drinking water quality may change abruptly, particularly in surface water sources, and therefore one should never make assumptions about drinking water safety based on past analysis. Any unusual changes in smell, clarity, taste of water, or changes in animal eating or drinking habits, loss of performance, or health problems should immediately trigger the need for water testing.

Drinking water quality for farm animals must comply with local regulations. The acceptable levels of chemical and biological contaminants may vary significantly between different jurisdictions. In most jurisdictions, the sanitary quality of water is assessed by counting numbers of coliform bacteria. The mere presence of any coliform bacteria, regardless of their pathogenicity, is a very sensitive indicator of poor sanitary status. It is commonly assumed that when coliforms are present, there is a high risk that other infectious bacteria and viruses may be present in the water.

When the need for water testing due to biosecurity concerns arises, the scope of analytical objectives for water contaminants, either chemical or biological, may be very broad, and therefore it is advisable that producers seek the assistance of a veterinarian in selecting specific tests depending on circumstances and risk analyses. Water quality and safety standards vary between different jurisdictions, so it is also important to seek assistance from local authorities for interpreting the water test results.

8 Risk Associated with Drinking Water Contaminants

In considering the adverse effects associated with drinking water contaminants, any risk analysis should always take into consideration two fundamental variables: 1) the concentration of hazardous agents in drinking water and 2) the volume of water consumed by the host.

In this context, an important factor in exposure assessment that must be carefully considered is that the water intake in farm animals may vary significantly depending on species, breed, animal age, production mode, environment, season, and climatic zone in which the animals are raised. It is worth noting that animals reared in a hot environment and high-production animals have higher water requirements so they may be at higher risk of adverse effects associated with drinking water contaminants.

As a general rule, the probability of exposure to toxic levels of waterborne chemicals is probably small, but exposure to low and moderate levels may be common and widespread. Although water contaminants may cause severe responses, including death, in practice the risk of significant adverse effects associated with chemical contaminants is rather low and would be mostly limited to those compounds with a strong toxicity potential.

On the other hand, there is probably a very high risk that drinking water for animals is contaminated with pathogens under most circumstances. The probability that drinking water from central sources can be contaminated with microorganisms is extremely low, as the quality of drinking water supplied by municipalities for human consumption is strictly regulated and water hygiene guidelines are diligently enforced. However, even though water delivered from central distribution points to the farm may be pathogen free, the probability of cross-contamination through on-farm water distribution systems is high. In practice, there is a rather high probability that drinking water at the watering point is contaminated with pathogens.

There is also a high probability that local farm water sources are contaminated with pathogenic microorganisms (Galanis et al., 2014; Butler et al., 2016). The risk of contamination is greatest in surface water (rivers, streams, lakes, dugouts, dams, reservoirs, channels, etc.) that are directly accessible by stock or that receive runoff or drainage from intensive livestock operations or human waste.

Historically, the risk of groundwater contamination by pathogens has generally been considered to be low, but with the expansion of intensive animal operations, contamination of ground water has become a concern (Li et al., 2014). Shallow groundwater sources, particularly those in sandy soils, run a high risk of being contaminated with pathogenic microorganisms from animal and human excrement.

Drinking water biosecurity is a significant challenge for the modern food animal industry, but it is important to remain mindful that one major threat to biosecurity from on-farm water sources is the animal industry itself. In the case of intensive livestock operations where large numbers of animals are reared in confined areas, the risk of local water source contamination with animal waste can be very high indeed.

Although the importance of drinking water biosecurity in the animal industry is widely recognised, a major challenge is the simple fact that eliminating all potential hazards associated with water contaminants does not appear to be a realistic goal. In reality, access to good quality water for farm animals remains problematic in many areas of the world, including in developed countries. The best practical approach to safeguarding drinking water biosecurity on the farm therefore is to apply prudent risk management.

9 Water Biosecurity and Risk Management

The concept of risk management is primarily based on risk-benefit analysis. When it comes to drinking water quality, risk management must take into account the economic aspect and the feasibility of risk options to ensure optimum security at the most efficient cost. The key variables which must be considered in risk management of drinking water contaminants are based on potential hazard assessment and exposure analysis weighed against the probability of adverse effects.

On a global scale the most significant likely threat to biosecurity in modern agriculture is continual contamination of water sources with microbial pathogens. Therefore, in the food animal industry, controlling risk associated with waterborne pathogens is of critical importance.

The main effort in addressing the problems associated with biotic contaminants should focus primarily on protecting water sources from contamination, and on taking preventive measures including effective methods of water disinfection. Adequate sanitation of drinking water beginning at the intake point would be an essential prerequisite for risk management, but a strict water hygiene protocol must be followed throughout the entire on-farm water distribution system.

A critical element of farm biosecurity is biocontainment in which risk management is defined as the strategy designed to control the spread of disease agents that have already occurred in a particular area. In this context, the success of biosecurity is strictly dependent on preventive measures designed to control dissemination of pathogens, particularly in situations where rapid responses are an absolute requirement in controlling the spread of contagious diseases, at the onset of an outbreak of infection for instance.

Monitoring pathogens in drinking water is a vital component of any risk management strategy, but in practice, the commonly used procedures for identifying infectious agent, which require at least 24-48 hours would not be an effective preventive tool. A real-time PCR technology offers specific detection, and requires less than 3 hours for analysis (Saxena et al., 2015), but this technology may not be commonly available. Therefore, early warning and prevention control at critical drinking water distribution points would be highly desirable in order to alert to putative problems in a timely manner, preferably before drinking water is offered to animals.

This can be accomplished by monitoring basic physicochemical changes in drinking water that are indicative of microbial proliferation (pH, free chlorine, dissolved oxygen, and turbidity) which can be readily measured in real time. Sudden deviations in any of these parameters could signal a problem within the system, which could probably be manageable in most cases before water is distributed to the drinkers. Undoubtedly, timely identification of changes in the drinking water sanitation status would offer many advantages in containing the spread of infectious agents.

A comprehensive, effective and functioning sanitation system must be in place, starting at the water source and extending throughout the entire drinking water distribution system. With a prudent approach to risk management strategy, threats to water biosecurity can be successfully mitigated, provided strict water hygiene measures are implemented and diligently followed.

10 Water Treatment

Source water treatment is an important tool in the arsenal for risk management, and under most practical circumstances, in order to ensure drinking water biosecurity, some specific water treatment is absolutely essential.

Common water treatment techniques used worldwide include physically removing chemical and biotic contaminants through filtration and/or inactivating pathogens by applying ultraviolet light or chemical oxidant disinfectants such as chlorine, chlorine dioxide, chloramines, and ozone.

Conventional coagulation and flocculation methods, along with simple filtration methods (sand, carbon filters) may be suitable for removing only major water insoluble contaminants, but are generally ineffective for removing all microorganisms in order to guarantee water biosecurity. Ultra-filtration, and nano-filtration in particular offer an effective means of removing the majority of biotic contaminants, but the most effective method for removal of both chemical contaminants and all biotic contaminants is reverse osmosis. A good reverse osmosis system can provide ==99.9% pure water, which is practically pathogen-free.

In recent years, filtration technology allowing physical removal of chemical and biological contaminants from any source of water has become universally available and affordable. However, one has to remain mindful that removal of biotic contaminants from source water does not safeguard on-farm water biosecurity. In reality, in order to maintain on-farm drinking water hygiene, disinfectants must be applied, even if source water is pathogen-free, as there is a high risk of cross-contamination at many points throughout the water distribution infrastructure, and especially at the drinking points.

There is a dearth of research on deactivation of waterborne toxins using water disinfection as a remedy. Although it has been shown that chlorine-based disinfection products such as sodium hypochlorite (Young 1972) and chlorine dioxide (Wilson et al., 2005) have the potential to neutralise some mycotoxins, the levels of active compounds in water required to achieve this goal are very high, and therefore the application of chlorine-based products for neutralising waterborne mycotoxins is not practical. Furthermore, water disinfection is totally ineffective in neutralising inorganic mineral waterborne toxins such as fluorine, nitrites, selenium, or heavy metals such mercury, arsenic, cadmium and lead. It is important therefore to remain mindful that water disinfection will not provide protection from waterborne toxins.

10.1 Water Sanitation

Treatment options such as ozonation or UV light are very effective for disinfecting drinking water as well as for controlling Cryptosporidium and Giardia (Korich et al., 1990; Betancourt and Rose, 2004). However, a major shortfall in this approach stems from the simple fact that neither of these methods leaves active residues in the water allowing the control of proliferation of pathogens after the process of sanitation has been completed.

In reality, although otherwise very effective for water sanitation, neither ozonation nor UV light treatments offer any protection against cross-contamination of drinking water at critical points of water distribution systems, in particular at the drinking points. Therefore, the best assurance in order to maintain proper hygiene of drinking water offered to animals is to add disinfectants capable of retaining residual microbiocidal activity throughout the entire on-farm water distribution system.

Chlorination is a widely used method of water sanitation throughout the world. When properly applied, chlorination inactivates bacteria and viruses, but is generally less effective or ineffective in controlling some parasitic contaminants, especially Cryptosporidium or Giardia.

However, not all chlorine based products will address complex problems when water lines and watering devices are colonised by biofilm. Removal of biofilm from the drinking water distribution system should be considered a high priority, as biofilm can form a very convenient scaffolding for proliferation of bacteria, and persistent "hiding places" for pathogens, which can be released continuously into water. This of course would increase the risk of waterborne infections. In situations like this therefore stronger oxidizing agents such as hydrogen peroxide or chlorine dioxide should applied (for details see next section).

Application of Disinfectants

When considering the application of chemical disinfectants, one has to remain mindful that the efficacy of disinfectants greatly depends on water chemistry. Generally, source water containing mineral contaminants and organic matter may require more disinfectant to ensure proper sanitation. However, excessive use of chlorine based disinfectants may be problematic because there is a real risk of toxicity associated with compounds resulting from the interaction of water contaminants with disinfectant. When water containing organic matter is treated with free chlorine, there is a particularly high risk that this will produce toxic disinfection by-products (DBPs). Because of their health hazard, DBPs content in drinking water is already regulated in some jurisdictions. The multi-stage approach to drinking water treatment using a combination of filtration technologies, ozonation, UV light, and application of disinfectants capable of maintaining residual presence at all points of the water distribution system is the best guarantee for controlling the risk of microbial contamination, and for avoiding potential health hazards associated with DBPs.

When animal houses are depopulated between production cycles, shock treatment of the entire water distribution system can be applied as required using high levels of chemical disinfectants to facilitate removal of biofilm from water lines and drinkers. Shock treatment is an effective strategy for dealing with stubborn biofilm residues, but it is important to remember that after this kind of treatment the water supply system must be flushed thoroughly to remove any toxic residues of the disinfectants used.

10.2 Practical Approach to Drinking Water Hygiene

On-farm drinking water biosecurity can be best safeguarded by strict adherence to hygiene principles. Properly designed sanitation systems will ensure that drinking water is free of pathogens, but if the sanitation system is not properly monitored and maintained the risk of biotic cross-contamination of drinking water will remain high. In most cases, the presence of pathogens in drinking water indicates poor hygiene, which is most probably associated with inadequate sanitation.

The best approach to controlling insufficient sanitation is to design a suitable end-stage drinking water disinfection treatment capable of maintaining a strong residual presence of microbiocidal activity throughout the drinking water distribution system, and in particular at the drinking points. With the currently approved chemical disinfectants, this goal can probably be best accomplished with a combination of free chlorine and mono-chloramine, where free chlorine would provide strength with respect to pathogen inactivation in the initial stage, and where mono-chloramine, in addition to its strong pathogen inactivation quality, would provide a more stable residual presence in water distribution systems. However, this strategy would need more research to optimise requisite dosages and obtain regulatory approval.

It is highly recommended that on-farm water hygiene protocol should be an integral component of the Hazard Analysis and Critical Control Points (HACCP) programme, which should be followed with due diligence as applied in the food industry to ensure biosecurity and quality control.

References

Amaral LA. (2004). Drinking Water as a Risk Factor to Poultry Health. *Brazilian Journal of Poultry Science* 6, 191- 199.

Baquero, F., Martínez, J.L. and Cantón, R. (2008). Antibiotics and antibiotic resistance in water environments. *Current Opinion in Biotechnology* 19, 260-265.

Bergeron, S., Boopathy, R., Nathaniel, R., Corbin, A. and LaFleur, G. (2015). Presence of antibiotic resistant bacteria and antibiotic resistance genes in raw source water and treated drinking water. *International Biodeterioration & Biodegradation* 102, 370-374

Bartelt-Hunt, S., Snow, D.D., Damon-Powell, T. and Miesbach, D. (2011). Occurrence of steroid hormones and antibiotics in shallow groundwater impacted by livestock waste control facilities. *Journal of Contaminant Hydrology* 123, 94-103.

Betancourt, W.Q. and Rose, J.B. (2004). Drinking water treatment processes for removal of Cryptosporidium and Giardia. *Veterinary Parasitology* 126, 219-234.

Brown, J.D., Swayne, D.E., Cooper, R.J., Burns, R.E. and Stallknecht, D.E. (2007). Persistence of H5 and H7 avian influenza viruses in water. *Avian Diseases.* 51(1 Suppl):285-289.

Bruce, G.M., Pleus, R.C. and Snyder, S.A. (2010). Toxicological relevance of pharmaceuticals in drinking water. *Environmental Science and Technology* 4, 5619-5626.

Burke, V., Richter, D., Greskowiak, J., Mehrtens, A., Schulz, L. and Massmann, G. (2016). Occurrence of Antibiotics in Surface and Groundwater of a Drinking Water Catchment Area in Germany. *Water Environment Research* 88, 652-659.

Butler, A.J, Pintar, K.D. and Thomas, M.K. (2016). Estimating the Relative Role of Various Subcategories of Food, Water, and Animal Contact Transmission of 28 Enteric Diseases in Canada. *Foodborne Pathogens Disease* 13, 57-64.

Cabello, F.C. (2006). Heavy use of prophylactic antibiotics in aquaculture: a growing problem for human and animal health and for the environment. *Environmental Microbiology* 8, 1137-1144.

Cabral, J.P.S. (2010). Water Microbiology. Bacterial Pathogens and Water. *International Journal of Environmental Research and Public Health* 7, 3657-3703.

Carvalho, I.T. and Santos L. (2016). Antibiotics in the aquatic environments: A review of the European scenario. *Environment International* 94, 736-757.

DEFRA Report. (2011). Review of Fungi in Drinking Water and the Implications for Human Health. http://dwi.defra.gov.uk/research/completed-research/reports/dwi70-2-255.pdf.

Doggett, M.S., (2000). Characterisation of fungal biofilms within a municipal water distribution system. *Applied and Environmental Microbiology* 66, 1249-1251.

Domanska-Blicharz, K., Minta, Z., Smietanka, K., Marche, S. and van den Berg, T. (2010). H5N1 high pathogenicity avian influenza virus survival in different types of water. *Avian Diseases* 54(1 Suppl),734-737.

Done, H.Y., Venkatesan, A.K. and Halden, R.U. (2015). Does the Recent Growth of Aquaculture Create Antibiotic Resistance Threats Different from those Associated with Land Animal Production in Agriculture? *American Association of Pharmaceutical Scientists Journal* 17,513-524.

EPA Report (2009) Review of Zoonotic Pathogens in Ambient Waters. EPA 822-R-09-002. Washington, DC: Health and Ecological Criteria Division, Office of Water.

EPA Report (2013). Literature Review of Contaminants in Livestock and Poultry Manure and Implications for Water Quality. EPA 820-R-13-002. Washington, DC: Health and Ecological Criteria Division, Office of Water. Office of Water (4304T).

FAO. (2016). Drivers, dynamics and epidemiology of antimicrobial resistance in animal production. http://www.fao.org/documents/card/en/c/d5f6d40d-ef08-4fcc-866b-5e5a92a12dbf/

Fram, M. S. and Belitz, K. (2011) Occurrence and Concentrations of Pharmaceutical Compounds in Groundwater Used for Public Drinking Water Supply in California. *Science of the Total Environment* 409, 3409-3417.

Galanis, E., Mak, S., Otterstatter, M., Taylor, M., Zubel, M., Takaro, T.K., Kuo, M. and Michel P. (2014). The association between campylobacteriosis, agriculture and drinking water: A case-case study in a region of British Columbia, Canada, 2005-2009. *Epidemiology and Infection* 142, 2075-2084.

Gall, A.M., Mariñas, B.J., Lu, Y. and Shisler, J.L. (2015). Waterborne Viruses: A Barrier to Safe Drinking Water. *PLoS Pathogens* 11(6):e1004867.

Hughes, S.R., Kay, P. and Brown, L.E. (2013). Global synthesis and critical evaluation of pharmaceutical data sets collected from river systems. *Environmental Science and Technology* 47,661-677.

Iglesias, A., Nebot, C., Miranda, J. M., Vazquez, B. I. and Cepeda, A. (2012) Detection and Quantitative Analysis of 21 Veterinary Drugs in River Water Using High-Pressure Liquid Chromatography Coupled to Tandem Mass Spectrometry. *Environmental Science and Pollution Research* 19, 3235-3249.

Jadhav, S.H., Sarkar, S.N., Ram, G.C. and Tripathi, H.C. (2007). Immunosuppressive effect of subchronic exposure to a mixture of eight heavy metals, found as groundwater contaminants in different areas of India, through drinking water in male rats. *Archives of Environmental Contamination and Toxicology* 53, 450-458.

Karesh, W.B., Dobson, A., Lloyd-Smith, J/O., Lubroth, J., Dixon, M.A., Bennett, M., Aldrich, S., Harrington, T., Formenty, P., Loh, E.H., Machalaba, C.C., Thomas, M.J. and Heymann, D.L. (2012). Ecology of zoonoses: natural and unnatural histories. *Lancet* 380(9857), 1936-1945.

Khan, S., Knapp, C.W. and Beattie, T.K. (2016). Antibiotic Resistant Bacteria Found in Municipal Drinking Water. *Environmental Processes* 3, 541-552.

Kolpin, D.W., Furlong, E. T., Meyer, M. T., Thurman, E. M., Zaugg, S. D., Barber, L. B. and Buxton, H. T. (2002) Pharmaceuticals, Hormones, and Other Organic Wastewater Contaminants in U.S. Streams, 1999_2000: A National Reconnaissance. *Environmental Science and Pollution Research* 36, 1202-1211.

Korich DG, Mead JR, Madore MS, Sinclair NA, Sterling CR. 1990. Effects of ozone, chlorine dioxide, chlorine, and monochloramine on Cryptosporidium parvum oocyst viability. *Applied and Environmental Microbiology* 56, 1423-1428.

Kotila, S.M., Pitkänen, T., Brazier, J., Eerola, E., Jalava, J., Kuusi, M., Könönen, E., Laine, J., Miettinen, I.T., Vuento, R. and Virolainen, A. (2013). Clostridium difficile contamination of public tap water distribution system during a waterborne outbreak in Finland. *Scandinavian Journal of Public Health* 41,541-545.

Kozul, C.D., Ely, K.H., Enelow, R.I. and Hamilton, J.W. (2009). Low-dose arsenic compromises the immune response to influenza A infection in vivo. *Environmental Health Perspective* 117, 1441-1447.

LeJeune, J., Besser, T.E. and Hancock, D.D. (2001). Cattle water troughs as reservoirs of *Escherichia coli* O157. *Applied and Environmental Microbiology* 67, 3053-3057.

Levantesi, C., Bonadonna, L., Briancesco, R., Grohmann, E., Toze, S. and Tandoi, V. (2012_. Salmonella in surface and drinking water: Occurrence and water-mediated transmission. *Food Research International* 45, 587-602.

Li, X., Watanabe, N., Xiao, C., Harter, T., McCowan, B., Liu, Y. and Atwill, E.R. (2014). Antibiotic-resistant E. coli in surface water and groundwater in dairy operations in Northern California. *Environmental Monitoring and Assessment* 186, 1253-1260.

Liu, X., Steele, J.C. and Meng, X.Z. (2017). Usage, residue, and human health risk of antibiotics in Chinese aquaculture: A review. *Environmental Pollution* 223, 161-169.

Lupo, A., Coyne, S. and Berendonk, T. U. (2012). Origin and evolution of antibiotic resistance: the common mechanisms of emergence and spread in water bodies. *Frontiers in Microbiology* 3, 18.

Magnusson, U. and Persson, S. (2015). Endocrine Disruptors in Domestic Animal Reproduction: A Clinical Issue? *Reproduction in Domestic Animals* 50 (Suppl. 3), 15-19.

Mata, A.T., Ferreira, J.P., Oliveira, B.R., Batoréu, M.C., Barreto Crespo, M.T., Pereira, V.J. and Bronze, M.R. (2015). Bottled water: analysis of mycotoxins by LC-MS/MS. *Food Chemistry* 176,455-464. .

Meijer, G.A.L., de Bree, J.A.,Wagenaar, J.A. and Spoelstra, S.F. (1999). Sewerage overflows put production and fertility of dairy cows at risk. *Journal of Environmental Quality* 28, 1381-1383.

Ogden, I.D., MacRae, M., Johnston, M., Strachan, N.J., Cody, A.J., Dingle, K.E. and Newell, D.G. (2007). Use of multilocus sequence typing to investigate the association between the presence of Campylobacter spp. in broiler drinking water and Campylobacter colonization in broilers. *Applied and Environmental Microbiology* 73, 5125-5129.

Oliveira, H.M., Santos, C., Paterson, R.R., Gusmão, N.B. and Lima, N. (2016). Fungi from a Groundwater-Fed Drinking Water Supply System in Brazil. *International Journal of Environmental Research and Public Health* 13(3), 304.

Paterson, R.R.M. and Lima, N. (2005). Fungal contamination of drinking water. In Water Encyclopedia; Lehr, J., Keeley, J., Lehr, J., Kingery, T.B., III, Eds.; JohnWiley & Sons: New York, NY, USA, 2005; pp. 1-7.

Pitkänen T. (2013). Review of Campylobacter spp. in drinking and environmental waters. *Journal of Microbiological Methods* 95,39-47.

Puschner, B., Galey, F.D., Johnson, B., Dickie, C.W., Vondy, M., Francis, T. and Holstege, D.M.

(1998). Blue-green algae toxicosis in cattle. *Journal of the American Veterinary Medical Association* 213, 1605-1607.

Sapkota, A.R., Curriero, F.C., Gibson, K.E. and Schwab, K.J. (2007). Antibiotic-resistant enterococci and fecal indicators in surface water and groundwater impacted by a concentrated swine feeding operation. *Environmental Health Perspective* 115, 1040-1045.

Saxena, T., Kaushik, P. and Krishna Mohan, M. (2015). Prevalence of E. coli O157:H7 in water sources: an overview of associated diseases, outbreaks and detection methods. *Diagnostic Microbiology and Infectious Diseases* 82, 249-64.

Siqueira, V.M., Oliveira, H.M., Santos, C., Paterson, R.R, Gusmão, N.B. and Lima, N. (2013). Biofilms from a Brazilian water distribution system include filamentous fungi. *Canadian Journal of Microbiology* 59,183-188.

WHO 2012. Pharmaceuticals in drinking-water. WHO Library Cataloguing-in-Publication Data. http://apps.who.int/iris/bitstream/10665/44630/1/9789241502085_eng.pdf

Wilson SC, Brasel TL, Martin JM, Wu C, Andriychuk L, Douglas DR, Cobos L, Straus DC. 2005. Efficacy of chlorine dioxide as a gas and in solution in the inactivation of two trichothecene mycotoxins. *International Journal of Toxicology*. 24, 181-186.

Xi, C., Zhang, Y., Marrs, C.F., Ye, W., Simon, C., Foxman, B. and Nriagu, J. (2009). Prevalence of Antibiotic Resistance in Drinking Water Treatment and Distribution Systems. *Applied and Environmental Microbiology* 75, 5714-5718

Yao, L., Wang, Y., Tong, L., Deng, Y., Li, Y., Gan, Y., Guo, W., Dong, C., Duan, Y. and Zhao, K. (2017). Occurrence and risk assessment of antibiotics in surface water and groundwater from different depths of aquifers: A case study at Jianghan Plain, central China. *Ecotoxicology and Environmental Safety* 135, 236-242.

Yang, S. and Healey, M.C. (1993). The immunosuppressive effects of dexamethasone administered in drinking water to C57BL/6N mice infected with Cryptosporidium parvum. *Journal of Parasitology* 79, 626-630.

Yang CY. 1972. Comparative studies on the detoxification of aflatoxins by sodium hypochlorite and commercial bleaches. *Applied Microbiology*. 24, 885-890.

You, Y. and Silbergeld, E.K. (2014). Learning from agriculture: understanding low-dose antimicrobials as drivers of resistome expansion. *Frontiers in Microbiology,* 5.

Zuccato, E., Calamari, D., Natangelo, M. and Fanelli, R. (2000). Presence of therapeutic drugs in the environment. *Lancet*.355(9217):1789-90.

9

CHAPTER 10

PROMOTING BIOSECURITY THROUGH INSECT MANAGEMENT AT ANIMAL FACILITIES

Alec C. Gerry

Amy C. Murillo

Department of Entomology, University of California, Riverside, CA 92521

1 Introduction

Insects and related terrestrial arthropods (including mites and ticks) are incredibly diverse groups of invertebrate animals found almost everywhere on Earth. Insects alone comprise approximately 75% of the total animal species on Earth (Samways, 2005). While not as species-diverse as insects, mites can be very abundant in some habitats. Fortunately, few insect and mite species directly harm animals. In contrast to insects and mites, all tick species have the potential to cause harm to animals because all ticks feed on animal blood. The insects, mites, and ticks that do harm animals can severely impact animal health and welfare, often resulting in considerable economic loss to domestic animal production.

2 Damage caused by insects

With few exceptions, the insects, mites, and ticks that harm animals feed on blood, skin, hair, feathers, or body exudates (e.g., tears, mucus) on the external body surface of their animal host and are therefore often collectively described as external parasites or 'ectoparasites.' These ectoparasites can negatively impact animal health and productivity in many ways, ranging from reduced feed consumption, growth, and economic output (e.g., in meat, milk, or eggs) to severe health consequences or even death of parasitized animals. Negative impacts include (1) physical damage to the animal host caused by insect feeding, (2) expression of unproductive animal behaviour in response to animal disturbance caused by the painful bites of some biting insects, and (3) transmission of viruses, parasites and other pathogens from infected animals to susceptible animals. Even when ectoparasites cause no obvious physical damage to their animal host, painful or irritating bites can negatively impact animal production due to increased host metabolic activity and behavioural responses that lower feed conversion efficiency or feed consumption of the animal host. Additionally, some insects and mites cause economic damage to animal producers as a result of nuisance to facility employees or neighbours.

2.1 Insects and animal disease

Of the negative impacts described above, the transmission of pathogens among animals is perhaps of greatest concern for many veterinarians and animal producers. In some cases, an arthropod is a necessary intermediary for the transfer of pathogens among animals, and disease transmission would not occur but for the presence and activity of the ectoparasite. These ectoparasites are called 'biological vectors' identifying their required role in transmission of the pathogen. In these cases, the arthropod is as much a host of the pathogen as is the vertebrate animal; the pathogen being adapted for life in both the arthropod and the vertebrate animal. Ectoparasites that feed on animal blood can acquire pathogens from an infected animal host, subsequently transferring these pathogens to susceptible animals during later feeding events. For example, biting midges in the genus *Culicoides* are biological vectors of several viruses that infect cattle, sheep, and horses. Within the biting midge, the virus must escape the digestive system, amplify, and spread to the insect salivary glands where the virus is then positioned to be introduced to a new host when the biting midge feeds again. The time required for the virus to amplify and reach the salivary glands is called the 'extrinsic incubation period' and a biting midge that feeds on a new host before the extrinsic incubation period is completed cannot pass on the virus. The extrinsic incubation period is typically dependent upon environmental temperature, with higher temperatures resulting in a shorter incubation period (Reisen, 2009). A higher environmental temperature typically also increases the insect development rate. These temperature effects are the reason that many insect transmitted diseases show a seasonal transmission pattern with greater disease incidence during warmer months of the year (e.g., see Gerry et al., 2001). A few biological vectors transmit pathogens to vertebrate animals through more unconventional associations. The lesser mealworm beetle (*Alphitobius diaperinus*) is a biological vector of chicken tapeworm, though this beetle does not bite or feed on chickens. Rather, these beetles acquire tapeworms when burrowing through poultry faeces contaminated with tapeworm from infected birds. The tapeworm then undergoes development within the body of the beetle before being passed to a susceptible bird that eats the infected beetle. Often, targeted control of these biological vectors will lead to a reduction in disease incidence in the vertebrate animal population.

In some cases, insects are not required intermediate hosts for animal pathogens. Rather, pathogens may be acquired from the environment and distributed among susceptible animal hosts as the insect moves about the landscape. These 'mechanical vectors' may act to some extent as fomites, simply carrying the pathogen as a contaminant on external body surfaces and depositing pathogens wherever they go. Insects that develop in or feed on animal faeces are often mechanical vectors of animal pathogens shed in the animal faeces. Susceptible animals become infected with the pathogen when they consume feed or water contaminated with a pathogen as a result of insect contact, or susceptible animals may simply consume a contaminated insect. For example, house flies are proven mechanical vectors of pathogenic *Escherichia coli* bacteria to cattle presumably through these mechanisms (Ahmad et al., 2007). Recent evidence suggests that some insects that serve as mechanical vectors may be more than simple fomites. For example, flies that feed on animal faeces may harbour some pathogens within their digestive system, with pathogen amplification occurring within the insect digestive tract or even in the excreted insect faeces (Wasala et al., 2013; Nayduch & Burrus, 2017).

2.2 Insects and biosecurity

Biosecurity traditionally includes those preventive measures employed at animal facilities to limit the spread of pathogens among animals or to/from other animal facilities. Because insects, mites, and ticks can transmit numerous pathogens to wild and domestic animals, measures to prevent the spread of these pests among animal facilities is a critical part of an effective biosecurity programme. However, given the direct harm that ectoparasites can cause to animals, even in the absence of disease transmission, a more comprehensive understanding of biosecurity also includes those measures intended to reduce pest numbers on animal facilities and prevent pest movement among animal facilities. It should be noted that most insects are winged as adults, resulting in a considerable challenge to preventing their movement and dispersal among nearby animal facilities. Instead, the focus of insect biosecurity should be on reducing the number of insects on animal facilities and limiting the contact of insects with infectious animals. In contrast, mites and ticks lack wings and dispersal among facilities generally occurs by movement of infested animals or by sharing machinery and supplies, though movement of facility employees among animal facilities can also pose a risk. Mite and tick biosecurity is thus best accomplished by quarantine and treatment of parasitized animals, exclusion of wild animals that may carry ectoparasites, and limiting the activities and movement of facility employees to reduce the accidental transport of ectoparasites to other susceptible animals.

2.3 Integrated pest management

Animal producers should implement the integrated pest management (IPM) concept to control insect pests and ectoparasites as part of a biosecurity programme. IPM is a coordinated strategy to reduce arthropod damage, including pathogen transmission, through application of a combination of techniques aimed at keeping pest abundance at levels below which damage is expected to occur. While it may be more difficult to determine a threshold of pest abundance when risk of disease transmission is involved, using an IPM strategy nevertheless provides a proactive focus on pest management ensuring that pests are held to low abundance levels thereby minimizing impacts on animal production. Lacking an IPM strategy, many animal producers respond to high pest numbers through application of pesticides for immediate reduction of the offending pest; but at these high pest numbers, disease transmission and economic damages have likely already occurred.

An IPM strategy focuses first on reducing opportunities for immature development of pest species. Reducing or manipulating the available pest development habitat may alone provide the desired level of control. Where immature development habitat cannot be reduced or manipulated sufficiently, judicious use of pesticides on insect development sites may reduce pest production and keep numbers of damaging pests low. In some situations, application of pesticides for control of adult insects will be needed and may form part of an IPM strategy. When pest numbers reach damaging levels, or when pathogen transmission has been detected, immediate control of adult insects is warranted. In these situations, pesticides may be applied directly to the host animal or to animal facility structures to target insects resting on these structures. A searchable, online database of pesticides registered by the U.S. Environmental Protection Agency for control of arthropod pests of animals is maintained by veterinary entomologists in the United States as part of a U.S. Department of Agriculture (USDA) sponsored multistate research project, and is available at https://www.veterinaryentomology.org/vetpestx (Ferguson et al., 2015). However, if pesticides are often used for emergency pest control due to failure of proactive IPM measures, facility managers should re-evaluate their IPM program. Frequent application of pesticides is unsustainable, and pests will quickly develop resistance to the chemicals used. When applying pesticides, care must be given to maximise control of the damaging pest while minimising pesticide impact to useful insects, such as pollinators or any insect predators and parasitoids that naturally prey on the damaging pest.

An IPM strategy necessarily includes a mechanism for monitoring pest abundance, with increasing abundance triggering additional control measures aimed at keeping pest numbers from reaching damaging levels. Monitoring pest abundance is also important to note if control measures applied have been effective in decreasing pest populations. Effective pest monitoring methods will differ by pest species based upon the biology and behaviour of each pest species as well as differences in the location of immature development sites and adult resting sites. In general, a weekly count of the number of individual ectoparasites on a representative number of host animals is a useful way to monitor changing pest abundance for many ectoparasites, including ticks and some of the larger biting flies. Animals can also be observed for certain behaviour or an appearance that is indicative of pest activity or pest abundance. For example, cattle will stamp their legs, toss their heads, or bunch together in a group to avoid the painful bites of some biting flies, and an animal's 'mangy' appearance is an indicator of possible infestation by a mite species. Other pest species can be monitored using attractive traps (baited with a host or food odour) or by using traps that passively capture pests as they move about their environment. Appropriate methods for monitoring relevant pest species will be discussed in each animal commodity section below.

3 Insect pests of cattle

Since the 1980s, the production of milk worldwide has increased more than 50% to 769 million tons of milk produced in 2013 (FAOSTAT, 2017). The increase in milk production is attributed to growth of the industry in developing countries throughout south Asia where milk is often produced on smallholder or family farms. Major milk producing countries are India, the United States, China, Pakistan, and Brazil. Countries with the highest milk surpluses are New Zealand, the United States, Germany, France, Australia, and Ireland. In developed countries, dairy farms are growing larger and are increasingly mechanised. Cow nutrition is now often carefully controlled through supplemental feed to increase milk production per animal. In contrast to milk production, beef production and consumption worldwide is increasing slowly with beef consumption increasing primarily in developing countries (FAO, 2016a). Beef production is limited by declining rangeland availability in most countries due to encroachment of other land uses and degradation of available rangelands. Further increases in beef production are likely to result from increasing animal density on available lands, with animals provided supplemental feeds where forage is no longer sufficient (Bruinsma, 2003). Modern cattle feedlots, where cattle have no access to pasture and are fed entirely on supplemental feed, are an extreme example of beef cattle intensification.

10

As cattle operations continue to move towards a more intensive operational model with increasing cattle density and reduced pasture availability, insect and tick species that impact cattle in open pasture settings are being eclipsed in importance by pest species that develop in cattle manure and feed waste. These often accumulate in great quantities on intensive operations (Gerry, in press).

3.1 Permanent ectoparasites

Some ectoparasites spend their entire life on a single host ('permanent ectoparasites'), with the host providing the necessary habitat and food for each life stage of the ectoparasite. There are five species of lice and four species of mites common to cattle as permanent ectoparasites. The more damaging blood feeding lice are the long-nosed cattle louse (*Linognathus vituli*), short-nosed cattle louse (*Haematopinus eurysternus*), cattle tail louse (*H. quadripertusus*), and little blue louse (*Solenopotes capillatus*). A single species of chewing louse, the cattle biting louse (*Bovicola bovis*), feeds on skin rather than blood. Cattle mites feed on skin debris or lymph within the dermal tissues, and include the important scabies or 'mange' mites *Psoroptes ovis*, *Sarcoptes scabiei* and *Chorioptes bovis*, as well as the cattle follicle mite (*Demodex bovis*). Feeding by lice and mites can be quite irritating to the host, and may result in considerable physical damage due to dermatitis, tissue destruction, and hair loss. Lice and mites can also cause damage to hides, particularly as animals rub and scratch against objects in their environment to alleviate the itching caused by ectoparasite feeding. Heavy infestations of lice and/or mites can reduce weight gain and milk yield (Wright, 1985). Additionally, poor physical condition of heavily infested animals, often coupled with substantial hair loss, can result in death of young calves and older cattle when exposed to severe weather conditions or low nutritional levels.

Surveillance for both lice and mites is by routine observation of animal health, with obvious signs of mange or other hide damage indicative of louse or mite infestation.

Management of lice and mites is commonly achieved by treating all cattle within a herd with a topically-applied insecticide (lice) or acaricide (mites), and by limiting contact among infested and uninfested animals or herds. Any animals left untreated in the herd, even if they appear to be free of lice or mites, will almost certainly result in treated cattle soon being infested again with lice and mites. Injection of ivermectin or related parasiticides may also provide control of lice and mites. For lice, two insecticide treatments 10-14 days apart are needed, as lice in the egg stage are protected from the insecticide and may survive the first treatment (Campbell, 1985).

3.2 Ticks

There are many tick species that feed on cattle. Ticks can be categorised as 'hard ticks' (Family Ixodidae) due to the presence of a rigid plate on the back that makes them difficult to crush between the fingers (Fig.10.1), or 'soft ticks' (Family Argasidae) which lack this rigid dorsal plate.

Most hard ticks have three life stages (larva, nymph, adult) and feed on a different vertebrate host during each life stage (3-host ticks), living off the host in the surrounding habitat between feeding periods. Attachment to hosts for feeding often lasts for at least several days. Where cattle are kept on pasture, 3-host ticks can be abundant due to the presence of off-host refuge and alternate hosts in this habitat. These ticks are less abundant on more intensive cattle operations where cattle access to pasture is limited, with ticks essentially absent on dairy and feedlot facilities where cattle have no access to pasture (Gerry, in press). While these ticks can cause economic damage from blood loss, irritation by tick feeding, and even toxic paralysis, their more important impact is as vectors of several bacterial and protozoal diseases of cattle. A few hard ticks will feed on the same cattle

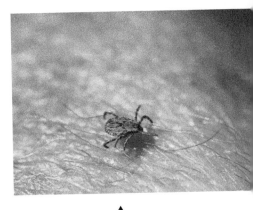

▲
Fig. 10.1: Hard ticks in several genera (including *Dermacentor*, shown) can impact livestock, especially as vectors of pathogens.

host during all life stages (1-host ticks). Cattle ticks (*Rhipicephalus* spp.) are a particularly important group of 1-host ticks that are biological vectors of the *Babesia* parasites that cause bovine babesiosis or 'cattle fever' (Pérez de León et al., 2012).

Soft ticks tend to be more common in arid environments and can have quite variable life histories, often including several nymph stages before reaching the adult stage. During each life stage, soft ticks will feed on a host for only a few minutes after which they typically leave the host to moult to the next life stage. One unusual soft tick, the spinose ear tick (*Otobius megnini*), will spend its immature life feeding within the ear canal of a single host animal (Fig. 10.2; cattle and non-cattle), before dropping to the ground to complete a non-feeding adult stage. Due to this unusual life history, the spinose ear tick can be abundant in both pasture-based and confined cattle facilities.

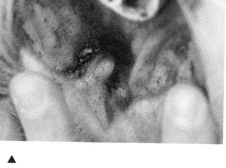

▲

Fig. 10.2: Spinose ear ticks (*Otobius megnini*) are soft ticks that feed and develop in the ear canal of several animals including cattle and swine. They are more commonly found on animals held in confinement.

Tick numbers on cattle can be reduced by application of acaricides to adult tick feeding sites on the animal or in some cases by immersion of the entire animal into a dipping vat containing acaricide (Wright, 1985). Management of ticks in pasture settings is quite challenging, as many ticks will also feed on non-cattle hosts, and will thus avoid the treatment or will be reintroduced with trespassing wildlife arriving from outside the cattle pasture. To address this, several novel methods to treat non-cattle hosts for ticks have been introduced in recent years, including the USDA '4-Poster' device for deer to self-treat with an acaricide while accessing food bait (Carroll et al., 2009).

3.3 Cattle grubs and screwworm flies

Cattle grubs (*Hypoderma bovis* and *H. lineatum*) and screwworm flies, both New World screwworm fly (*Cochliomyia hominivorax*) and Old World screwworm fly (*Chrysomya bezziana*), are intermittent parasites of cattle that feed on internal body tissues of cattle only during their immature life stages. The adult flies of these species do not feed on the animal, but seek cattle on which they will lay their eggs. Cattle grubs are parasites only of cattle, while screwworm flies will attack many warm-blooded animals (including humans). Neither fly is a vector of cattle pathogens, but the damage caused by the feeding of these flies on internal tissues can be severe, resulting in considerable economic cost to producers. Feeding damage by immature screwworm flies (maggots) can be particularly devastating. This often leads to the death of the animal as feeding wounds become infected which attracts additional egg-laying by tissue-consuming flies (Alexander, 2006).

Where the adult cattle grub (called a heel fly) is active, cattle often exhibit behaviour called 'gadding' where they run madly with their tails raised in the air in an apparent effort to prevent these flies from depositing eggs on the cattle body. Parasitized cattle will show swellings along the back ('warble') where the cattle grub has cut a breathing hole in the animal hide to complete its immature development. In geographic regions where screwworm is present, cattle should be routinely observed for wounds within which immature flies may be developing.

Cattle grubs are readily treated using systemic insecticides applied to cattle in late summer to kill the developing immature flies as they migrate though the body of cattle. Management of screwworm flies is more difficult and relies on early treatment of screwworm infested wounds with insecticides and culling of severely infested animals to prevent fly development to the adult stage. New World screwworm fly has been eradicated throughout North and Central America by sustained releases of sterile male screwworm flies initiated by the USDA in 1958.

3.4 Flies that develop in cattle faecal pats

Pest flies that require fresh, undisturbed cattle faeces (faecal pats) to complete their immature development are the horn fly (*Haema-*

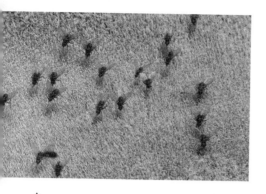

▲

Fig. 10.3: Horn flies (*Haematobia irritans*) feed on blood from cattle and occasionally horses. They spend most of their time on the host, and tend to orient themselves facing downward.

tobia irritans) and face fly (*Musca autumnalis*). During the adult stage, both fly species feed on cattle, but the horn fly feeds on blood (Fig. 10.3) while the face fly feeds primarily on exudates, particularly nasal and eye secretions (Fig. 10.4). Horn flies spend most of their adult life resting or feeding on cattle, taking many small blood meals each day (Cupp et al., 1998). Horn flies are easily disturbed by cattle activity, and readily move among nearby animals throughout the day. Face flies feed only briefly on cattle before leaving the host animal to rest in the surrounding habitat. Face flies are recognized vectors of a bacterium (*Moraxella bovis*) causing bovine pinkeye, and of filarial nematodes (*Thelazia* spp.) that parasitize the cattle eye (Wall & Shearer, 1997). Horn flies are not recognized as vectors of a cattle disease, but their painful bites irritate cattle and can greatly impact production efficiency.

Both flies can be monitored by visual observation of fly numbers on cattle. Flies should be counted during mid-morning when horn

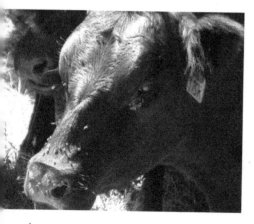

flies are typically resting on the back and sides of cattle and face flies are actively feeding around the eyes and face. When daytime temperatures are high, horn flies can be difficult to accurately count as they retreat to the shaded lower regions of the cattle body to escape direct sun exposure (Lysyk, 2000). A weekly count of horn flies and face flies on 15 randomly selected animals in a herd is suitable for showing changes in fly abundance over time.

▲

Fig. 10.4: Face flies (*Musca autumnalis*) congregate near the eyes of cattle where they feed on exudate. Face flies are vectors of pathogens including bovine pinkeye and eyeworms of cattle and horses.

Management of these flies is best achieved by disturbance of freshly deposited cattle faecal pats. Where cattle are held in confinement at high density, faecal pats rarely remain intact as cattle disturb the pats as they move about their pen. For this reason, horn flies and face flies are usually not abundant on intensive cattle operations where cattle lack access to pasture. However, where cattle density is low or where cattle have at least some access to pasture, these flies can be abundant unless facility workers manually or mechanically disturb the fresh faecal pats. Where disturbance of faecal pats is impractical, cattle can be given feed additives containing an insect growth regulator (IGR) that will pass through the animal digestive system and into the faeces to prevent immature fly development. However, some IGRs can also prevent development of dung beetles and other insects that assist with the breakdown of cattle faeces, so these products should be used judiciously. Where faecal pats cannot be disturbed or treated to prevent development of these flies, adult flies can be controlled using insecticides applied to cattle as insecticide-treated ear tags, or as topical pour-ons, sprays, oils, and dusts (Wright, 1985). Insecticide applications have been particularly useful in reducing adult horn flies as these flies only rarely leave their cattle host. However, over-use of insecticides for adult horn fly management has led to the inevitable development of horn fly resistance to some insecticides (Foil & Hogsette, 1994). There has recently been increased interest in using low toxicity botanical extracts and essential oils primarily as repellents applied to cattle to reduce biting by horn flies (Showler, 2017; Mullens et al., 2017a).

3.5 Flies that develop in fermenting organic matter

Fermenting organic matter including animal faeces, cattle bedding, and wet animal feed is often plentiful on most modern dairies and feedlots, with increasing animal density and mechanisation associated with greater quantities of these materials. Important pest flies that develop in fermenting organic materials are the stable fly (*Stomoxys calcitrans*) and the house fly (*Musca domestica*). The adult stable fly feeds on animal blood (Fig.10.5) while the adult house fly feeds on any number of carbohydrate or protein-rich foods available in the environment, including feeding on cattle faeces. Adult stable flies typically feed on cattle or other animals once per day. The bites are quite painful causing cattle to exhibit bite avoidance behaviour includ-

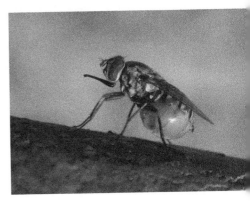

Fig. 10.5: Resting female stable fly (*Stomoxys calcitrans*) after taking a blood meal. Note the rigid proboscis.

▼

ing leg stamping and tail switching to dislodge biting stable flies (Mullens et al., 2006). When biting pressure is high, cattle gather into groups ('bunching') to avoid these biting flies. This unproductive cattle behaviour can result in reduced weight gain and milk production for animals molested by stable flies (reviewed by Gerry et al., 2007). Somewhat surprisingly, the stable fly is not known to transmit important cattle diseases. In contrast, house flies do not feed on blood but are mechanical vectors of a number of viral and bacterial pathogens which they acquire from contact with animal faeces and subsequently distribute throughout the environment. Pathogen deposition by house flies onto human food crops is of particular concern (Talley et al., 2009).

Stable fly abundance and activity can be determined by counting flies on cattle, by using traps such as the Alsynite trap that target adult stable flies, or by observing animal behaviour in response to the painful biting of these flies (Gerry et al., 2007). If monitoring stable flies by counting flies on cattle, counts are performed by approaching the animal from one side and visually observing the number of stable flies on the outside of the front leg nearest to the observer and the inside of the opposite front leg (Lysyk, 1995) (Fig. 10.6). A count of 5 stable flies per leg is considered the threshold for economic impact on cattle. Some cattle behaviour is associated with stable fly biting activity, and can be used as a means to monitor fly activity. When stable fly activity is high, cattle bunching may be noted and is certainly an indication that stable fly management is needed. At lower stable fly abundance, the number of cattle tail flicks within a 2-minute period can be used as a measure of fly activity, with an average of 10 tail flicks per animal considered the economic threshold (Mullens et al., 2006). It should be noted that high numbers of horn flies will also affect cattle behaviour, including increasing tail flicks (Boland et al., 2008), making it difficult to distinguish which fly species are responsible for observed behaviour when both flies are abundant

Fig. 10.6: On cattle, stable flies (*Stomoxys calcitrans*) prefer to feed on the lower legs. While feeding, they generally position themselves facing upward.

▼

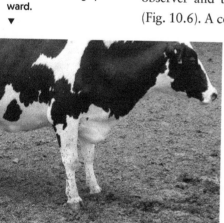

on cattle. All cattle observations should be performed on a minimum of 15 randomly selected animals for statistical validity.

House fly activity can be determined by capturing flies using sticky traps or traps baited with food attractants, or by using 'spot cards', paper cards placed at fly resting sites on which flies deposit faecal and regurgitation spots. For a reliable monitoring programme, 5 traps or 12 spot cards are usually sufficient (Gerry et al., 2011). There has been recent interest in using computational technologies to improve fly monitoring, with development of software (Fly Spotter©) to automate counting fly spots on spot cards (Fig. 10.7) (Gerry et al., 2011). Monitoring systems that identify wingbeat frequency of flying insects passing through a sensor array are currently under development and may soon greatly simplify pest monitoring by identifying and counting several pest fly species simultaneously without the need to capture the insects (Chen et al., 2014).

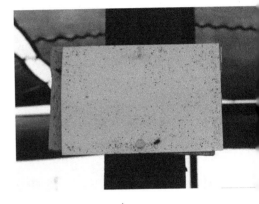

▲
Fig. 10.7: House fly monitoring can be accomplished via placing white cards in likely fly resting areas. When flies land (shown) they regurgitate and/or defecate leaving 'fly spots'. Spots can be hand counted or software such as FlySpotter© can be utilized to track relative populations over time.

Management of both the stable fly and house fly can be challenging on modern intensive cattle operations. Substantial quantities of cattle faeces collected from animal housing areas are often stored on-site and long-term storage of animal feed including hay, straw, grains, and fermenting feed additives including fruit and nut waste is also common. For both fly species, management is best achieved by applying sanitation measures to rapidly dry cattle faeces, to prevent wetting of stored dry cattle feeds, and to limit fly access to cattle feed that is intentionally fermented. Cattle pens should be regularly scraped or harrowed to break up and dry faecal accumulations within the pen. If faeces cannot be dried this way due to high animal density or pen characteristics, cattle faeces should instead be collected and piled to compost in a location where it will not be rewetted. Composting of cattle faeces can greatly reduce fly development as internal pile temperatures increase to exceed lethal temperatures for developing flies while simultaneously drying the outer portion of the compost pile to make it unsuitable for egg-laying by female flies. Hay, grains, and other dry animal feeds should be stored in a manner to prevent wetting and subsequent fermentation of these materials. Flies will not develop on dry animal feed. Where fermentation of animal feed is desired or necessary, animal feed should be fermented within enclosed fermentation bags to prevent fly access. When sanitation measures fail and adult fly numbers reach damaging levels, insecticides used for immediate control of adult flies are best applied as sprays, fogs, or mists of a long-lasting or residual chemical such as a synthetic pyrethroid to facility structures near cattle where adult flies are noted to rest. However, insecticide application alone will not provide sustainable control of adult flies, and over-reliance on pesticides has resulted in the development of resistance to many available insecticides in both species (e.g., see Keiding, 1999).

3.6 Biting midges

Biting midges in the genus *Culicoides* are small, blood-feeding flies that are important vectors of several viruses that impact cattle, including bluetongue virus and the recently isolated Schmallenberg virus (Mellor et al., 2000; Rasmussen et al., 2012). These flies can be produced in substantial numbers in semi-aquatic habitats, moist leaf litter or even moist manure, depending on the species of biting midge. Developmental sites are difficult to identify for many species and are often widespread in the habitat surrounding animal facilities. *Culicoides* that bite cattle are usually active during crepuscular periods near both sunrise and sunset (Mellor et al., 2000), though activity may shift toward daylight periods in cooler weather. Risk of bluetongue virus transmission to cattle is primarily determined by *Culicoides* abundance and their cattle biting rate (Gerry et al., 2001; Mayo et al., 2016).

Culicoides activity is commonly measured using traps baited with UV light or carbon dioxide, though there are a number of limitations associated with these traps, including the inability of light traps to capture diurnally active midges and the poor efficiency of carbon dioxide traps for capturing a number of important midge vectors of bluetongue virus (reviewed by Mullens et al., 2015). Collection of biting midges by aspiration directly from animals would provide better surveillance outcomes, but is certainly more difficult and is rarely done (e.g., see Gerry et al., 2009; Cohnstaedt et al., 2012).

Even when *Culicoides* development sites are known, manipulation of these developmental sites is often impractical, making management of biting midges challenging. Application of insecticides or insect repellents directly to animals may provide some level of protection from biting midges (Mullens et al., 2010; Griffioen et al., 2011) and might be particularly useful when transporting small numbers of animals through quarantine zones, but insecticide applications to cattle herds may not be successful in reducing virus transmission to treated herds overall (Mullens et al., 2001). Stabling of animals indoors can reduce biting by some *Culicoides* that are reluctant to enter structures (Meiswinkel et al., 2000).

3.7 Biosecurity for cattle pests

Biosecurity measures for cattle pests should focus on (1) sanitation measures to reduce fly development in cattle faeces and stored cattle feed, (2) limiting movement of cattle among herds and particularly among cattle facilities to reduce transfer of lice, mites, and ticks, (3) restricting deer and related wildlife access to cattle facilities to limit tick introductions, and 4) routine observation of cattle to monitor for pest introductions and increasing pest abundance to drive management efforts. The main biosecurity concerns will differ by geographic region, habitat, and the level of intensification of the cattle operation. In pasture-based cattle systems, management efforts should focus on ticks, cattle grub, horn fly, and face fly, while in more intensive confined dairy and feedlot systems management efforts should focus on house fly and stable fly, with biosecurity efforts applied to other pests when noted on cattle.

4 Insect pests of sheep

In the United States, sheep production has declined rapidly in the last 50 years as the use of synthetic fibres has replaced the need for wool (Jones, 2004). While meat production has replaced wool production as the primary emphasis for the sheep industry, the industry continues to decline in the United States and other countries due to increased regulatory pressures, reduced access to grazing lands, and increased costs for raising sheep (Shiflett, 2017). However, sheep production in Australia and New Zealand has adjusted to the shrinking wool industry, and export of sheep meat from these countries is increasing. Top producers of sheep meat today are China, Australia, New Zealand, the United Kingdom, and Turkey (FAOSTAT, 2017). Sheep are particularly suited for the conversion of many different types of forage vegetation into wool and meat, and for this reason are rarely held in intensive confined animal production systems.

4.1 Permanent ectoparasites

There are four species of lice found on sheep. Blood-feeding sheep lice are the sucking body louse (*Linognathus ovillus*), the sucking foot louse (*L. pedalis*), and the African blue louse (*L. africanus*). A single species of chewing louse, the sheep biting louse (*Bovicola ovis*), feeds on skin rather than blood. The sheep biting louse can be very irritating, causing sheep to pull at their fleece and rub against objects to alleviate the itching. These actions can result in considerable fleece damage as large areas of fleece can be completely rubbed off. Lice are transferred among animals by direct contact.

Sheep mites include *Psoroptes ovis* which causes a condition called 'sheep scab', the scabies mite (*Sarcoptes scabiei*), the sheep leg mite (*Chorioptes ovis*), and the Australian itch mite (*Psorergates ovis*). Of these mites, *Psoroptes ovis* is of most concern as this mite causes intense itching so that sheep scratch their bodies against objects in their environment, often to the point of causing physical damage to their fleece and hide. *Psoroptes ovis* has been eradicated from the United States, Australia, New Zealand, Scandinavia, and Canada (Spickler, 2009).

The sheep ked (*Melophagus ovinus*) is a wingless, blood-feeding fly that spends its entire life in the fleece of sheep. Female sheep ked develop larvae one at a time within their body, periodically depositing a fully developed larva onto the fleece. Populations of sheep ked therefore build up more slowly than for most ectoparasites. Like lice and mites, sheep ked are transferred among sheep by direct contact between animals. Sheep ked cause damage from their irritating bites which can result in the formation of nodules or 'cockles' on the skin, which reduces the value of sheep skin.

Permanent ectoparasites are monitored by direct observation of animals, with poor fleece or skin conditions indicative of ectoparasite presence. Management of lice and mites on sheep is similar to their management on cattle (see above). Sheep ked can be eradicated by shearing of sheep before lambing in spring, followed by application of insecticides to all animals in the herd. To prevent reinfestation of the herd, new animals should be quarantined, inspected and treated with insecticide prior to introduction to the herd.

4.2 Ticks

Ticks described in the cattle section above will also feed on sheep, and management is similar for ticks on both animals.

4.3 Sheep bot fly

The sheep bot fly (*Oestrus ovis*) is a worldwide pest of sheep and goats. Adult flies deposit first instar larvae in the nostrils of sheep where the larvae (maggots) consume the nasal mucosa. Feeding by sheep bot maggots can be irritating to the sheep and can increase the opportunity for bacterial infection of the nostrils. The mere presence of adult flies can also irritate sheep, and they will attempt to avoid the flies by running in short bursts and by snorting, behaviour which affects sheep grazing and reduces animal weight gains. There are no management recommendations for this fly, though individual animals can be treated with ivermectin or other antihelminthics if infestation is deemed to be problematic for the animal.

4.4 Wool maggots

Wool maggots are the generic name for the larvae of any fly species that lay their eggs on sheep fleece that is soiled with urine, faeces, or blood due to wounding. Most of these flies belong to the blow fly family (Calliphoridae) and are typically carrion-feeding flies. Wool maggots consume bacteria associated with the soiled fleece and may also readily feed on infected skin wounds or lesions. Where an infestation becomes severe, sheep mortality may occur.

Preventive measures include shearing pregnant ewes to prevent soiling of fleece during lambing, and scheduling lambing for early spring before flies are abundant. Fleece that is soiled by urine or faeces should be clipped to reduce the opportunity for fly strike (egg laying by flies). Animals infested with wool maggots can be spot treated with insecticide at the site of infestation to eliminate maggots.

4.5 Biting midges

Sheep are a suitable host for many *Culicoides* species that will attack cattle. Sheep are particularly at risk of *Culicoides* transmitted bluetongue virus, which can often result in death of infected sheep.

Surveillance and management for biting midges is described in the cattle section above.

4.6 Biosecurity for sheep pests

Biosecurity measures for sheep pests includes limiting movement of sheep among herds to reduce transfer of lice, mites, sheep ked, and ticks, and monitoring sheep for the presence of other pests with increasing pest abundance driving management efforts. The main biosecurity concerns will differ by geographic region and by habitat, with viruses transmitted by biting midges perhaps of greatest concern for sheep health in most countries.

5 Insect pests of swine

Pork is the most consumed animal protein worldwide and accounts for 35% of the world's meat intake (FAO, 2016b). China is the world's leading pork producer, which over 50 million metric tons produced in 2016; this is followed by the European Union (> 23 million MT) and the United States (> 11 million MT). Over 780 million pigs were stocked for consumption in 2016, 68 million in the United States alone (USDA, 2017). Most swine are housed indoors, with modern confinement facilities in Europe and the U.S. housing a high density of swine within environmentally controlled facilities (Plain & Lawrence, 2003). However, pasture-based swine production has increased recently in response to animal welfare interests (e.g., Edwards, 2005; Honeyman et al., 2006).

5.1 Permanent ectoparasites

The hog louse (*Haematopinus suis*) is a large (ca. 6 mm) blood-feeding louse specific to pigs. Eggs are glued to hair near the skin and typically require 2-3 weeks to hatch (Williams, 1985). Lice are typically found on pigs in the area around the tail and upper inside of the legs. Blood-feeding causes irritation, which can indirectly lead to hair loss and skin damage as animals rub against objects to alleviate itching. Hog lice are also recognized as important vectors of the swine pox virus, though this virus can also be transmitted

10

by direct contact among pigs. Lice do not survive more than a few days off host and are more noticeable during the winter months.

Like many other animals, swine may get sarcoptic mange caused by the mite *Sarcoptes scabiei*. In pigs, mange usually appears first around the head but can occur anywhere. Damage to swine due to the irritating bites of lice and mites and the management of these pests is similar to that described for lice and mites of cattle.

5.2 Ticks and fleas

Like cattle or sheep, swine with access to pasture may become hosts for many of the 3-host ticks commonly encountered in the pasture environment. Also like cattle and sheep, swine can host the spinose ear tick (*Otobius megnini*), a soft tick that may be found feeding in the ear canal of pigs. Soft ticks in the genus *Ornithodoros* are known to vector African swine fever virus (Kleiboeker & Scoles, 2001), an often fatal viral disease among pigs. While African swine fever virus is not currently in the U.S. or Europe, an outbreak of this virus on the eastern edge of Europe that started in 2013 is threatening to expand into Eastern Europe, perhaps distributed by infected wild boars (FAO, 2017). In the past, African swine fever virus was also transmitted to pigs by soft ticks endemic in the Caribbean and in Brazil. Should this virus spread to the main pig raising regions of Europe or North America, soft ticks in both regions are capable of transmitting the virus.

Swine may also become infested with several species of fleas, including the cat flea (*Ctenocephalides felis*), the dog flea (*C. canis*), and the human flea (*Pulex irritans*). Adult fleas take blood meals from the host. Larvae develop and feed on organic material near vertebrate hosts. Adult fleas are dark brown and may be spotted periodically feeding on pig bodies; larvae are too small to easily find in the environment. Flea bites are quite irritating to swine who will scratch continuously in response to the bites.

Fleas that attack swine will also attack their handlers as well. Observation of fleas or flea bites on handlers is often the first indication of a flea problem in a swine facility. Fleas are controlled by removal of animal bedding and application of insecticides to the floor, lower walls, and other structures in the swine facility before replacement of bedding. Insecticides may be applied directly to pigs as well for immediate control of fleas on the animals.

5.3 Flies and mosquitoes

House flies (*Musca domestica*) and stable flies (*Stomoxys calcitrans*) can develop in and around swine facilities where manure and other organic material accumulate and are left relatively undisturbed. To address animal welfare concerns, swine producers often add enrichment devices to swine pens. Enrichment devices can range from balls to teeter-totter type structures with devices fixed to the ground. Faeces can accumulate beneath and around such devices creating additional challenges for sanitation of swine pens. House flies are mechanical vectors of *Salmonella* and classical swine fever virus, and there is evidence that they may also be involved in the transmission of porcine reproductive and respiratory virus (PRRSV) in swine facilities (Otake et al., 2003).

Monitoring of flies is described in the cattle section above. Fly control in swine facilities is achieved primarily through sanitation measures aimed at interrupting fly development in swine faeces and bedding. All bedding and accumulated faeces should be removed and pens cleaned each week, or twice per week if weekly cleanouts are insufficient to achieve the desired level of control. Immediate control of adult flies can be achieved by using long-lasting insecticides applied by sprayer to facility walls and structures.

Mosquitoes are typically produced in waste water lagoons or other bodies of standing water, though some pestiferous mosquito species can develop in small, temporary water sources such as pails or other objects that can fill with rainwater. At least one mosquito species (*Aedes vexans*) has been shown to vector PRRSV (Otake

10

et al., 2002). Mosquitoes are controlled by eliminating aquatic development sites or by treatment of sites with insecticides, oils, or bacteria that kill some strains of mosquitoes.

5.4 Biosecurity for swine pests

Limiting the movement of animals and humans among groups of swine will help to prevent the direct spread of permanent ectoparasites. Proper manure management can limit house fly and stable fly development. Developmental sites for fleas or soft ticks near animals should be eliminated or treated. Tick prevention will be more difficult if swine are on pasture. Measures for pastured swine would reflect biosecurity for pastured cattle (above).

6 Insect pests of horses

Worldwide horses and other equines are kept for recreation, sport, and as work animals. Indirect economic impact of the equine industry is over $100 billion in both the United States and in Europe, with horse riding in Europe reported to be increasing by 5% each year (FEI Sports Forum, 2013). While horses are still used in some parts of the world as work animals for farming or herding, in many countries they are predominantly used for recreation and competitive sport. Horse meat is consumed in some countries, but is generally unavailable or even taboo, especially in many English-speaking countries where horses are considered more as pets than food animals. Horses are perhaps the most exported animal worldwide, for example accounting for 57% of all U.S. live livestock exports (including cattle, poultry, swine, sheep, and goats; USDA, 2015). The United State is the world leader in horse population followed by Mexico, China, Brazil, and Argentina (FAOSTAT, 2017). There is also an exceptionally active international equine sporting industry with worldwide horse movement to attend international competitions. Horse travel has increased the risk of movement of horse pathogens from endemic areas to non-endemic areas.

6.1 Permanent ectoparasites

Horses host two lice species; the horse biting louse (*Bovicola equi*) and the horse sucking louse (*Haematopinus asini*). Eggs of the horse biting louse are laid on fine hairs of the neck and flank of animals, but can spread to the entire body. Adult biting lice are 1-2 mm in length. Horse sucking lice prefer coarse hair and are found on the mane, base of the tail, and above hooves. Adult sucking lice are 2-3 mm in length. Lice can be spread by direct contact or by contaminated equipment or blankets. Lice infestations tend to be heaviest in winter months when longer coats offer better habitat. Horses can be infested with various species of scabies or mange mites and will exhibit similar scratching behaviour as cattle (see above).

Management of lice and mites on horses is similar to that described for cattle.

6.2 Ticks

Many of the ticks that negatively impact cattle will also infest horses. Ticks can transmit a suite of protozoan, viral, and bacterial pathogens to horses, including those that cause anaplasmosis, piroplasmosis, Lyme disease, tularemia, and Q-fever (Granström, 1997).

Management of ticks on horses is similar to that described for cattle.

6.3 Bot flies

The main species of bot fly that can affect horses are the common horse bot fly (*Gasterophilus intestinalis*), the throat bot fly (*G. nasalis*), and the nose bot fly (*G. haemorrhoidalis*). Eggs are laid onto the fur of horses and are ingested during grooming. First instar larvae attach to the mucosa of the mouth or gastrointestinal tract where they feed on tissue. This process takes several months,

10

and when larvae reach the 3rd instar they detach and are excreted. Bots will then pupate in soil or dried manure. Damage to the host occurs when the gastrointestinal lining becomes inflamed or 1st instar larvae burrow into the mouth lining. As for cattle, the presence of adult flies attempting to lay eggs can panic horses leading to horse self-injury.

6.4 Flies and mosquitoes

Horses are affected by many of the same fly species that impact cattle, including the stable fly, horn fly, face fly and house fly. While horse faeces is typically less productive for flies relative to cattle faeces, both stable fly and house fly can be produced in large numbers when horse faeces and urine is mixed with straw bedding for stabled horses. Horn flies and stable flies will bite horses and stable flies in particular have painful bites. Horn flies prefer bovine hosts, but will feed on horses and cause irritation to animals despite not reaching high populations on them (Fig. 10.8). Face flies feed on eye secretions and annoy animals. They are also vectors of eye worms (*Thelazia* spp.) House flies do not directly affect horses, but may be a nuisance to animals, workers, and neighbours. House flies are also vectors of numerous pathogens and parasites of animal health importance, including roundworms of horses (*Habronema microstoma*).

Fig. 10.8: Horn flies blood-feeding on a horse. While cattle are the preferred host, horses in proximity to cattle may be also be attacked.

▼

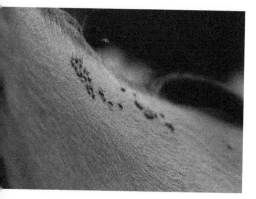

Mosquitoes develop in aquatic environments in and around horse facilities. Mosquitoes are vectors of several important viruses of horses, including eastern equine encephalitis (EEEV), western equine encephalitis (WEEV), West Nile virus (WNV), St. Louis encephalitis (SLEV), and Venezuelan equine encephalitis (VEEV). These viruses can cause significant disease in horses, with mortality as high as 90% for EEEV (Knapp, 1985). A vaccine is available to protect horses against WNV, and should be considered for horses in geographic regions where this virus is actively transmitted.

Other flies that negatively affect horses and develop in aquatic or semi-aquatic habitats include black flies (Family: Simuliidae), biting midges (*Culicoides* spp.), and horse flies (Family: Tabanidae). The adults of both black flies and biting midges are small (≤ 15 mm) but in large numbers they can severely depress animals due to their painful and irritating bites. Biting by these flies can also result in pronounced itching and tissue irritation as a result of host allergic reaction to salivary compounds injected into the bite wound by these flies (Knapp, 1985). Biting midges are also of concern as vectors of African horse sickness virus (AHSV), a severe disease of horses which is currently limited to sub-Saharan Africa but has the potential to spread to other geographic regions. Horse flies are large (10-30 mm) blood-feeding flies that will readily attack horses. Horse flies have painful bites that can cause horses to display defensive behavior including panicked running which may cause horse self-injury. Horse flies are vectors of equine infectious anaemia and trypanosomes (Knapp, 1985).

Monitoring for flies and management of flies and mosquitoes is described in the cattle and swine sections above.

10

6.5 Biosecurity for horse facilities

Horse facilities present a unique challenge in terms of biosecurity because of their inherent purpose. Rather than being kept for livestock or as work animals, most horses are kept for recreation, meaning that limiting contact among animals or between humans and animals is not feasible. It may be much more important, therefore, to monitor for insect pests on animals more closely, especially those that could spread to uninfested animals by direct contact (e.g., lice and mites) and to keep horse stalls clean to prevent insect breeding. Guidelines outlined for pastured cattle (above) also apply to horses kept on pasture

7 Insect pests of poultry

Poultry is one of the most important sources of protein found around the world (Vaarst et al., 2015). Commercial poultry raised for food include chickens or related birds that lay eggs and birds raised for meat. Worldwide, poultry meat production is increasing with worldwide consumption expected to increase 19% by 2025 (Conway, 2016a). An estimated 110 million metric tons of poultry meat were produced worldwide in 2016 with the United States as the world leader followed by China, Brazil, and the European Union. China is the leading producer of eggs at 30 million metric tons in 2015, followed by the United States (5.8 million MT), India (4.4 million MT) and Mexico (2.6 million MT) (Conway, 2016b). A variety of insect and arthropod pests and ectoparasites can negatively impact commercial birds. Egg-laying chickens (layers) are generally raised for longer periods of time than chickens for meat (broilers), which can influence the type and severity of insect pests. Additionally, poultry housing can influence the prevalence and severity of poultry pests (reviewed in Mullens & Murillo, 2017). As animal welfare concerns influence poultry housing (e.g., cage-free eggs) arthropod pest complexes will be affected.

7.1 Permanent ectoparasites

There are several species of lice and mites that infest chickens and other poultry as permanent ectoparasites. Common species include, the chicken body louse (*Menacanthus stramineus*), the shaft louse (*Menopon gallinae*), the northern fowl mite (*Ornithonyssus sylviarum*) and the scaly leg mite (*Knemidocoptes mutans*) (McCrea et al., 2005). Lice are generally host-specific, able to feed on a single host species or very closely related host species. In contrast, poultry mites can often feed on a range of avian hosts (Baker et al., 1956). With a rapid life cycle and high reproductive rate, both lice and mites can reach high numbers on layers, which have a productive life of 1-3 years. However, broilers rarely have high infestations of lice or on-host dwelling mites due to their limited lifespan (6-14 weeks).

Louse nymphs and adults feed on feathers and sometimes blood of poultry, causing irritation to birds (Fig.10.9). Eggs are laid singly or in clumps in bird feathers, and the location of the life stages will vary by louse species. Lice can only survive for short periods of time off-host. For example, chicken body louse adults can survive off-host for only up to 2-3 days in favourable conditions (Chen & Mullens, 2008).

The northern fowl mite is the most common mite that lives on poultry (Fig. 10.10). It is primarily found in the vent region of birds due to a favourable microclimate in this location. Eggs are laid in these feathers, and protonymphs and adult mites blood feed in this area. Mite blood feeding results in irritation to birds and can result in decreased egg production. These mites are not important vectors of disease. Adult northern fowl mites can survive nearly a month off-host when temperatures are cooler (<33 °C) and relative humidity is high (85%) (Chen & Mullens, 2008). The northern fowl mite can feed on a range of poultry and wild bird hosts making it difficult to prevent introduction of these mites into a new poultry flock (Knee & Proctor, 2007). The scaly leg mite looks similar to scabies and lives in the skin under foot and leg scales where they can cause irritation, inflammation, and in severe cases, foot deformation or lameness.

Monitoring for lice or mites that live on-host will rely on direct inspection of animals periodically. Lice may be found all over the body, but mites will be primarily in the vent area (Axtell & Arends, 1990). The presence of mites on eggs is also an indicator of high mite populations and has been used as a threshold for treatment, though ideally treatment would occur before mite populations reach such levels (Mullens et al., 2000).

Control of permanent ectoparasites has traditionally relied on insecticidal sprays applied directly

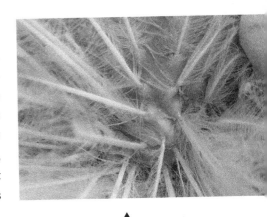

▲
Fig. 10.9: Chicken body lice (*Menacanthus stramineus*) on a chicken (dark brown near the base of the feather). Several species of chewing lice infest poultry. Most are feather-feeding, but *Menacnathus* spp. also sometimes feed on blood.

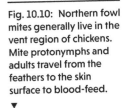

10

Fig. 10.10: Northern fowl mites generally live in the vent region of chickens. Mite protonymphs and adults travel from the feathers to the skin surface to blood-feed.
▼

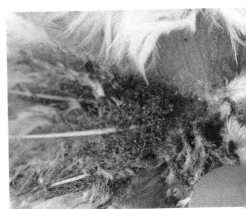

to the birds (Axtell & Arends, 1990). These chemicals must be sprayed at high pressures to penetrate the feather layer to reach where the ectoparasites live. Chemical resistance, increasing organic production, and the shift from caged to cage-free birds has limited the use and effectiveness of insecticides in recent years (Mullens & Murillo, 2017; Mullens et al., 2017b). Alternatives to traditional insecticides include the use of inorganic dusts such as kaolin clay or diatomaceous earth in dustboxes (Martin & Mullens, 2012) or the application of sulphur dust directly to birds or by dustboxes or bags (Martin & Mullens, 2012; Murillo & Mullens, 2016).

7.2 Nest parasites

Some ectoparasites require poultry blood for development and reproduction, but spend most of their time living off their poultry host in the nest area ('temporary ectoparasites'). Common temporary ectoparasites of poultry include the bed bug (*Cimex lectularius*), poultry red mite (*Dermanyssus gallinae*), sticktight flea (*Echidnophaga gallinacea*), and several soft ticks (*Argas* spp.). These temporary ectoparasites can be problematic for both layers and broilers as long as suitable off-host harbourage is available.

Fig. 10.11: Adult sticktight fleas (*Echidnophaga gallinacea*) attach to the host to blood-feed. They prefer to attach to combs, wattles, and areas around the eyes (shown).

▼

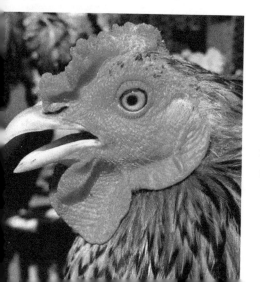

The eggs of bed bugs, poultry red mites, and soft ticks are laid in protected cracks and crevices near poultry, such as in nest boxes. Other life stages of these ectoparasites also live within cracks and crevices and other harbourage locations near birds, emerging at night to blood feed on nearby birds. Bed bugs can take 1-4 months to develop from egg to adult depending on environmental conditions, and they survive for weeks to months without feeding. Bed bugs cause irritation by feeding but have not been found to vector poultry disease (Krinsky, 2009). Poultry red mites can develop from egg to adult in as little as 10 days (Maurer & Baumgärtner, 1992). Red mites have been implicated as vectors of numerous poultry pathogens including bacteria and viruses (Moro et al., 2005). Soft ticks can transmit spirochetes and cause tick paralysis (Proctor & Owens, 2000).

Sticktight flea adults blood feed by attaching to hosts on the head or face area for extended periods of time (Fig. 10.11) (Axtell, 1985). Sticktight flea adults lay eggs without detaching from birds. Eggs fall to the litter, where immatures develop on organic material and adult flea faeces. Sticktight fleas have not been implicated in disease transmission.

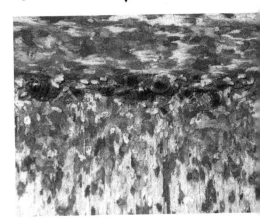

Fig. 10.12: Bed bugs (eggs, immatures, and adults) in a wooden nest box on a commercial poultry facility. The dark spots are caused by bed bug defecation of digested blood and can be indicative of an infestation. ▼

Monitoring for off-host dwelling ectoparasites should target likely harbourage near animals. Nest boxes should be examined periodically for various life stages of ectoparasites, including eggs, or signs of ectoparasites such as blood-faecal spots (Fig. 10.12). Traps made from corrugated cardboard create harbourage for ectoparasites and can be used for monitoring presence and relative abundance. The combs of birds should be examined directly for the presence of sticktight fleas.

While it can be difficult to locate the often numerous harbourage sites of these temporary ectoparasites, application of insecticide or acaricide sprays to these harbourages near birds can provide control. Sprays must be thorough for effective control. Dusts or silica gels or entomopathogenic fungi can likewise be applied directly to cracks and crevices, though environmental conditions may affect their efficacy.

7.3 Insects that develop in poultry faeces and litter

Insects that develop in poultry faeces and poultry litter include the lesser mealworm (*Alphitobius diaperinus*) and several species of flies, notably the house fly and the little house fly (*Fannia canicularis*). Lesser mealworm immatures require months to develop, then burrow into soft wood or poultry housing insulation to pupate

(Axtell, 1985). Besides causing structural damage, beetles are also reservoirs and vectors of numerous poultry diseases. They can also be nuisance pests of humans if large numbers of these beetles are removed from poultry houses with manure cleanout, leaving the adult beetles to disperse into the surrounding area. House flies and little house flies develop in nutrient-rich moist environments that include poultry litter, manure, and spilled feed.

House flies can develop from egg to adult in as little as 7-10 days. Little house flies, in contrast, require 20-30 days to develop from egg to adult (Axtell, 1985). Adult flies can mechanically transfer pathogens, though flies are primarily nuisance pests of humans.

Various traps can be used to monitor for immature and adult beetles (Axtell & Arends, 1990). Tube traps can be constructed out of short (ca. 15 cm) pieces of PVC pipe filled with corrugated cardboard. These traps should be placed along the poultry house perimeter and checked weekly to track relative beetle abundance. Fly monitoring and control as described for cattle (above) apply here. In poultry housing, moist manure or litter should be inspected directly for the presence of developing beetles and fly larvae, which may then be targeted for control.

Control of these pests is best achieved by sanitation efforts applied to poultry manure and litter. Moist areas, such as under leaking water lines, may be hot spots of development. Every effort should be made to dry manure quickly, which will make it unsuitable for fly development. In addition, insecticides or insect growth regulators (prevent insects from maturing to adults) may be applied to manure or other immature development habitat where these pests are noted. Control of adult flies includes insecticidal spray to resting areas, granular fly baits, or fly traps, though this should be secondary to reducing immature development sites.

7.4 Biosecurity for poultry pests

Biosecurity can impact how insect pests get into poultry flocks, how insects and disease are spread among flocks, and the dispersal of insect pests from commercial poultry facilities to nearby properties. Permanent and temporary pests can be limited or prevented entirely with good biosecurity because they are so dependent on poultry hosts for survival. Excluding wild birds and their nests and excluding or limiting rodent activity can limit introduction and spread of mites and lice. Humans may act as incidental carriers of poultry ectoparasites and move them from infested to uninfested flocks. Cleaning boots and equipment in between flocks can limit the spread of insects. Limiting movement between poultry houses will also reduce the risk of spreading ectoparasites.

Lice and northern fowl mites do not infest humans, but poultry red mites may feed on people causing irritation. The bed bug species that feeds on humans can also infest poultry flocks, though the importance of humans to introducing bed bugs to poultry facilities is unknown.

Insects that develop in poultry manure are not as dependent on the presence of poultry, and the way in which manure is stored or managed is much more important for their survival during the time between flocks. Manure and litter can be composted or treated with insect growth regulators or insecticides to limit the spread of nuisance pests and potential vectors. Flies in particular may be able to transmit pathogens to or from poultry facilities. House flies and little house flies can potentially mechanically transmit exotic Newcastle disease, and the vector potential for avian influenza is currently unknown.

10

8 Conclusion

Biosecurity measures employed to protect animal health must include control of insects, mites, and ticks that negatively impact animals by direct feeding damage or as vectors of animal pathogens. Control of these pests should follow the general principles and practices of an integrated pest management (IPM) programme, including pest monitoring and focusing on proactive measures to limit pest production.

Insect biosecurity is best achieved by (1) reducing fly abundance through appropriate sanitation practices to limit fly development habitat, (2) quarantining and treating animals infested with lice or mites to prevent direct transfer of these pests to other animals, (3) separating farm animals from wild animals that may carry and transfer lice, mites, and ticks, (4) monitoring pest abundance and activity regularly to identify new pest introductions and to determine whether pests are nearing damaging levels, and (5) training facility employees to avoid accidental transfer of ectoparasites from infested facilities to non-infested facilities.

The pests that need to be monitored and managed will depend upon the production animal, the operational characteristics of the facility (e.g., pasture-based or confinement), the geographic region where animals are located, the season, and the presence or absence of pathogens within the region. As discussed in the sections above, pests of importance often differ among the different species of vertebrate hosts, so monitoring efforts should focus on relevant pests for each animal commodity.

References

Ahmad, A., Nagaraja, T.G., and Zurek, L. (2007). Transmission of *Escherichia coli* O157: H7 to cattle by house flies. *Preventive Veterinary Medicine* 8, 74-81.

Alexander, J.L. (2006). Screwworms. *Journal of American Veterinary Medical Association* 3, 357-367.

Axtell, R.C. (1985). Arthropod pests of poultry. In: Williams, R.E., Hall, R.D., Broce, A.B., Scholl, P.J. (Eds.) *Livestock Entomology*, pp. 269-295. Wiley-Interscience Publication.

Axtell, R.C., and Arends, J.J. (1990). Ecology and management of arthropod pests of poultry. *Annual Review of Entomology* 35, 101-126.

Baker, E.W., Evans, T.M., Gould, D.J., Hull, W.B., & Keegan, H.L. (1956). *A manual of parasitic mites of medical or economic importance*. National Pest Control Association.

Boland, H.T., Scaglia, G., and Umemura, K. (2008). Impact of horn flies, *Haematobia irritans* (L.) (Diptera: Muscidae), on the behavior of beef steers. *The Professional Animal Scientist* 24, 656-660.

Bruinsma, J. ed. (2003). *World Agriculture: Towards 2015/2030 An FAO Perspective*.

Campbell, J.B. (1985). Arthropod pests of confined beef. In: Williams, R.E., Hall, R.D., Broce, A.B., Scholl, P.J. (Eds.) *Livestock Entomology*, pp. 207-221. Wiley-Interscience Publication.

Carroll, J.F., Hill, D.E., Allen, P.C., Young, K.W., Miramontes, E., Kramer, M., Pound, J.M., Miller, J.A., and George, J.E. (2009). The impact of 4-poster deer self-treatment devices at three locations in Maryland. *Vector-Borne and Zoonotic Diseases* 9, 407-416.

Chen, B.L., and Mullens, B.A. (2008). Temperature and humidity effects on off-host survival of the northern fowl mite (Acari: Macronyssidae) and the chicken body louse (Phthiraptera: Menoponidae). *Journal of Economic Entomology* 101, 637-646.

Chen, Y., Why, A., Batista, G., Mafra-Neto, A., and Keogh, E. (2014). Flying insect classification with inexpensive sensors. *Journal of Insect Behavior* 27, 657-677.

Cohnstaedt, L.W., Rochon, K., Duehl, A.J., Anderson, J.F., Barrera, R., Su, N.Y., Gerry, A.C., Obenauer, P.J., Campbell, J.F., Lysyk, T.J., and Allan, S.A. (2012). Arthropod surveillance programs: basic components, strategies and analysis. *Annals of the Entomological Society of America* 105, 135-149.

Conway, A. (2016a). Poultry makes up most meat production growth by 2025. *Poultry Trends 2016*. 24-30.

Conway, A. (2016b). Egg Production breaks record 70-million-metric-ton mark in 2015. *Poultry Trends 2016*. 32-38.

Cupp, E.W., Cupp, M.S., Ribeiro, J.M., and Kunz, S.E. (1998). Blood-feeding strategy of *Haematobia irritans* (Diptera: Muscidae). *Journal of Medical Entomology* 35, 591-595.

Edwards, S.A. (2005). Product quality attributes associated with outdoor pig production. *Livestock Production Science* 94, 5-14.

FAO. (2016a). Meat & meat products. Accessed September 18, 2017. http://www.fao.org/ag/againfo/themes/en/meat/home.html

FAO. (2016b). Animal production and health – Pigs. Accessed September 11, 2017. http://www.fao.org/ag/againfo/themes/en/pigs/home.html

FAO. (2017). EMPRESTADs African swine fever. Accessed September 18, 2017. http://www.fao.org/ag/againfo/programmes/en/empres/disease_asf.asp

FAOSTAT Database. (2017). Food and Agriculture Organization of the United Nations. Accessed September 2017. http://faostat3.fao.org/home/E

FEI Sports Forum (2013). Fédération Equestre Internationale. Accessed September 13, 2017. https://inside.fei.org/system/files/1_Trends_in_Growth_of_Equestrian_Sport_GCO.pdf

Ferguson, H.J., Gerry, A.C., Talley, J.L., and Smythe, B. (2015). VetPestX: Finally! An online, searchable, pesticide label database just for pests of animals. *Journal of Extension* 53, 3TOT7.

Foil, L.D., and Hogsette, J.A. (1994). Biology and control of tabanids, stable flies and horn flies. *Revue scientifique et technique (International Office of Epizootics)* 13, 1125-1158.

Gerry, A.C., Mullens, B.A., MacLachlan, N.J., and Mecham, J.O. (2001). Seasonal transmission of bluetongue virus by *Culicoides sonorensis* (Diptera: Ceratopogonidae) at a southern California dairy and evaluation of vectorial capacity as a predictor of bluetongue virus transmission. *Journal of Medical Entomology* 38, 197-209.

Gerry, A.C., Peterson, N.G., and Mullens, B.A. (2007). Predicting and controlling stable flies on California dairies. *UC ANR Publication* 8258.

Gerry, A.C., Monteys, V.S.I., Vidal, J.O.M., Francino, O., and Mullens, B.A. (2009). Biting rates of *Culicoides* midges (Diptera: Ceratopogonidae) on sheep in northeastern Spain in relation to midge capture using UV light and carbon dioxide-baited traps. *Journal of Medical Entomology* 46, 615-624.

Gerry, A.C., Higginbotham, G.E., Periera, L.N., Lam, A. and Shelton, C.R. (2011). Evaluation of surveillance methods for monitoring house fly abundance and activity on large commercial dairy operations. *Journal of Economic Entomology* 104, 1093-1102.

Gerry, A.C. *In press.* Cattle ectoparasites in extensive and intensive cattle systems. In: T. Engle, D. Klingborg, and B. Rollin (eds). *Cattle Welfare in North America* CRC Press/Taylor & Francis.

Granström, M. (1997). Tick-borne zoonoses in Europe. *Clinical Microbiology and Infection* 3, 156-169.

Griffioen, K., Van Gemst, D.B., Pieterse, M.C., Jacobs, F., and van Oldruitenborgh-Oosterbaan, M.M.S. (2011). *Culicoides* species associated with sheep in the Netherlands and the effect of a permethrin insecticide. *The Veterinary Journal* 190, 230-235.

Honeyman M.S., Pirog, R.S., Huber, G.H., Lammers, P.J., and Hermann, J.R. (2006). The United States pork niche market phenomenon. *Journal of Animal Science.* 84, 2269-2275.

Jones, K.G. (2004). Trends in the US sheep industry. *USDA Economic Research Service Bulletin* 787.

Keiding, J. (1999). Review of the global status and recent development of insecticide resistance in field populations of the housefly, *Musca domestica* (Diptera: Muscidae). *Bulletin of Entomological Research* 89, 1-67.

Kleiboeker, S.B., and Scoles, G.A. (2001). Pathogenesis of African swine fever virus in *Ornithodoros* ticks. *Animal Health Research Reviews* 2, 121-128.

Knapp, F.W. (1985). Arthropod pests of horses. In: Williams, R.E., Hall, R.D., Broce, A.B., Scholl, P.J. (Eds.) *Livestock Entomology*, pp. 297-313. Wiley-Interscience Publication.

Knee, W., and Proctor, H. (2007). Host records for *Ornithonyssus sylviarum* (Mesostigmata: Macronyssidae) from birds of North America (Canada, United States, and Mexico). *Journal of Medical Entomology* 44, 709-713.

Krinsky, W.L. (2009). True bugs (Hemiptera). In: Mullen, G.R., Durden, L.A. (Eds.) *Medical and Veterinary Entomology*, pp. 83-99 second ed. Oxford: Academic Press.

Lysyk, T.J. (1995). Temperature and population density effects on feeding activity of *Stomoxys calcitrans* (Diptera: Muscidae) on cattle. *Journal of Medical Entomology* 32, 508-514.

Lysyk, T.J. (2000). Comparison of sample units for estimating population abundance and rates of change of adult horn fly (Diptera: Muscidae). *Journal of Medical Entomology*. 37, 299-307.

Martin, C.D., Mullens, B.A. (2012). Housing and dustbathing effects on northern fowl mites (*Ornithonyssus sylviarum*) and chicken body lice (*Menacanthus stramineus*) on hens. *Journal of Medical and Veterinary Entomology* 26, 323-333.

Maurer, V., and Baumgärtner, J. (1992). Temperature influence on life table statistics of the chicken mite *Dermanyssus gallinae* (Acari: Dermanyssidae). *Experimental and Applied Acarology* 15, 27-40.

Mayo, C., Courtney, S., MacLachlan, N.J., Gardner, I., Hartley, D., and Barker, C. (2016). A deterministic model to quantify risk and guide mitigation strategies to reduce bluetongue virus transmission in California dairy cattle. *PloS One* 11, e0165806.

McCrea, B., Jeffrey, J.S., Ernst, R.A., and Gerry, A.C. (2005). Common lice and mites of poultry: identification and treatment. *UC ANR Publications* 8162.

Meiswinkel, R., Baylis, M., and Labuschagne, K. (2000). Stabling and the protection of horses from *Culicoides bolitinos* (Diptera: Ceratopogonidae), a recently identified vector of African horse sickness. *Bulletin of Entomological Research* 90, 509-515.

Mellor, P.S., Boorman, J., and Baylis, M. (2000). *Culicoides* biting midges: their role as arbovirus vectors. *Annual Review of Entomology* 45, 307-340.

Moro, C.V., Chauve, C., and Zenner, L. (2005). Vectorial role of some dermanyssoid mites (Acari, Mesostigmata, Dermanyssoidea). *Parasite* 12, 99-109.

Mullens, B.A., Hinkle, N.C., and Szijj, C.E. (2000). Monitoring northern fowl mites (Acari: Macronyssidae) in caged laying hens: feasibility of an egg-based sampling system. *Journal of Economic Entomology* 93, 1045-1054.

Mullens, B.A., Gerry, A.C., and Velten, R.K. (2001). Failure of a permethrin treatment regime to protect cattle against bluetongue virus. *Journal of Medical Entomology* 38, 760-762.

Mullens, B.A., Lii, K., Mao, Y., Meyer, J.A., Peterson, N.G., and Szijj, C.E. (2006). Behavioural responses of dairy cattle to *Stomoxys calcitrans* in an open field environment. *Medical and Veterinary Entomology* 20, 122-137.

Mullens, B.A., Gerry, A.C., Monteys, V.S.I., Pinna, M., and Gonzalez, A. (2010). Field studies on *Culicoides* (Diptera: Ceratopogonidae) activity and response to deltamethrin applications to sheep in northeastern Spain. *Journal of Medical Entomology* 47, 106-110.

Mullens, B.A., McDermott, E.G., and Gerry, A.C. (2015). Progress and knowledge gaps in *Culicoides* ecology and control. *Veterinaria Italiana* 21, 313-323.

Mullens, B., and Murillo, A. (2017). Parasites in laying hen systems. In: P. Hester (Ed.) *Egg Production: Innovations and Strategies for Improvement*, pp. 597-606. Oxford: Academic Press.

Mullens, B.A., Watson, D.W., Gerry, A.C., Sandelin, B.A., Soto, D., Rawls, D., Denning, S., Guisewite, L., and Cammack, J. (2017a). Field trials of fatty acids and geraniol applied to cattle for suppression of horn flies, *Haematobia irritans* (Diptera: Muscidae), with observations on fly defensive behaviours. *Veterinary Parasitology* 245, 14-28.

10

Mullens, B., Murillo, A., Zoller, H., Heckeroth, A., Jirjis, F., and Flochlay-Sigognault, A. (2017b). Comparative in vitro evaluation of contact activity of fluralaner, spinosad, phoxim, propoxur, permethrin, and deltamethrin against the northern fowl mite, *Ornithonyssus sylviarum*. *Parasites & Vectors* 10, 358.

Murillo, A.C., and Mullens, B.A. (2016). Sulfur dust bag: a novel technique for ectoparasite control in poultry systems. *Journal of Economic Entomology* 109, 2229-2233.

Nayduch, D., and Burrus, R.G. (2017). Flourishing in filth: house fly–microbe interactions across life history. *Annals of the Entomological Society of America* 110, 6-18.

Otake, S., Dee, S.A., Rossow, K.D., Moon, R.D., and Pijoan, C. (2002). Mechanical transmission of porcine reproductive and respiratory syndrome virus by mosquitoes, *Aedes vexans* (Meigen). *Canadian Journal of Veterinary Research* 66, 191.

Otake, S., Dee, S.A., Rossow, K.D., Moon, R.D., Trincado, C., and Pijoan, C. (2003). Transmission of porcine reproductive and respiratory syndrome virus by houseflies (*Musca domestica*). *The Veterinary Record* 152, 73-76.

Pérez de León, A.A., Teel, P.D., Auclair, A.N., Messenger, M.T., Guerrero, F.D., Schuster, G., and Miller, R.J. (2012). Integrated strategy for sustainable cattle fever tick eradication in USA is required to mitigate the impact of global change. *Frontiers in Physiology* 3, 195.

Plain, R.L., and Lawrence, J.D. (2003). Swine production. *Veterinary Clinics of North America: Food Animal Practices* 19, 319-337.

Proctor, H., and Owens, I. (2000). Mites and birds: diversity, parasitism and coevolution. *Trends in Ecology & Evolution* 15, 358-364.

Rasmussen, L., Kristensen, B., Kirkeby, C., Rasmussen, T., Belsham, G. J., Bødker, R., and Bøtner, A. (2012). Culicoids as vectors of Schmallenberg virus. *Emerging Infectious Diseases*, 18, 1204-1206.

Reisen, W.K. (2009). Epidemiology of vector-borne diseases In: Mullen, G.R., Durden, L.A. (Eds.) *Medical and Veterinary Entomology*, 2nd Ed. Elsevier.

Samways, M.J. (2005). *Insect Diversity Conservation*. Cambridge University Press.

Shiflett, J.S. (2017). Sheep Industry Economic Impact Analysis – 2017. Accessed September 18, 2017. https://d1cqrq366w3ike.cloudfront.net/http/DOCUMENT/SheepUSA/Sheep%20Industry%20Impact%20Analysis%208-10-17%20with%20Logo.pdf

Showler, A.T. (2017). Botanically based repellent and insecticidal effects against horn flies and stable flies (Diptera: Muscidae). *Journal of Integrated Pest Management* 8, 1-11, https://doi.org/10.1093/jipm/pmx010.

Spickler, A.R. (2009). Sheep scab. Accessed September 18, 2017. http://www.cfsph.iastate.edu/Factsheets/pdfs/psoroptes_ovis.pdf

Talley, J.L., Wayadande, A.C., Wasala, L.P., Gerry, A.C., Fletcher, J., DeSilva, U., and Gilliland, S.E. (2009). Association of *Escherichia coli* O157: H7 with filth flies (Muscidae and Calliphoridae) captured in leafy greens fields and experimental transmission of *E. coli* O157: H7 to spinach leaves by house flies (Diptera: Muscidae). *Journal of Food Protection*, 72, 1547-1552.

USDA. (2015). Equine 2015: Changes in the U.S. Equine Industry 1998-2015. *USDA APHIS Veterinary Services National Animal Health Monitoring Systems* Report 2, 1-85.

USDA. (2017). Livestock and Poultry: World Markets Trade. *USDA Foreign Agricultural Service*

Vaarst, M., Steenfeldt, S., and Horsted, K. (2015). Sustainable development perspectives in poultry production. *World's Poultry Science Journal*. 71, 609-620.

Wall, R. and Shearer, D. (1997). *Veterinary Entomology*. Chapman & Hall, London.

Wasala, L., Talley, J.L., DeSilva, U., Fletcher, J., and Wayadande, A. (2013). Transfer of *Escherichia coli* O157: H7 to spinach by house flies, *Musca domestica* (Diptera: Muscidae). *Phytopathology* 103, 373-380.

Williams, R.W. (1985). Arthropod pests of swine. In: Williams, R.E., Hall, R.D., Broce, A.B., Scholl, P.J. (Eds.) *Livestock Entomology*, pp. 239-251. Wiley-Interscience Publication.

Wright, R.E. (1985). Arthropod pests of beef cattle on pasture or range land. In: Williams, R.E., Hall, R.D., Broce, A.B., Scholl, P.J. (Eds.) *Livestock Entomology*, pp. 191-206. Wiley-Interscience Publication.

Photo credits

Alex Gerry: figures 10.1, 10.2, 10.4, 10.7, 10.8

Amy Murillo: figures 10.9, 10.10, 10.11

B.A. Mullens: figures 10.3, 10.5, 10.6

Cornell Vet Entomology: figure 10.12

10

CHAPTER 11

RODENT CONTROL IN ANIMAL PRODUCTION

Trees Loncke[1]

Jeroen Dewulf[2]

[1] Alphatac, 8940 Wervik, Belgium

[2] Faculty of Veterinary Medicine, Department of Obstetrics, Reproduction and Herd Health, Veterinary Epidemiology Unit, University of Ghent, 9820 Merelbeke, Belgium

1 Introduction

Animal production facilities are highly attractive to rodents as the conditions, such as an easily accessible abundance of food, plenty of shelter, and protection from variable and harsh climate conditions, are extremely beneficial to them. Unfortunately, the uncontrolled presence of rodents on farms can cause a lot of problems. First of all they are a potential source of infectious disease transmission acting as both a biological as well as mechanical vector (Amass and Baysinger, 2006). Rodents are recognised carriers of at least 35 diseases, including the major zoonoses such as campylobacteriosis, salmonellosis, and yersiniosis, pasteurellosis, leptospirosis, swine dysentery, trichinosis, toxoplasmosis Hepatitis E, EMC virus, PCV2 virus and rabies (Backhans and Fellstrom, 2012; Lapuz et al., 2008, 2012; Friedman et al., 2008; Pinheiro et al., 2013; CDC, 2017). Mice and rats can carry disease-causing organisms on their feet and fur thus increasing the spread of disease. Rodents may roam the countryside looking for new food sources when animal houses are emptied, and return when they are repopulated. As a consequence they may not only be responsible for the spread of infectious agents within the farm, but they may also transmit diseases between farms or re-contaminate incoming animals. In addition to transmitting diseases, rodents can also cause substantial damage to building infrastructures, by eating the casing of electric wires (Fig. 11.1) for instance and consequentially causing electric short circuit which can cause a fire hazard (Lang et al., 2013).

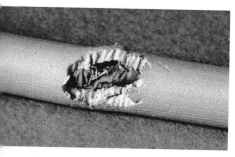

▲
Fig. 11.1: Wire that has been damaged by rats

They will also frequently damage insulation material as this is one of their preferred locations for nesting. The presence of rodents may also stress animals (pigs, birds, etc.). As most rodents are nocturnal, they are generally very active during the night and they may scare off the housed animals. And finally the rodents may also consume a substantial amount of animal feed and spoil the remainder of the feed. By way of example, 100 rats can eat up to

2 kilos of animal feed per day. When measured over one year, this results in a loss of up to 700 kilos of feed (Lang et al., 2013).

For all of these reasons it is highly advisable to try to keep rodents out of farms and animal housings as much as possible. If they are present, it is essential to control them and to try to eliminate them as quickly as possible.

2 Rodents and the reasons for their success

The rodents we encounter the most in animal facilities are rats and mice.

The black rat (*Rattus rattus*) (Fig. 11.2), also known as the ship rat, roof rat, house rat, is a common long-tailed rat. An adult black rat weighs between 150 and 250 grams, measures around 18 centimetres and has a long tail of around 22 cm. The black rat is a very good climber and very often lives in ceilings therefore. The black rat is very shy and hard to seduce with bait. They prefer to eat grains or fruit and do not like a meat diet. They require the presence of fresh water.

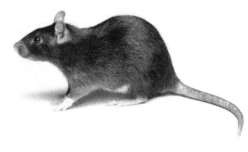

▲
Fig. 11.2: Black rat

The brown rat (Fig. 11.3), also referred to as common rat, street rat, sewer rat, Norwegian rat (*Rattus norvegicus*) is one of the best-known and most common rats. The brown rat is a little taller than the black rat and weighs between 150 and 500 grams. They often nest under surfaces. They are very good swimmers and eat just about anything they can find (including meat). They also dig burrows for instance in insulation material.

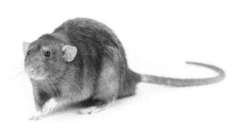

▲
Fig. 11.3: Brown rat

The mice encountered in stables are mainly house mice (*Mus musculus*) (Fig. 11.4). They are found in and around animal facilities. They generally search for warm locations and make their nests in warm, dry locations. They require very little drinking water. The house mouse eats around 3 grams of food a day and is omnivo-

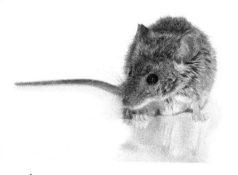

▲

Fig. 11.4: Mice

rous. They never eat large volumes at once but generally eat small amounts continuously.

Rats and mice have poor eyesight but an excellent sense of smell, taste, touch and hearing. They do not like open areas and prefer contact with walls and other objects. They do not range far from the nest. The range for rats is up to 45 metres and 9 metres for mice.

In addition to the reasons stated above (food, climate, shelter), there are several other reasons for the successful presence of rodents in stables. First of all they are relatively small which means they are able to hide in very small surfaces and to move through very narrow gaps. Secondly they are smart and flexible so that they are able to adapt easily to varying circumstances. They are also very athletic which allows them to move very fast, to climb walls, jump over obstacles and swim. And finally, and probably most importantly, they are highly reproductive. A female rat for instance starts to be reproductive from the age of 2-3 months (mice are reproductive from the age of 6-8 weeks) and they can produce around 6-8 litters a year, producing up to 10 young per litter. As a result, one female rat is capable of producing another 22 breeding females in one year (assuming a 50:50 male/female ratio of offspring), which mature within 3 months. In ideal conditions this means that a pair of rats and their offspring can produce 20,000,000 offspring in the space of three years. The size of the population in a stable will largely depend of course on the available hiding and nesting places (in ceilings, under feeding troughs, in wall cavities) and the availability of food and water.

3 Monitoring: how to identify a rodent problem?

Monitoring is an important step in preventing and/or controlling rodent populations. Traditional rodent control methods such as baiting and trapping can also be used as a monitoring tool. Thorough record-keeping of bait disappearance can warn farmers if

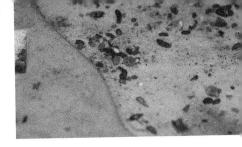

Fig. 11.5: Rat droppings

their rodent population is increasing. This is especially important in the autumn when rodents start to look for suitable wintering sites.

The following are signs of rodent infestation (Lang et al., 2013):

- Sounds: gnawing, climbing noises in walls, squeaking.
- Droppings: found along walls, behind ob-jects and near food supplies (Fig. 11.5).
- Burrows: rat burrows are indicated by fresh diggings along foundations, through floorboards into wall spaces (Fig. 11.6 and 11.7).
- Runs: look for dust-free areas along walls and behind storage material.
- Gnawing marks: look for wood chips around boards, bins and crates. Fresh gnawing marks will be pale in colour.
- Rodent odours: persistent musky odours are a positive sign of infestation.
- Visual sightings: daylight sightings of mice are common. Rats will only be visible in daylight if populations are high (Fig. 11.8). Enter your barn quietly at night, wait in silence for five minutes and listen for the sound of rodent activity. Look around with a powerful flashlight; rat eyes will reflect the light.
- Smudge marks: these may be found on pipes or rafters where dirt and oil from their fur leave a greasy film.

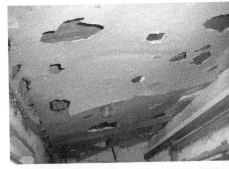

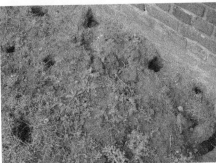

Fig. 11.6 & 11.7:
Rat burrows in ground or in roof insulation material

It is a generally accepted rule of thumb that there are approximately 25 mice or rats for every one that is visible. If rats and mice are seen during daylight hours, it may indicate a severe infestation, as the population and feeding pressure are so high that juveniles are forced to forage during the day.

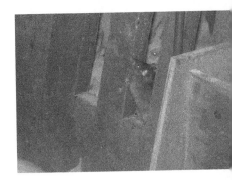

Fig. 11.8: Rat observed during day time herd visit

4 How to control rodents

A good rodent control plan will always consist of at least two components: control outside the animal houses to prevent the rodents from entering the animal facilities and control inside the stables to control the rodents that have entered the buildings.

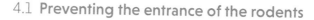

Fig. 11.9: Rodent proof exterior where rats and mice have no places to shelter ▼

4.1 Preventing the entrance of the rodents

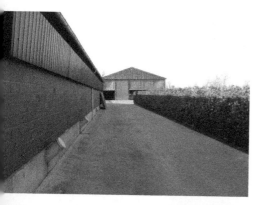

To prevent rats and mice from entering animal facilities as much as possible, it is advisable to make the outside of the farm rodent-proof. This can be done by making sure that there are as few places as possible where rodents can shelter or settle (Fig. 11.9).

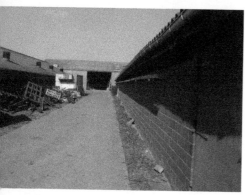

In other words, no equipment, weeds or waste should be piled up against the stable walls (Fig. 11.10). It is important to understand that rodents don't have good vision so they don't rely on their eyes, but on their sense of touch (whiskers) when they are moving. For this reason, they always run alongside the wall. Moreover, they are extremely shy and will continuously search for places to hide. As a result, a first step in rodent control is to clean up the surroundings of the stables and remove all possible shelter options.

▲

Fig. 11.10: Waste piled up along the stable walls

Secondly, the animal houses should be sealed off as much as possible. This means that all possible entrances (e.g. windows, air inlets, spaces under the roof) should be either fully closed or equipped with gratings that prevent rodents from entering. With regards doors it is important to ensure that they fit well, are always closed and that there is no space under the door allowing rodents to enter. Buildings should be inspected at least once a year for possible entryways for rodents. As mice only need a hole the size of a finger, and as rats can enter through a hole the size of a thumb, entryways can be small. Cracks around door frames, under doors, broken windows, water and utility hook-ups, vents and holes surrounding feed augers are potential points of entry. Coarse steel wool, hardware cloth or sheet metal can be used to cover/fill any entrances. Plastic, wood or insulation material should not to be used, as rodents simply gnaw their way through them.

Finally, it is important to place bait outside the buildings (Fig. 11.11) to ensure that any rodents that do attempt to enter come into contact with the bait first and have eaten poison before they manage to enter the stables. When using bait stations it is important that the rodenticides are well covered (not accessible to children and/or non-targeted species) and that they are fixed inside the bait station to avoid them being carried out by the rodents.

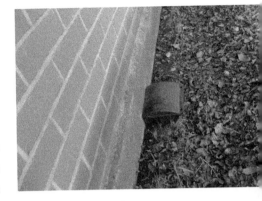

▲
Fig. 11.11: Baits placed at the outside of the building
___

4.2 Control of rodents inside the animal houses

Once all possible measurements have been taken to avoid rodents entering the buildings, the next step is to ensure a good control strategy inside the stables. This is based, first of all, on prevention, by avoiding conditions that favour nesting, feeding and reproduction (see above). Secondly the control should be based on a combination of chemical and mechanical control measures.

4.2.1 Chemical control

Chemical control is based on the use of rodenticides. The most frequently used rodenticides are anticoagulantia (table 11.1). They work by preventing blood coagulation. They are vitamin K precursor analogues that inhibit the production of vitamin K as the enzymes that are needed to produce vitamin K use the precursors analogues as substrate Vitamin K is essential for the production of precursors of coagulation factors. This results in internal bleeding and shock that cause death among rodents 3 to 4 days after intake.

The slow action of the products is the result of a gradual decrease in body reserves of vitamin K. The carcasses of these rodents will slowly dry out and will not spread a bad smell. As mentioned before rodents are very suspicious and very clever, and if the connection between eating a rodenticide and death is noticed, they will very quickly refrain from eating the poison. It is important therefore that they do not die immediately after eating the rodenticide.

Table 11.1: Most frequently used rodenticides

1st generation	2nd generation	
	Group A	Group B
Chlorophancinon	Difenacoum	Brodifacoum
Warfarin	Bromadiolone	Difethialon
Coumatetralyl		Flocoumafen
Diphacinone		

The toxicity of a rodenticide is expressed in terms of LD50. This is the dose needed to kill 50% of the rodents that have eaten it. A frequently used rodenticide is brodifacoum which has an LD50 of 0.26 mg/kilo for the brown rat and 0.70 mg/kilo for the black rat. More rodenticide is needed therefore to kill a black rat than a brown rat. First generation and second generation group A anticoagulants require rodents to feed over several days in order to acquire a lethal dose of the active ingredient whereas second-generation group B anti-coagulants may only require a single feeding to acquire a lethal dose. Both are slow-acting products which is essential in order to avoid the animals associating the consumption of the poison with death.

In addition to the toxicity, the formulation of the rodenticide is also of importance. Depending on the circumstances paraffin blocs, foam, gel, wheat, malt, oaks, or other formulations can be used (Fig. 11.12). In any case, rodents, and especially the black rats, are very selective about what they eat making it important that the rodenticide and its vector are fresh and tasty, to

Fig. 11.12: Different formulations of rodenticides: a) paste; b) grain mixture; c) sticky foam; d) grains
▼

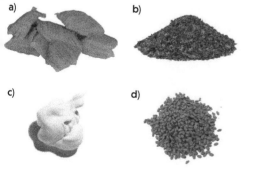

a)
b)
c)
d)

avoid the rodents ignoring it. When using bait stations outside the stables it is advisable to use paraffin blocks as they are more resistant to humidity, although they are a little less attractive than grains.

The location of the baits is important as rodents tend to use the same runs all the time (Fig. 11.13). The easiest time to identify the runs is at night as this is when there is the highest likelihood of seeing the animals walking around. Rodents will not make a detour to reach the rodenticides, even if they smell attractive. It is important therefore to check the location of their runs very carefully and install the mechanical traps (see below) or the rodenticide along these runs. Moreover, rats are extremely apprehensive about new objects and will avoid them for several days. Leaving a trap or bait station out for about five days is necessary to ensure acceptance. Mice quickly accept new objects. These tendencies are very important when designing baiting or trapping programmes.

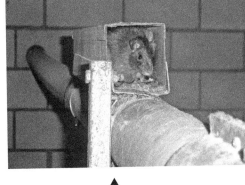

Fig. 11.13: Make sure you place the baits along the rat runs

It is highly recommendable to put the rodenticide in a bait station, not only for safety of personnel, pets, and animals, but also because this keeps it away from dust and it remains more attractive. Moreover, rodents feel comfortable hidden in a bait station and will eat more of the rodenticide. Mice have a small territory, so rodent bait stations should be placed about every five metres. Rodents may occasionally develop bait shyness after being made sick, but not killed, by a rodenticide. The shyness is towards the bait carrier, e.g., grain, and not to the rodenticide. In this event another formulated product or a different attractant can be used.

4.2.2 Mechanical control

In combination with chemical control, it is advisable to use mechanical control measures. This consists mainly of using traps. They are efficient as a monitoring tool in circumstances where the rodent infestation is under control and for monitoring potential reintroductions.

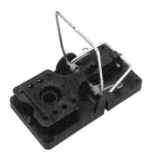

▲

Fig. 11.14: A rodent trap

The best mechanical control devices are traps (Fig. 11.14). These should be placed on rodent runs. It is also advisable to place two traps one behind each other to avoid rats jumping over them. It is also advisable to use plastic trays rather than wooden ones as they are easier to clean and absorb less of the smell of rat urine and faeces. Whenever a trap catches a rodent it is important to empty and clean the trap as quickly as possible. Cages are less suitable as the animals in the cage are not killed immediately and they _might tart to panic and scare away the others rodents. The rats will consequently quickly learn to avoid the cages.

Sound and ultrasound devices are not advised in animal facilities. Rodents may be frightened by strange noises in the first few days but then quickly become accustomed to them. Sound devices may cause distress among commercial poultry flocks, as well as result in decreased production and increased injury/mortality.

Fig. 11.15 & 11.16: Rodents should not be controlled by cats or dogs

▼

Pets such as cats and dogs are not good partners in rodent control. They may catch a few mice or rats however they do not comply with biosecurity measures themselves either. In this instance therefore you are replacing one potential vector of disease transmission with another.

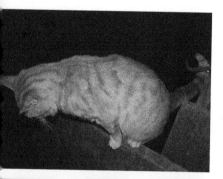

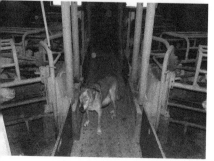

5 When to control rodents

Rodent control should be a continuous focus in all animal facilities. Even if there are no visible signs of rodent infestation, prevention is still required in order to avoid new entries that may result in large infestations before the problem has been detected.

If an important rodent problem is encountered, a very good time to control the infestation is when the stables are emptied. Any remains of animal feed should be removed so that there is no more feed for the rodents to eat. If attractive rodenticides are placed after feed removal, at sites where the rodents have been accustomed to feeding (e.g. animal feeding troughs), it is very likely that they will eat large volumes of the rodenticides. This is especially true of rats living under the floors above dung and which are hard to reach as long as the animal house is populated. To avoid having rats living above the dung it is also important to make sure that no crusts form on the slurry as these are ideal hiding and nesting locations for rats.

Common mistakes in rodent control

Rodent control programmes often produce disappointing results and this may be due to a number of frequently made mistakes such as:

1. Insufficient control outside the stables and/or too many entrances to the stables from the outside. In these cases control methods are inefficient as there will be a continuous influx of new rodents from outside.
2. The rodenticide is placed at the wrong place, at a location where the rodents don't pass for instance. As mentioned before rodents stick very closely to their habits and runs and will not make a detour. It is important therefore to make frequent checks to see whether rodenticides have been eaten. If not, new locations should be found.
3. Fresh rodenticide is not put down sufficiently frequently. As rodents prefer fresh food they will ignore rodenticide that has become stale and mouldy. It is important therefore to replenish the baits frequently even if they have not been touched.
4. Insufficient follow-up of pest control after a while because the farmer has the impression that the infestation is under control. This is often when new animals enter the buildings and a new episode of heavy infestation may start.

11

6 Conclusions

Rodent infestations can cause huge damage and may be important disease transmitters. An efficient rodent control programme is an indispensable component of a biosecurity plan therefore. It should be based on a combination of efficient prevention of entrance and good chemical and mechanical control inside the stables.

References

Amass S.F and Baysinger A., 2006. Swine disease transmission and prevention. In: Straw B.E., Zimmerman J.J., D'Allaire S., Taylor D.J. (editors). Diseases of Swine. 9th edition Blackwell Publishing Ltd., Oxford, UK, 1075-1098.

Backhans A. and Fellstrom C., 2012. Rodents on pig and chicken farms – a potential threat to human and animal health. Infection Ecology & Economy 2, 17093.

Center for disease control and prevention, 2017, Diseases directly transmitted by rodents https://www.cdc.gov/rodents/diseases/direct.html

Friedman M., Bednář V., Klimeš J., Smola J., Mrlík V., Literák I., 2008. Lawsonia intracellularis in rodents from pig farms with the occurrence of porcine proliferative enteropathy. Letters in Applied Microbiology 47, 117-121.

Lang, B. Dam, A., Taylor, K. 2013. Rodent Control in Livestock and Poultry Facilities, Ontario Ministry of agriculture, food and rural affairs, http://www.omafra.gov.on.ca/english/livestock/dairy/facts/13-057.htm

Lapuz R, Umali DV, Suzuki T, Shirota K, Katoh H. 2012. Comparison of the prevalence of Salmonella infection in layer hens from commercial layer farms with high and low rodent densities. Avian Dis. 56(1):29-34.

Lapuz, R., Tani, H. Sasai K., Shirota, K. Katoh H., and Baba E., 2008. The role of roof rats *(Rattus rattus)* in the spread of *Salmonella* Enteritidis and *Salmonella* Infantis contamination in layer farms in eastern Japan. Epidemiol. Infect. 136:1235-1243.

Pinheiro A.L.B.C., Bulos L.H.S., Onofre T.S., de Paula Gabardo M., de Carvalho O.V., Fausto M.C., Guedes R.M.C., de Almeida M.R., Silva Júnior A., 2013. Verification of natural infection of peridomestic rodents by PCV2 on commercial swine farms. Research in Veterinary Science 94, 764-768.

CHAPTER 12

TRANSMISSION OF PIG DISEASES AND BIOSECURITY IN PIG PRODUCTION

Jeroen Dewulf [1]

Merel Postma [1]

Bo Vanbeselaere [1,2]

Dominiek Maes [1]

Maria Eleni Filippitzi [1]

[1] Faculty of Veterinary Medicine, Department of Obstetrics, Reproduction and Herd Health, Veterinary Epidemiology Unit, University of Ghent, 9820 Merelbeke, Belgium
[2] CID LINES NV, 8900 Ieper, Belgium

1 Introduction

Pigs are susceptible to a wide range of endemic and epidemic diseases, including zoonotic infections, which can affect health, welfare and productivity, and thereby have a major economic impact. The implementation of biosecurity measures along the production chain presents itself as one of the major solutions for minimising the risk of introduction of these diseases into farms (external biosecurity), as well as their spread within farms (internal biosecurity) (Anonymous, 2010). Probably as a consequence of its role in disease prevention and control, biosecurity has been shown to have a positive impact in reducing the amount of antimicrobials used in Belgian pig production (Laanen et al., 2013; Postma et al., 2016). This is a promising finding considering that antimicrobial use in pig production has been identified as one of the highest among livestock sectors in European Union (EU) countries (Filippitzi et al., 2014; Carmo et al., 2017).

Recently, several studies have demonstrated a positive association between biosecurity and production parameters (Laanen et al., 2013; Postma et al., 2016) and between biosecurity and farm profitability (Corrégé et al., 2012; Siekkinen et al., 2012; Rojo Jimeno et al., 2016; Collineau et al., 2017). Despite these documented associations and the recognised importance of biosecurity measures, there are still major shortcomings in the implementation of these measures among European pig farms (Laanen et al., 2013; Backhans et al., 2015, Filippitzi et al., 2017). There are several examples of spread of diseases due to insufficient implementation of biosecurity measures, such as the porcine epidemic diarrhoea (PED) (Scott et al., 2016), the highly pathogenic strain of porcine reproductive and respiratory syndrome (HP-PRRS) (Brookes et al., 2015) and the foot-and-mouth disease (FMD) epidemic in the United Kingdom in 2001 (Ellis-Iversen et al., 2011). It is highly necessary therefore to continue emphasising the importance of biosecurity in disease prevention.

In this chapter, the routes of direct and indirect transmission of the most common pig diseases are described and translated into biosecurity measures. These measures might help in preventing infectious agents from moving between and within pig farms via these routes.

2 Review of pig disease transmission

In order to identify the disease transmission routes of the most important pig diseases we first studied a table by Amass (2005). This table included the routes of indirect transmission of 19 important pig pathogens. We then reviewed more recent literature published between 2005 and 2016 on transmission of the same pathogens in order to retrieve additional information and to update this table. Additionally, based on the opinion of three experts in swine health, biosecurity and epidemiology, the list of pathogens selected by Amass (2005) was extended to include five important diseases for pig production in Europe. Finally, the direct disease transmission route was also added. For each disease, a rapid structured literature search was carried out in PubMed and Web of Science (Thomson Reuters) using a search string formulated as the combination of (the name of the pathogen) AND (pig OR swine) AND transmission. The book *Diseases of Swine* (Wiley-Blackwell® 2012) was also used as reference. The results are summarised in Table 12.1 (see p. 298-301).

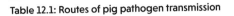

Table 12.1: Routes of pig pathogen transmission

Pathogen	Direct contact	Indirect contact — People	Semen	Manure	Domestic/feral animals
	Biosecurity measures (in sub-categories) preventing each route of disease transmission				
	Purchasing policy, Transport/removal of animals/manure/cadavers, All sub-categories of internal biosecurity [a]	Access check Indirectly: Transport/removal of animals/manure/cadavers; Supply of fodder, water and equipment; Cleaning and disinfection	Purchasing policy	Transport/removal of animals/manure/cadavers	Vermin and bird control
Actinobacillus pleuropneumoniae	O (Gottschalk, 2012a; Tobias et al., 2014)				O (Gottschalk, 2012a; Baroch et al., 2015; Marinou et al., 2015)
Bordetella bronchiseptica	O (Nicholson et al., 2012; Brockmeier et al., 2012)				X
Brachyspira hyodysenteriae	O (Desrosiers, 2011; Hampson, 2012)	O (Hampson, 2012)		X	X
Brucella suis	O (Wu et al., 2012; Olsen et al., 2015)	X	X	O (Olsen et al., 2015)	X
Classical swine fever virus	O (Muñoz-González et al., 2015; Anonymous, 2014)	O (Ribbens et al., 2007; Anonymous, 2014)	X	X	X
Clostridium perfringens	O (Songer et al., 2012; Allaart et al., 2013)			O (Songer et al., 2012; Allaart et al., 2013)	
Erysipelothrix rhusiopathiae [c]	O (Opriessnig et al., 2012)			O (Opriessnig et al., 2012)	
Escherichia coli	O (Cornick et al., 2008; Fairbrother et al., 2012; Callens et al., 2015)	X		X	O (Fairbrother et al., 2012; Pearson et al., 2016)
Foot-and-mouth disease virus	O (Desrosiers, 2011; Dekker, 2011; Anonymous, 2011; Pacheco et al., 2012)	X	X	X	O (Mohamed et al., 2011; Fukai et al., 2015)
Haemophilus parasuis [c]	O (Aragon et al., 2012; Brockmeier et al., 2013)				O (Aragon et al., 2012)
Lawsonia intracellularis [c]	O (McOrist et al., 2012)			O (McOrist et al., 2012)	O (Baroch et al., 2015; Pearson et al., 2016)

a As described in Biocheck.UGentTM; b Transmitted to distances >2 km; c Added to the original list of Amass (2005).

Rodents	Insects (Vectors)	Aerosol	Animal feed	Water	Fomites
Vermin and bird control	Location, environment	Purchasing policy, Transport/ removal of animals/manure/cadavers, Location, environment, All sub-categories of internal biosecurity	Supply of fodder, water and equipment	Supply of fodder, water and equipment	Cleaning and disinfection, Indirectly: Transport/removal of animals/manure/cadavers; Supply of fodder, water and equipment; Access check; Vermin and bird control
		X		O (Gottschalk, 2012a; Assavacheep et al., 2013; Loera-Muro et al., 2013)	O (Assavacheep et al., 2013)
X	O (Brockmeier et al., 2012)	X		X	O (Brockmeier et al., 2012)
X	O (Desrosiers, 2011)		O (Hampson, 2012)	X	O (Hampson, 2012)
	O (Olsen et al., 2015)	O (Olsen et al., 2015)	O (Olsen et al., 2015)		
	X	X	O (Anonymous, 2014b)		X
	O (Allaart et al., 2013)	X		X	O (Allaart et al., 2013)
X	X	X	O (Fairbrother et al., 2012)	X	X
		X[b]	O (Schembri et al., 2010; Hernández-Jover et al., 2011)	O (Schijven et al., 2005)	X
O (Friedman, et al., 2008; McOrist et al., 2012; Pearson et al., 2016)	O (McOrist et al., 2012)				O (McOrist et al., 2012)

'X' represents possible transmission routes described by Amass (2005). 'O' describes new possible transmission routes based on studies published between 2005 and January 2016.

	Direct contact	Indirect contact			
		People	Semen	Manure	Domestic/feral animals
Pathogen	Biosecurity measures (in sub-categories) preventing each route of disease transmission				
	Purchasing policy, Transport/removal of animals/manure/cadavers, All sub-categories of internal biosecurity [a]	Access check Indirectly: Transport/removal of animals/manure/cadavers; Supply of fodder, water and equipment; Cleaning and disinfection	Purchasing policy	Transport/removal of animals/manure/cadavers	Vermin and bird control
Leptospires	O (Ellis, 2012)	X	O (Althouse and Rossow 2011, Maes, 2016)		X
Mycoplasma hyopneumoniae	O (Thacker and Minion, 2012)	O (Nathues et al. 2012)			O (Baroch et al. 2015, Marinou et al. 2015, Pearson et al. 2016)
Pasteurella multocida	O (Fablet et al. 2011, Desrosiers, 2011, Register et al. 2012)	O (Desrosiers, 2011)		X	O (Desrosiers 2011, Register et al. 2012)
Porcine circovirus type 2 [c]	O (Segalés et al. 2005)		O (Althouse and Rossow 2011, Maes, 2016, Segalés et al. 2012, Woeste and grosse Beilage 2007)	O (Patterson et al. 2011)	O (Baroch et al. 2015, Boadella et al. 2012, Segalés et al. 2012, Corn et al. 2009)
Porcine epidemic diarrhoea virus [c]	O (Saif et al. 2012)	O (Scott et al. 2016)		O (Scott et al. 2016)	O (Scott et al. 2016)
Porcine parvovirus	O (Miao et al. 2009, Truyen and Streck, 2012)				
Porcine reproductive and respiratory syndrome virus	O (Zimmerman et al. 2012, Thakur et al 2015)	X	X	X	O (Baroch et al. 2015, Boadella et al. 2012, Corn et al. 2009, Zimmermann et al. 2012)
Pseudorabies virus	O (Mettenleiter et al. 2012)		X	X	X
Salmonella spp.	O (Carlson et al. 2012, Andres and Davies 2015)	X		X	X
Streptococcus suis	O (Fablet et al. 2011, Gottschalk 2012b)	X		X	X
Swine influenza virus	O (Van Reeth et al. 2012)	X		X	X
Swine vesicular disease virus	O (Alexandersen et al. 2012)	X	X	O (Alexandersen et al. 2012)	O (Alexandersen et al. 2012)
Transmissible gastroenteritis virus	O (Saif et al 2012)	X		X	X

a As described in Biocheck.UGentTM; b Transmitted to distances >2 km; c Added to the original list of Amass (2005).

Rodents	Insects (Vectors)	Aerosol	Animal feed	Water	Fomites
Vermin and bird control	Location, environment	Purchasing policy, Transport/ removal of animals/manure/cadavers, Location, environment, All sub-categories of internal biosecurity	Supply of fodder, water and equipment	Supply of fodder, water and equipment	Cleaning and disinfection, Indirectly: Transport/removal of animals/manure/cadavers; Supply of fodder, water and equipment; Access check; Vermin and bird control
X				X	
		X[b]		X	X
		X		X	O (Desrosiers, 2011, Register et al. 2012)
O (Pinheiro et al. 2013, Cságola 2008)	O (Blunt et al. 2011)		O (Opriessnig et al. 2009)	O (Woeste and grosse Beilage 2007, Fablet et al. 2011, Segalés et al. 2005)	
	X		X	O (Truyen and Streck, 2012, Sliz et al. 2015)	O (Truyen and Streck, 2012)
O (Marinou et al. 2015, Zimmermann et al. 2012)	X	X[b]	O (Brookes et al. 2015)	X	X
X	X	X		O (Mettenleiter et al. 2012)	X
X	X	X[b]	X	X	X
	X	X		X	X
		X			
		X	O (Alexandersen et al. 2012)		X
	X				X

'X' represents possible transmission routes described by Amass (2005). 'O' describes new possible transmission routes based on studies published between 2005 and January 2016.

3 Biosecurity measures in pig production

Based upon the described disease transmission routes biosecurity measures are described that aim to prevent either the introduction or spread of these pathogens in pig herds. For the sake of clarity, these measures are subdivided into external biosecurity measures aimed at prevention of disease introduction, and internal biosecurity measures aimed at the prevention of disease spread within herds.

3.1 External Biosecurity

3.1.1 Purchasing policy

The introduction of non-proprietary animals or genetic material (e.g. semen) is a possible source of the introduction of pathogens against which there is no farm immunity. Pathogen transmission occurs very effectively via direct contact between infected and susceptible animals (Filippitzi et al., 2017). The importance of biosecurity in purchasing policy therefore is great in ensuring the protection of farms from many pathogens as listed in Table 12.1. As a consequence, the primary aim should be to avoid purchasing animals or genetic material as much as possible (Amass and Baysinger, 2006; Dewulf, 2014; Filippitzi et al., 2017). A fully closed herd or production system has a substantially lower risk of disease introduction. Moreover, in addition to the risk of disease introduction, the frequent addition of 'naïve' animals may also favour the continuous circulation of herd-specific pathogens, which may in turn hamper the control and eradication of certain pathogens in herds. Yet, in modern pig production facilities, avoiding the introduction of new animals or semen is often very difficult because farms want to keep up with the genetic progress made by breeding companies. Therefore, whenever new animals are introduced, a number of precautionary measures should be taken.

3.1.1.1 Limit the frequency of introduction

Both the frequency of introduction and the number of animals purchased will influence the risk of disease introduction (Fèvre et al., 2006; Laanen et al., 2013). In both, the maxim from a biosecurity point of view is 'the less, the better'. However, sometimes it can be advisable to increase the size of the group of purchased animals (e.g. new gilts) as this may enable a reduction in the frequency of new introductions. It is believed to be less risky to buy twenty gilts five times a year than 10 gilts 10 times a year.

3.1.1.2 Limit the number of sources

It is very important to limit the number of source herds, both for animals and semen, as much as possible (Dewulf, 2014). Several studies have shown that introducing animals from different source herds increases the risk of disease introduction (Hege et al., 2002; Lo Fo Wong, 2004). Moreover, source herds should preferably have a documented high health status (Pritchard et al., 2005; Kirwan, 2008; Dewulf, 2014). This status may include the certified absence of a number of infectious diseases (e.g. specific pathogen free status) thus avoiding the unintended introduction of new pathogens in the receptor herd (Laanen et al., 2010; Filippitzi et al., 2017).

3.1.1.3 Implement good quarantine measures

Newly purchased animals should always be introduced first into a quarantine stable. A good quarantine stable is fully isolated from the other animal facilities and should be accessed through a separate entry with its own hygiene lock (Fig. 12.1). During the quarantine period, animals should be clinically inspected to ensure that no symptoms of disease are present or will emerge. Animals can also be sampled in order to detect any current infections and to identify the immune status of the animals. Moreover the quarantine period can also be used to vaccinate the newly introduced animals to ensure a sufficient level of immunity when they are brought into contact with the resident animals (Barceló

12

and Marco, 1998; Corréegée, 2002; Pritchard et al., 2005; Calvar et al., 2012; Dewulf, 2014). A quarantine period should last at least four weeks and for some diseases longer periods are required (PRRSV and PCV2 – 6 to 8 weeks; M. *hyopneumoniae* – 8 to 10 weeks) (Eijck, 2003; Pritchard et al., 2005).

Fig. 12.1: Design of a good quarantine stable

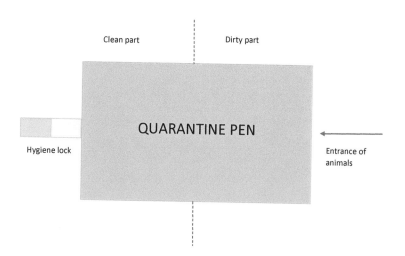

3.1.2 Transport of animals, removal of manure and carcasses

Pathogens can spread through the transport of live animals and/or the removal of cadavers or manure. This spreading of infectious germs can be achieved directly (via se- and excreta of diseased animals and cadavers) or indirectly (via fomites of cadavers, the rendering truck, humans and their equipment, rodents, domestic animals and manure) (Table 12.1).

3.1.2.1 Use clean animal transport vehicles

Epidemiological field studies have highlighted contagious livestock lorries as a main source of contamination for many disease-causing agents, including classical swine fever (CSF) (Fritzemeier et al., 2000), *Mycoplasma hyopneumoniae* (Hege et al., 2002), *Actino-*

bacillus pleuropneumoniae (Fussing et al., 1998 and Hege et al., 2002), *Brachyspira hyodysenteriae* (Windsor and Simmons, 1981) and *Salmonella* (Rajkowski et al., 1998). They should be empty, cleaned and disinfected at all times therefore before entering the premises (Pritchard et al., 2005; Dewulf, 2014). Although this is a well-known principle, there are many occasions when this is not sufficiently respected. Very cold weather conditions may hamper thorough cleaning and disinfection for example. Moreover, trucks that collect culled breeding sows are not always fully empty upon arrival at the farm. Some recommendations state that a livestock transport lorry should be empty for at least a couple of hours or days before it can enter the farm. This might provide an additional reduction in risk, however it is clear that thorough cleaning, disinfection and drying are the principal measures that cannot be replaced by a certain 'downtime'. Pigs that have been in contact with the lorry during loading, should not be moved back to the stable in order to minimise the chance of introducing pathogens through an inadequately cleaned lorry. For the same reason, the lorry-driver should not be allowed to enter the stables either. The loading bay should also be cleaned and disinfected after every load of animals (Pritchard et al., 2005; Backhans et al., 2015).

3.1.2.2 Make a separation between the clean and the dirty area

The principle of the clean and dirty road in a pig farm guarantees a clear separation between the clean and the dirty (risky) sections of the premises (Hémonic et al., 2010; Anonymous, 2010; Neumann, 2012; Filippitzi et al., 2017). All inbound and outbound traffic that serves multiple companies (e.g. feed, liquid manure, external transportation of animals, etc.) should always go via the 'dirty road'. The 'clean road' is preserved for the delivery of animals and harmless products, but only in fully cleaned and disinfected lorries.
Only the 'dirty road' should be of relatively easy access to visitors, suppliers and consumers. The collection of cadavers should, for obvious reasons, be part of the dirty section. Barrels, wheelbarrows and other tools used for this, should only be returned to the clean section after they have been thoroughly cleaned and disinfected.

Liquid manure must always be conveyed via the dirty road. Furthermore, it is advisable that farmers use farm-specific discharge pipes in order to prevent pipes belonging to the manure removal company, which recently have been in contact with manure on other farms, also being used on your farm.

Recent studies have indicated that the clean-dirty area principle is not always completely observed by manure removal and supply companies in a number of EU countries (Filipitzi et al., 2017). This indicates that the farmers should ensure that the clean-dirty areas are clearly defined with signs illustrating how to adhere to these rules. Making reminders could also help influence behaviour in these kinds of problems (e.g. Reddy et al., 2016).

3.1.2.3 Management of cadavers

Cadavers are always a major source of infectious material. Animals often die due to infections and cadavers thus have the great potential to spread a lot of infectious material. It is strongly advisable therefore to remove the cadavers from the stables as soon as possible and to store them in a well-insulated place (Meroz et al., 1995; Pritchard et al., 2005). Make sure that no vermin can reach the cadavers as they could spread the infectious material.

After the collection of the cadavers the cadaver storage room should be thoroughly cleaned and disinfected. The people handling the cadavers should always wear disposable gloves for their own safety as well as in order to avoid further spread of pathogens (Pritchard et al., 2015; Filippitzi et al., 2017).

The cadaver storage room should be located in a place where the rendering company can collect the cadavers without entering the farm to avoid disease introduction through these potentially high-risk cargos (Evans and Sayer, 2000; McQuiston et al., 2005; Pritchard et al., 2005; Anonymous, 2010; Maes, 2016). It is also advisable to have a cooled cadaver storage room both to avoid the smell and to reduce the frequency of visits by the rendering company (by achieving a higher storage capacity) (Fig. 12.2). Moreover, these

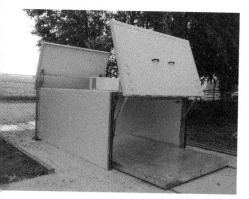

Fig. 12.2: Cooled cadaver storage
▼

cooled systems are generally also fully sealed and are very effective in preventing contact with vermin.

3.1.3 Supply of feed, water and equipment

Feed itself should generally not pose a risk due to the strict hygienic conditions in the production thereof. However swill feeding (banned for decades under EU law) is a practice that was previously associated with major outbreaks of infectious diseases, among others CSF (Horst et al., 1997; Fritzemeier et al., 2000; Filippitzi et al., 2017). Pig drinking-water quality often leaves much to be desired. The water may originate from different sources (surface, wells, etc.) after which it is stored most of the time in a tank and then supplied to the animals. At the source, in the reservoir or in the pipes, the water may be contaminated and biofilms may form. Regular (at least once a year) examination of drinking water quality both at the entrance and at the nipples is therefore definitely advisable, as well as the systematic cleaning of the pipes (see also chapter on quality of drinking water).

The introduction of all sorts of equipment such as floating panels or shovels, which comes into contact with the animals and their manure may also introduce pathogens. It is preferable therefore to avoid the introduction of new equipment as much as possible or if any is introduced, it is advisable to carry out a disinfection step first.

3.1.4 Access of personnel and visitors

Humans can act as a mechanical vector of pathogens if they have been in contact with infected animals and subsequently come in to contact with susceptible animals without taking any preventive measures. This type of transmission has been proven through experiments on several pathogens, among which the transmissible gastroenteritis virus (Alvarez et al., 2001), *Escherichia coli* (Amass et al., 2003) and CSF (Ribbens et al., 2007). The transmission occurs mainly through remains of excreta from infected animals on footwear and clothing. The possibility of biological transmission of pathogens between humans and pigs exists and these can infect both humans and pigs, such as the H1N1 influenza virus

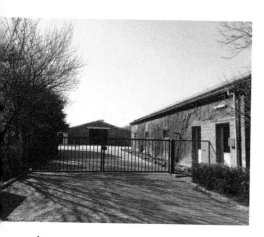

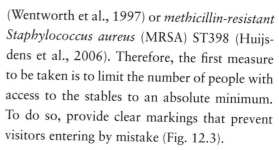

(Wentworth et al., 1997) or *methicillin-resistant Staphylococcus aureus* (MRSA) ST398 (Huijsdens et al., 2006). Therefore, the first measure to be taken is to limit the number of people with access to the stables to an absolute minimum. To do so, provide clear markings that prevent visitors entering by mistake (Fig. 12.3).

When visitors and personnel enter the stables, they should always wear clean, herd-specific clothes and footwear. They should also wash their hands properly (Pritchard et al., 2005; Hémonic et al., 2010; Dewulf, 2014; Maes, 2016). The latter is a simple and very useful measure, which is often omitted. Pathogens are efficiently transferred by the hands of animal carers via direct contact with the animals (Vangroenweghe et al., 2009; Hémonic et al., 2010; Backhans et al., 2015). A study by Lo Fo Wong et al. (2004) reveals that the chance of testing positive for *Salmonella* is reduced as a result of consistent hand washing before entering a section with pigs.

▲
Fig. 12.3: Clear entrance control at the farm to avoid unwanted visitors

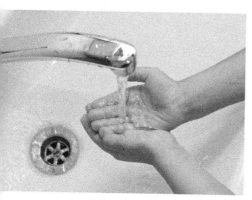

▲
Fig. 12.4: Proper washing of hands

To ensure a change of clothing and allow people and visitors to wash their hands, a good hygiene lock should be available (Vangroenweghe et al., 2009). In this hygiene lock, a clear physical separation (e.g. bench) between the dirty and the clean areas should be provided. When entering the hygiene lock the following steps should be observed (Maes, 2016):

1. When entering the lock, take off your jacket and shoes.
2. Wash your hands with disinfecting soap.
3. Step over the bench and put on a clean overalls and boots.
4. Disinfect the boots with the boot washer before entering the stable.

5. When returning to the hygiene lock, clean and disinfect the boots with the boot washer
6. Put the boots on the appropriate shelf
7. Take off the dirty overalls and put them in the laundry basket
8. Step over the bench and wash your hands before you put on your own jacket and shoes again.

In companies with high health standards, visitors and personnel are often obliged to shower before entering the farm. The main benefit of this obligation is the certainty that all possibly contaminated clothing is exchanged for farm-specific clothing and that hands are washed thoroughly. It also discourages less urgent visits (Moore, 1992; Amass and Clark, 1999).

A pig free downtime of 24 or even 48 hours is also often required for visitors before they can gain access to the farm. This is based on the argument that germs excreted by pigs could survive on humans for a specific period. During this period, people can secrete germs passively and transfer them to susceptible animals. Yet, in scientific literature there is very little proof of the true risk related to this transmission route. As far as we are aware, there is only one study that dates back to 1970, in which it was noted that FMD could be isolated from the nose and mouth of people who had been in contact with animals infected with the FMD-virus. On one person the virus could be isolated 28 hours after contact with the infected pigs. After 48 hours this was no longer possible (Sellers et al. 1970). If all required precautionary measures are taken as described above, the downtime probably has little additional value.

3.1.5 Vermin and bird control

A number of pathogens can be directly or indirectly transmitted from outside the farm or between different compartments within the farm by rodents, birds, dogs and cats (Table 12.1). They can act as reservoirs for herd-specific pathogens that will continue to circulate in the farm (Andres et al., 2015). Rodents and birds can also cause damage to the equipment and the farm buildings or they can be a cause of food wastage if they have access to it (Backhans and Fellstrom, 2010).

To control vermin an efficient control programme is required. This is often developed in collaboration with specialised companies (Amass, 2005; Lister, 2008; Hémonic et al., 2010; Dewulf, 2014; Backhans et al., 2015; Filippitzi et al., 2017). It is important to prevent vermin taking up residence in the proximity of the stables. This can be achieved by avoiding the presence of all types of hiding places close to the stables (e.g. plants, piles of dirt, etc.). Feed should also be stored in closed reservoirs with no access for rodents or birds (Lister, 2008; Anonymous, 2010).

The entrance of birds into the stables can be prevented by covering all air inlets with nets. Pets should also be kept out of the stables as they can act as mechanical vectors of pathogens. The use of cats or dogs to control rats and mice therefore is not a good policy (Vangroenweghe et al., 2009).

The measures required for controlling vermin in stables are described in more detail in chapter 11 Of this book

3.1.6 Location and environment

The location of the farm and the density of pig farming in the proximity are important factors for airborne and vector-borne disease transmission. Wild boars may also act as a reservoir for swine diseases (Table 12.1).

3.1.6.1 Airborne transmission diseases

Usually, transmission through the air is particularly important within short distances (< 2 kilometres (km)), hence the importance of distance to the nearest neighbour. Rose and Madec (2002) concluded that the number of farms within a range of 2 km had significantly increased the frequency of respiratory disorders in a farm. As for the chance of transmission of *Mycoplasma hyopneumoniae* through the air of e, the distance to neighbouring farms proved to be the most determining factor (Goodwin, 1985, Dee et al., 2009). Maes et al. (2000a) reported increased seroprevalences for *M. hyo-pneumoniae*, swine influenza viruses and Aujeszky's disease virus in herds located in pig-dense areas. Mintiens et al. (2003) showed that the combination of distance to a neighbouring farm and pig herd density in an area are major risk factors for the spread of CSF. When planning the building of a new pig farm, the distance to the nearest neighbour pig farm should be a determining factor for the choice of location. The predominant direction of the wind should also be taken into account. Knowledge of the presence of diseases in neighbouring farms is equally important. The spread of liquid manure, originating from other farms, in the neighbourhood of the farm should also be avoided. It has become possible to equip stables with highly performant air filtration systems that can prevent the entrance of pathogens through the air. This might be worth evaluating in densely populated livestock areas, especially if the animals at the farm are free of a number of endemic diseases in the area. It has been demonstrated that filtration of incoming air, in combination with standard biosecurity procedures, can prevent transmission of PRRSV into susceptible herds (Alonso et al., 2013). The authors showed that air filtration reduced the risk of introduction of novel PRRSV by approximately 80%, indicating that on large sow farms with good biosecurity in pig-dense regions, approximately four out five PRRSV outbreaks may be attributable to aerosol transmission. Air filtration may also be helpful in preventing airborne transmission of other pathogens such as swine influenza and *M. hyopneumoniae*.

3.1.6.2 Wild animals

Direct or indirect contact with wild boars may cause disease transmission (e.g. CSF (Fritzemeier et al., 2000) and Aujeszky's disease (Artois et al., 2002)). Therefore, in regions where free ranging wild boar are present, it is important to keep them out of the farm by setting up a solid fence (Amass and Clark, 1999) with a depth of 30 to 40 cm under the ground (Hartung, 2005). Even if pigs are kept indoors, wild boars should not have access to the vicinity of the farm in order to avoid the indirect transmission of infections (e.g. airborne transmission, through vectors, trough contact with stored feed).

3.2 Internal Biosecurity

3.2.1 Management of diseases

Disease management concerns all actions related to the correct handling and treatment of diseased animals. This includes proper diagnostics, isolation of the sick animals and disease registration as well as the improvement of the immunity status of susceptible animals, in particular through vaccination. Correct disease management should provide a good insight into the specific health status of the herd and should result in the application of the required preventive treatments to avoid disease (Table 12.1) and any subsequent losses.

3.2.1.1 Returning to younger age group

In the case of a slower growth rate among some piglets compared to the rest of the group, it is of crucial importance to avoid these animals that are lagging behind, being returned to a batch of younger piglets. It is very likely that these slower growing piglets suffer from one or more infectious diseases. By transferring these pigs to a younger age group, potential carriers of germs are introduced into a susceptible population (Vangroenweghe et al., 2009; Dewulf, 2014; Filippitzi et al., 2017). When a piglet demonstrates a low probability of becoming a profitable fattening pig, euthanasia is a better choice to avoid the piglet, and subsequently the whole litter, becoming a permanent source of infection. Its litter will also be a permanent source of infection. If euthanasia is not believed to be the right option, these animals should be isolated in the sick bay.

3.2.1.2 Sick bay

Diseased pigs should be isolated in a sick bay in order to protect other animals from exposure to pathogens through infected excretions and secretions. A good sick bay should be completely separated from the rest of the animals in a separate house. (Hémonic et al., 2010; Dewulf, 2014). Once an animal has been in the sick bay, it should never return to the regular stables as it is very likely that it will transmit remaining pathogens to the healthy animals. Therefore, the sick bay should also be accessed separately by farm workers and the necessary hygienic measures (e.g. changing of overalls, footwear, washing hands, etc.) should be implemented when entering and leaving this place. The sick bay should preferably only be visited at the end of the working round (Vangroenweghe et al., 2009; Backhans et al., 2015).

3.2.1.3 Use of needles and medicines

Extensive literature on the spread of germs via injection equipment (needles and syringes) (Hémonic et al., 2010; Filippitzi et al., 2017) exists. On pig farms the same needles are often used, and are only replaced when they become blunt! These needles may become contaminated by numerous environmental germs through use and storage. Moreover, injecting sick animals may cause the needle (and consequently the bottle) to become contaminated with a pathogen. Injecting multiple animals with the same needle increases the risk of the spread of germs. Ideally, single-use needles should be used (Hémonic et al., 2010). If this is unfeasible, it is highly advisable to use one needle per group (e.g. pen). Avoid the use of the same needles for different age groups and do not wait to replace needles until they become blunt, both for hygiene and animal welfare reasons. Previously opened bottles should be stored in a hygienic environment at the recommended temperature.

3.2.2 Farrowing and suckling period

Pathogens can be transmitted from sows to piglets vertically, via the placenta or via contaminated colostrum and milk. They can also be transmitted horizontally through the skin for example or the nipples and the udder. Cross-fostering in particular increases the risk of transmission from infected or carrier sows to susceptible piglets without maternal antibodies (e.g. of PRRSV as indicated by Zimmerman et al., 2012). Returning piglets to younger age groups is also a risky practice, since it can introduce pathogens to a susceptible population as discussed in the previous paragraph. Nursery pigs are a vulnerable age group due to their temporary

12

lower immunity status, the higher presence of diverse pathogens in this life period (Johnson et al., 2012) and the fighting or biting when the pigs are mixed (Cameron et al., 2012). Another route of pathogen transmission in the farrowing unit is the use of materials (e.g. castration blades, elastrator for tail docking, ear-tagger, iron injection needles) from one piglet to another without intermediate cleaning and disinfection thereof.

3.2.2.1 Washing the sows

Before the sows are placed in the farrowing pen, they should be dewormed and washed in order to prevent the transmission of germs from the sow barn to the farrowing pen. It is important that sows are washed before they enter the farrowing pen, to avoid the contamination of these pens during the washing process.

3.2.2.2 Cross-fostering

Mixing litters in the farrowing pen is an important way of spreading infection to different animal groups. Sows carrying *Streptococcus suis* may already infect their piglets during parturition (Amass et al., 1996). A further spread of *S. suis* may take place if piglets are moved to other litters. This principle applies to other germs as well. If 5 % of the piglets are moved between pens more than 48 hours after birth, there is an increased probability of problems with PRRS (Duinhof et al., 2006). It is advisable therefore to avoid cross-fostering as much as possible. If this is not possible, it is advisable to limit cross-fostering to one occasion and to perform it in the first 48 hours after birth.

3.2.2.3 Equipment for treatment of piglets

Equipment that is used in the farrowing pen, such as pliers for cutting the teeth and blades for castration, is exposed to secretions and excretions of the piglets. This allows germs to be transferred from one piglet to another. It is necessary to clean and disinfect the equipment when using it for different piglets (immerse in disinfectant). This will limit the chance of disease transmission (Vangroenweghe et al., 2009; Filippitzi et al., 2017).

3.2.3 Nursery and fattening unit

3.2.3.1 All in / all-out (also applies to the farrowing unit)

The all-in/all-out (AI/AO) principle helps to prevent cross-contamination and makes it possible to clean and disinfect the stables thoroughly between different consecutive rounds. The strict application of this AI/AO principle is a very important measure in breaking the infection cycle from one production round to another (Clark et al., 1991). It is of fundamental importance that the AO part in particular is fully respected. Sometimes this is only applied for 95% and a few (light-weight) animals are kept in the stables and mixed with the next round. These animals, albeit few in number, are a likely source of infection for the next groups (see above on returning to younger age groups; repetition of previous sections). When moving the animals from one production stage to the next (e.g. from the farrowing house to the nursery pen), it is advisable to keep the groups together as much as possible rather than sorting all animals according to size. The latter will result in a lot of mixing which substantially increases the likelihood of spread of infection (Maes et al., 2008; Hémonic et al., 2010).

3.2.3.2 Stocking density

A high stocking density induces stress which results in an increased sensitivity to infection and increased excretion of germs. Large numbers of infected pigs in a small area can cause a sharp rise in infection pressure. Various studies have shown that higher stocking density in the different production phases increases the occurrence of respiratory illnesses as well as digestive tract disorders (Pointon et al., 1985; Maes et al., 2000a; Maes et al., 2000b; Stärk, 2000; Laanen, 2011). In addition, it has been proven several times over that there is a positive connection between available space per animal and its daily growth (Dewulf et al., 2007). In many cases the norms, as prescribed in EU legislation, are based on outdated research and insights and have not evolved along with the recent developments in the industry. It is advisable therefore to consider these norms as the absolute minimum requirement rather

12

than ideal values (Dewulf et al., 2007). Studies have shown that the optimal average values for stocking density are 20 to 24 % above the legal requirements (Hamilton et al., 2003; Laanen et al., 2011). If we compare Belgium with the Netherlands, we see that the legal requirements in the Netherlands are closer to the optimal values. It is clear that a lower stocking density will result in better on-farm biosecurity.

Table 12.2: Legal and optimal standards of stocking density in a pig house (Dewulf et al., 2007; Council Directive 18 December 2008; Dutch Government, 5 June 2014)

Average animal weight (kg)	Required area EU, among which Belgium (in m²) per animal	Required area in the Netherlands (in m²) per animal		Optimal area (in m²) per animal
	Council Directive 18 December 2008	*Dutch Government 5 June 2014*		*Dewulf et al., 2007*
<10 kg	0.15	Up to 15 kg	0.20	0,17
10 to 20 kg	0.20	15 to 30 kg	0.30	0,27
20 to 30 kg	0.30			0,35
30 to 50 kg	0.40		0.50	0.49
50 to 85 kg	0.55		0.65	0.70
85 to 110 kg	0.65		0.80	0.83
>110 kg	1.00		1.00	

3.2.4 Compartmentalising, working lines and equipment

Animals of different ages may have different levels of sensitivity to certain pathogens and therefore it is crucial to keep different age groups separate and to work in a well-defined sequence. Equipment and materials (e.g. bedding material, feeders, drinking troughs, boots, spades, syringes, needles, etc.) may also play an important role in the transmission of a large number of diseases (Table 12.1).

3.2.4.1 Working lines and separate hygiene locks

An important basic rule for preventing the spread of disease between different age groups is to determine and uphold working lines within farms. A fixed route should be created and used at all times to visit and work in the stables. During the rounds to the stables the youngest animals should be visited first, followed by the pregnant sows, the older age groups, the quarantined and sick animals and finally the cadaver storage.

For each age category and especially for risk-bearing groups (e.g. quarantine stables, sick bay), it is advisable to provide an additional hygiene lock allowing proper changing of clothing, footwear and hand washing.

3.2.4.2 Equipment in the various compartments

Specially designated equipment should be foreseen along the working lines. A brush, a shovel or floating panels can easily be contaminated with faeces containing a great number of germs. It is t recommendable therefore to use different equipment in different sections. The equipment has to be clearly recognisable (different colours) (Fig. 12.5) to avoid moving it from one section to another (Vangroenweghe et al., 2009; Laanen, 2011; Gelaude et al., 2014). The same rule applies to clothing and footwear for exactly the same reason.

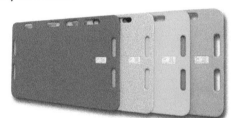

Fig. 12.5: Floating panels in different colours to be used in different compartments of the herd to avoid using the same material for different age groups

▼

12

3.2.4.3 Boot washers and disinfection baths

To avoid dragging germs on your footwear, boot washers and disinfection baths should be placed between the different production units. An efficient disinfection can only be achieved if dirt and faeces are removed from the boots in advance. This can be done with a boot washer and water (preferably with detergent added). The boots should then be placed in a visually clean solution with a disinfectant. This protocol requires that instructions for the concentration of the disinfectant and the duration of the cleaning as provided in the disinfectant manual, should be strictly adhered to

(Amass et al., 2000). Disinfection baths that are not used properly will inadvertently increase the number of germs on the boots. This results in a lot of wasted time and money and it even increases the risk of the spread of disease. However, having to stand for many minutes in a disinfection bath before being able to go to another section is not very practical. This inconvenience can be avoided by providing a pair of extra boots at each disinfection bath, so there's always a pair of boots ready to be used at each bath while the other boots are placed in the disinfection solution. Moreover, the presence of foot baths draws the attention of staff and visitors to the importance of biosecurity on farm grounds (Amass et al., 2000).

3.2.5 Cleaning and disinfection

Pens, feeding troughs and equipment infected by faeces can maintain an infection cycle because new animals keep getting infected. These animals will consequently secrete germs and will reinfect their environment. To break the infection cycle between consecutive litters pens should be thoroughly cleaned and disinfected.

A complete C&D protocol consists of seven steps:
1. Dry cleaning to remove all organic material.
2. Soaking of all surfaces, preferably with a detergent.
3. High-pressure cleaning with water to remove all dirt. This step will be much easier, faster and effective if a goad soaking step is performed before.
4. Drying the stable to avoid dilution of the disinfectant applied in the next step.
5. Disinfecting the stable to achieve a further reduction in the concentration of germs.
6. Drying the stable to ensure that animals cannot come into contact with pools of remaining disinfectant afterwards.
7. Testing the efficiency of the procedure through surface sampling.

(Vangroenweghe et al., 2009a; Hémonic et al., 2010; Laanen, 2011; Dewulf, 2014; Luyckx, 2016).

It is possible to check all surfaces simply and quickly for microbial contamination with the aid of pressure plates. These plates measure and quantify the presence of bacterial contamination (mostly: the presence of small parts of germs after cleaning and disinfection). The results are expressed in colony-forming units (CFU) per plate. Reference values used for such hygienograms in pig stables are provided in table 12.3 (Anonymous, 2017).

Table 12.3: Criteria for hygienograms (Anonymous, 2017)

Score	CFU per plate	Interpretation
0	0	Perfect
1	1-40	Very good
2	41-120	Good
3	121-400	Average
4	> 400	Poor
5	No count	Very poor

CFU= colony-forming unit

If all these steps are performed correctly it is not necessary to foresee an additional empty period to further reduce the infection load (Luycks et al., 2016).

For more details on cleaning and disinfection see chapter 6.

4 Conclusions

As illustrated above, biosecurity in pig production is a combination of many different measures aimed at preventing the introduction and spread of pathogens on farms. It forms the basis of any disease control programme. Although most of the measures to be implemented are logical and generally easy to apply, adhering to the measures in daily practice requires strong discipline. However, those who do so will surely see the benefits.

References

Alexandersen S., Knowles N.J., Dekker A., Belsham G.J., Zhang Z., Koenen F., 2012. Picornaviruses. In: Zimmermann J.J., Karriker L.A., Ramirez A., Schwartz K.J., Stevenson G.W. (Editors). Diseases of Swine. Wiley-Blackwell, Chichester, West Sussex, United Kingdom, 2150-2279.

Allaart J.G., van Asten A.J.A.M., Gröne A., 2013. Predisposing factors and prevention of Clostridium perfringens-associated enteritis. Comparative Immunology, Microbiology and Infectious Diseases 36, 449-464.

Alonso C., Murtaugh M., Dee S., Davies P., 2013. Epidemiological study of air filtration systems for preventing PRRSV infection in large sow herds. Preventive Veterinary Medicine 112, 109-117.

Althouse G.C. and Rossow K., 2011. The potential risk of infectious disease dissemination via artificial insemination in swine. Reproduction in Domestic Animals 46, 64-67.

Alvarez R.M., Amass S.F., Stevenson G.W., Spicer P.M., Anderson C., Ragland D., Grote L., Dowell C., Clark L.K., 2001. Evaluation of biosecurity protocols to prevent mechanical transmission of transmissible gastroenteritis virus of swine by pork production unit personnel. Pig Journal 48, 22-33.

Alvarez J., Goede D., Morrison R., Perez A., 2016. Spatial and temporal epidemiology of porcine epidemic diarrhoea (PED) in the Midwest and Southeast regions of the United States. Preventive Veterinary Medicine, 123, 155-160.

Amass S.F and Baysinger A., 2006. Swine disease transmission and prevention. In: Straw B.E., Zimmerman J.J., D'Allaire S., Taylor D.J. (editors). Diseases of Swine. 9th edition Blackwell Publishing Ltd., Oxford, UK, 1075-1098.

Amass S.F. and Clark L.K., 1999. Biosecurity considerations for pork production units. Journal of Swine Health and Production 7, 217-228.

Amass S.F., Clark L.K., Knox K., Wu C.C., Hill M.A., 1996. Streptococcus suis colonization of piglets during parturition. Journal of Swine Health and Production 4, 269-272.

Amass S.F., Halbur P.G., Byrne B.A., Schneider J.L., Koons C.W., Cornick N., Ragland D., 2003. Mechanical transmission of enterotoxigenic Escherichia coli to weaned pigs by people, and biosecurity procedures that prevented such transmission. Journal of Swine Health and Production 11, 61-68.

Amass S.F., Vyverberg B.D., Ragland D., Dowell C.A., Anderson C.D., Stover J.H., Beaudry D.J., 2000. Evaluating the efficacy of boot baths in biosecurity protocols. Journal of Swine Health and Production 8, 169-173.

Andres V.M. and Davies R.H., 2015. Biosecurity measures to control salmonella and other infectious agents in pig farms: a review. Comprehensive Reviews in Food Science and Food Safety 14, 317-335.

Anonymous, 2010. Food and Agriculture Organization of the United Nations/World Organisation for Animal Health/World Bank. Good practices for biosecurity in the pig sector – Issues and options in developing and transition countries. FAO Animal Production and Health Paper No. 169.

Anonymous, 2011. European Commission: Animals – Foot-and-mouth disease.

Anonymous, 2014. European Commission. Animals – Classical swine fever.

Anonymous, 2017. Diergezondheidszorg Vlaanderen: Hygiënogram varkensstal (in Dutch). Available at: http://www.dgz.be/hygi-nogram-varkensstal (accessed August 2017).

Aragon V., Segalés, J., Oliveira S., 2012. Glässer's disease. In: Zimmermann J.J., Karriker L.A., Ramirez A., Schwartz K.J., Stevenson G.W. (Editors). Diseases of Swine. Wiley-Blackwell, Chichester, West Sussex, United Kingdom, 2780-2805.

Artois M., Depner K.R., Guberti V., Hars J., Rossi S., Rutili D., 2002. Classical swine fever (hog cholera) in wild boar in Europe. Revue Scientifique et Technique 21, 287-303.

Assavacheep P. and Rycroft A.N., 2013. Survival of Actinobacillus pleuropneumoniae outside the pig. Research in Veterinary Science 94, 22-26.

Backhans A. and Fellstrom C., 2012. Rodents on pig and chicken farms – a potential threat to human and animal health. Infection Ecology & Economy 2, 17093.

Backhans A., Sjölund M., Lindberg A., Emanuelson U., 2015. Biosecurity level and health management practices in 60 Swedish farrow-to-finish herds. Acta Veterinaria Scandinavica 57, 14.

Barceló J. and Marco E., 1998. On-farm biosecurity. In: Proceedings of the 15th IPVS Congress, Birmingham, England, 5-9 July, 129-133.

Baroch J.A., Gagnon C.A., Lacouture S., Gottschalk M., 2015. Exposure of feral swine (Sus scrofa) in the United States to selected pathogens. Canadian Journal of Veterinary Research 79, 74-78.

Bender J.S., Shen H. G., Irwin C. K., Schwartz K. J., Opriessnig T., 2010. Characterization of Erysipelothrix species isolates from clinically affected pigs, environmental samples, and vaccine strains from six recent swine Erysipelas outbreaks in the United States. Clinical and Vaccine Immunology 17, 1605-1611.

Blunt R., McOrist S., McKillen J., McNair I., Jiang T., Mellits K., 2011. House fly vector for porcine circovirus 2b on commercial pig farms. Veterinary Microbiology 149, 452-455.

Boadella M., Ruiz-Fons J.F., Vicente J., Martín M., Segalés J., Gortazar C., 2012. Seroprevalence evolution of selected pathogens in Iberian wild boar. Transboundary and Emerging Diseases 59, 395-404.

Brockmeier S.L., Loving C.L., Mullins M.A., Register K.B., Nicholson T.L., Wiseman B.S., Baker R.B., Kehrli M.E., 2013. Virulence, transmission, and heterologous protection of four isolates of Haemophilus parasuis. Clinical and Vaccine Immunology 20, 1466-1472.

Brockmeier, S.L. Register K.B., Nicholson T.L., Loving C.L., 2012. Bordetellosis. In: Zimmermann J.J., Karriker L.A., Ramirez A., Schwartz K.J., Stevenson G.W. (Editors). Diseases of Swine. Wiley-Blackwell, Chichester, West Sussex, United Kingdom, 2446-2482.

Brookes V.J., Hernández-Jover M., Holyoake P., Ward M.P., 2015. Industry opinion on the likely routes of introduction of highly pathogenic porcine reproductive and respiratory syndrome into Australia from Southeast Asia. Australian Veterinary Journal 93, 13-19.

Callens B., Faes C., Maes D., Catry B., Boyen F., Francoys D., de Jong E., Haesebrouck F., Dewulf J., 2015. Presence of antimicrobial resistance and antimicrobial use in sows are risk factors for antimicrobial resistance in their offspring. Microbial Drug Resistance 21, 50-58.

Calvar C., Heugebaert S., Caille M.E., Roy H., 2012. La quarantaine. Des préconisations de techniciens diversifiés. Des conduits multiples chez de très bons éleveurs. Rapport d'étude, Chambres d'agriculture de Bretagne.

Cameron R., 2012. Integumentary system: Skin, hoof, and claw. In: Zimmermann J.J., Karriker L.A., Ramirez A., Schwartz K.J., Stevenson G.W. (Editors), Diseases of Swine. Wiley-Blackwell, Chichester, West Sussex, United Kingdom, 926-991.

12

Carlson S.A., Barnhill A.E., Griffith R.W., 2012. Salmonellosis. In: Zimmermann J.J., Karriker L.A., Ramirez A., Schwartz K.J., Stevenson G.W. (Editors). Diseases of Swine. Wiley-Blackwell, Chichester, West Sussex, United Kingdom, 3013-3058.

Carmo L.P., Schuepbach-Regula G., Muentener C., Chevance A., Moulin G., Magouras I., 2017. Approaches for quantifying antimicrobial consumption per animal species based on national sales data: a Swiss example (2006-2013). Eurosurveillance 22, 30458.

Clark L., Freeman M., Scheidt A., Knox K., 1991. Investigating the transmission of Mycoplasma hyopneumoniae in a swine herd with enzootic pneumonia. Veterinary Medicine 86, 543-550.

Collineau L., Rojo-Gimeno C., Léger A., Backhans A., Loesken, S., Okholm Nielsen, E., Postma M., Emanuelson, U., Grosse Beilage, E., Sjölund, M., Wauters, E., Stärk K.D.C., Dewulf J., Belloc C., Krebs S., 2017. Herd-specific interventions to reduce antimicrobial usage in pig production without jeopardising technical and economic performance. Preventive Veterinary Medicine 144, 167-178.

Corn J.L., Cumbee J.C., Barfoot R., Erickson G.A., 2009. Pathogen exposure in feral swine populations geographically associated with high densities of transitional swine premises and commercial swine production. Journal of Wildlife Diseases 45, 713-721.

Cornick N.A. and VuKhac H., 2008. Indirect transmission of Escherichia coli O157:H7 occurs readily among swine but not among sheep. Applied Environmental Microbiology 74, 2488-2491.

Corrégé I., 2002. Problématique de l'introduction des reproducteurs. Techniporc 25, 27-30.

Corrégé I., Fourchon P., Le Brun T., Berthelot N., 2012. Biosécurité et hygiène en élevage de porcs: état des lieux et impact sur les performances technico-économiques. Journées Recherche Porcine 44, 101-102.

Cságola A., Cadar D., Tuboly T., 2008. Replication and transmission of porcine circovirus type 2 in mice. Acta Veterinaria Hungarica 56, 421-427.

Dee S., Otake S., Oliveira S., Deen J., 2009. Evidence of long distance airborne transport of porcine reproductive and respiratory syndrome virus and Mycoplasma hyopneumoniae. Veterinary Research 40, 1-13.

Dekker A., 2011. Biosecurity and FMD transmission. Veterinary Record 168, 126-127.

Desrosiers R., 2011. Transmission of swine pathogens: different means, different needs. Animal Health Research Reviews 12, 1-13.

Dewulf J., 2014. An online risk-based biosecurity scoring system for pig farms. Veterinary Ireland Journal 4, 426-429.

Dewulf J., Tuyttens F., Lauwers L., Van Huylenbroeck G., Maes D., 2007. De invloed van de hokbezettingsdichtheid bij vleesvarkens op productie, gezondheid en welzijn. Vlaams Diergeneeskundig Tijdschrift 76, 410-416.

Duinhof T., Van de Ven S.C.G., Van Schaik G., 2006. A survey among veterinarians and pig farmers in the Netherlands: more focus needed on diagnostic approach and on-farm contact structures in the control of prrs. Proceedings of the 19th IPVS Congress, Copenhagen, Denmark, 2006 Volume 1 p. 234.

Dutch Government, Besluit houders van dieren, 05/06/2014. Accessed at 24/08/2017: http://wetten.overheid.nl/BWBR0035217/2017-01-01

Eijck I.A.J.M., 2003. Gezond starten, gezond blijven. Praktijkonderzoek veehouderij, Animal Science Group, Wageningen.

Ellis W.A., 2012. Leptospirosis. In: Zimmermann J.J., Karriker L.A., Ramirez A., Schwartz K.J., Stevenson G.W. (Editors). Diseases of Swine. Wiley-Blackwell, Chichester, West Sussex, United Kingdom, 2976-3012.

Ellis-Iversen J, Smith R.P., Gibbens J.C., Sharpe C.E., Dominguez M., Cook A.J., 2011. Risk factors for transmission of foot-and-mouth disease during an outbreak in southern England in 2007. Veterinary Record 168, 128.

Evans S.J. and Sayer A.R., 2000. A longitudinal study of Campylobacter infection of broiler flocks in Great Britain. Preventive Veterinary Medicine 46, 209-223.

European Commission, 2008. Council Directive 2008/120/EC of 18 December 2008 on laying down minimum standards for the protection of pigs. In European Commission (editors), 2008/120/EC. Official Journal of the European Communities, Brussels, Belgium.

Fablet C., Marois C., Kuntz-Simon G., Rose N., Dorenlor V., Eono F., Eveno E., Jolly J.P., Le Devendec L., Tocqueville V., Quéguiner S., Gorin S., Kobisch M., Madec F., 2011. Longitudinal study of respiratory infection patterns of breeding sows in five farrow-to-finish herds. Veterinary Microbiology 147, 329-339.

Fairbrother J.M. and Gyles C.L., 2012. Colibacillosis. In: Zimmermann J.J., Karriker L.A., Ramirez A., Schwartz K.J., Stevenson G.W. (Editors). Diseases of Swine. Wiley-Blackwell, Chichester, West Sussex, United Kingdom, 2649-2745.

Fèvre E.M., Bronsvoort B.M.C., Hamilton K.A., Cleaveland S., 2006. Animal movements and the spread of infectious diseases. Trends in Microbiology 14, 125-131.

Filippitzi M., Callens B., Pardon B., Persoons D., & Dewulf J., 2014. Antimicrobial use in pigs, broilers and veal calves in Belgium. Vlaams Diergeneeskundig Tijdschrift, 83, 215-224.

Filippitzi M.E., Kruse A.B., Postma M., Sarrazin S., Maes D., Alban L., Nielsen L.R., Dewulf J., 2017. Review of transmission routes of 24 infectious diseases preventable by biosecurity measures and comparison of the implementation of these measures in pig herds in six European countries. Transboundary and Emerging Diseases (Early View). DOI: https://doi.org/10.1111/tbed.12758.

Friedman M., Bednář V., Klimeš J., Smola J., Mrlík V., Literák I., 2008. Lawsonia intracellularis in rodents from pig farms with the occurrence of porcine proliferative enteropathy. Letters in Applied Microbiology 47, 117-121.

Fritzemeier J., Teuffert J., Greiser-Wilke I., Staubach Ch., Schlüter H., Moennig V., 2000. Epidemiology of classical swine fever in Germany in the 1990s. Veterinary Microbiology 77, 29-41.

Fukai K., Yamada M., Morioka K., Seiichi O., Yoshida K., Kitano R., Yamazoe R., Kanno T., 2015. Dose-dependent responses of pigs infected with foot-and-mouth disease virus O/JPN/2010 by the intranasal and intraoral routes. Archives of Virology 160, 129-139.

Fussing V., Barfod K., Nielsen R., Møller K., Nielsen J.P., Wegener H.C., Bisgaard M., 1998. Evaluation and application of ribotyping for epidemiological studies of Actinobacillus pleuropneumoniae in Denmark. Veterinary Microbiology 62, 145-162.

Gelaude P., Schlepers M., Verlinden M., Laanen M., Dewulf J., 2014. Biocheck.UGent: a quantitative tool to measure biosecurity at broiler farms and the relationship with technical performances and antimicrobial use. Poultry Science 93, 2740-2751.

Goodwin R.F.W., 1985. Apparent reinfection of enzootic-pneumonia-free pig herds: search for possible causes. The Veterinary Record 116, 690-694.

12

Gottschalk M., 2012a. Actinobacillosis. In: Zimmermann J.J., Karriker L.A., Ramirez A., Schwartz K.J., Stevenson G.W. (Editors), Diseases of Swine. Wiley-Blackwell, Chichester, West Sussex, United Kingdom, 2383-2445.

Gottschalk M., 2012b. Streptococcis. In: Zimmermann, J.J., Karriker, L.A., Ramirez, A., Schwartz, K.J., Stevenson, G.W. (Eds.), Diseases of Swine. Wiley-Blackwell, Chichester, West Sussex, United Kingdom, 3083-3141.

Hampson D.J., 2012. Brachyspiral colitis. In: Zimmermann, J.J., Karriker, L.A., Ramirez, A., Schwartz, K.J., Stevenson, G.W. (Editors). Diseases of Swine. Wiley-Blackwell, Chichester, West Sussex, United Kingdom, 2483-2549.

Hamilton D., Ellis M., Wolters B., Schninckel A., Wilson R., 2003. The growth performance of the progeny of two swine sire lines reared under different floor space allowances. Journal of Animal Science 81, 1126-1135.

Hartung J., 2005. Zur Abschirmung von Beständen aus tierhygienischer Sicht. Deutsche Tierärztliche Wochenschrift 112, 313-316.

Hege R., Zimmermann W., Scheidegger R., Stärk K.D.C., 2002. Incidence of reinfections with Mycoplasma hyopneumoniae and Actinobaillus pleuropneumoniae in pig farms located in respiratory-disease-free regions of Switzerland – identification and quantification of risk factors. Acta Veterinaria Scandinavica 43, 145-156.

Hémonic A., Corrégé I., Lanneshoa M., 2010. Quelles sont les pratiques de biosécurité et d'hygiène en élevages de porcs? TechniPorc 33, 7-13.

Hernández-Jover M., Cogger N., Marti P.A.J., Schembri N., Holyoake P.K., Toribio J.A.L.M.L., 2011. Evaluation of post-farm-gate passive surveillance in swine for the detection of foot-and-mouth disease in Australia. Preventive Veterinary Medicine 100, 171-186.

Horst H.S., Huirne R.R., Dijkhuizen A.A., 1997. Risks and economic consequences of introducing classical swine fever into the Netherlands by feeding swill to swine. Revue Scientifique et Technique 16, 207-214.

Huijsdens X.W., Van Dijke B.J., Spalburg E., Van Santen-Verheuvel M.G., Heck M.E., Pluister G.N., Voss A., Wannet W.J., De Neeling A.J., 2006. Community-acquired MRSA and pig-farming. Annals of Clinical Microbiology and Antimicrobials 5.

Johnson A.K., Edwards L.N., Niekamp S.R., Philips C.E., Sutherland M.A., Torrey S., Casey-Trott T., Tucker A.L., Widowski T., 2012. Behaviour and welfare. In: Zimmermann J.J., Karriker L.A., Ramirez A., Schwartz K.J., Stevenson G.W. (Editors), Diseases of Swine. Wiley-Blackwell, Chichester, West Sussex, United Kingdom, 180-249.

Kirwan P., 2008. Biosecurity in the pig industry – an overview. Cattle Practice 16, 147-154.

Laanen M., 2011. Waarop letten voor meer bioveiligheid? Varkensbedrijf 11, 30-33.

Laanen M., Beek J., Ribbens S., Vangroenweghe F., Maes D., Dewulf J., 2010. Bioveiligheid op varkensbedrijven: ontwikkeling van een online scoresysteem en de resultaten van de eerste 99 deelnemende bedrijven. Vlaams Diergeneeskundig Tijdschrift 79, 302-306.

Laanen M., Persoons M., Ribbens S., de Jong E., Callens B., Strubbe M., Maes D., Dewulf J., 2013. Relationship between biosecurity and production/antimicrobial treatment characteristics in pig herds. The Veterinary Journal 198, 508-512.

Lister S.A., 2008. Biosecurity in poultry management. M. Patisson, P. F. McMullin, J. M. Bradburry, Alexander D.J., ed. p. 48-65 in Poultry Diseases. 6th edition Saunders Elsevier, Beijing, China.

Lo Fo Wong D.M.A., Dahl J., Stege H., van der Wolf P.J., Leontides L., von Altrock A., Thorberg B.M., 2004. Herd-level risk factors for subclinical Salmonella infection in European finishing-pig herds. Preventive Veterinary Medicine 62, 253-266.

Loera-Muro V.M., Jacques M., Tremblay Y.D.N., Avelar-González F.J., Loera-Muro A., Ramírez-López E.M., Medina-Figueroa A., González-Reynaga H.M., GuerreroBarrera A.L., 2013. Detection of Actinobacillus pleuropneumoniae in drinking water from pig farms. Microbiology 159, 536-544.

Luyckx, K., 2016. Evaluation and implication of cleaning and disinfection of broiler houses and pig nursery units. Ghent University. Faculty of Veterinary Medicine, Merelbeke, Belgium.

Maes D., 2016. Bedrijfsdiergeneeskunde varken. Universiteit Gent, Faculteit Diergeneeskunde. Hoofstuk 8: Hygiëne, 377-395.

Maes D., Deluyker H., Verdonck M., Castryck F., Miry C., Vrijens B., de Kruif A., 2000a. Herd factors associated with the seroprevalences of four major respiratory pathogens in slaughter pigs from farrow-to-finish pig herds. Veterinary Research 31, 313-327.

Maes D., Deluyker H., Verdonck M., Castryck F., Miry C., Vrijens B., Ducatelle R., de Kruif A., 2000b. Non-infectious herd factors associated with macroscopic and microscopic lung lesions in slaughter pigs from farrow-to-finish pig herds. The Veterinary Record 148, 41-46.

Maes D., Segales J., Meyns T., Sibila M., Pieters M., Haesebrouck F., 2008. Control of Mycoplasma hyopneumoniae infections in pigs. Veterinary Microbiology 126, 297-309.

Marinou K.A., Papatsiros V.G., Gkotsopoulos E.K., Odatzoglou P.K., Athanasiou L.V., 2015. Exposure of extensively farmed wild boars (Sus scrofa scrofa) to selected pig pathogens in Greece. Veterinary Quarterly 35, 97-101.

McOrist S., Gebhart C.J., 2012. Proliferative enteropathy. In: Zimmermann J.J., Karriker L.A., Ramirez A., Schwartz K.J., Stevenson G.W. (Editors). Diseases of Swine. WileyBlackwell, Chichester, West Sussex, United Kingdom, 2976-3013.

McQuiston J.H., Garber L.P., Porter-Spalding B.A., Hahn F.W., Pierson S.H., Wainwright S.H., Senne D.A., Brignole T.J., Akey B.L., Holt T.J., 2005. Evaluation of risk factors for the spread of low-pathogenicity H7N2 avian influenza virus among commercial poultry farms. Journal of the American Veterinary Medical Association 226, 767-772.

Meroz M. and Samberg Y., 1995. Disinfecting poultry production premises. Revue Scientifique et Technique (Office International des Epizooties) 14, 273-291.

Mintiens K., Laevens H., Dewulf J., Boelaert F., Verloo D., Koenen F., 2003. Risk analysis of the spread of classical swine fever virus through 'neighbourhood infections' for different regions in Belgium. Preventive Veterinary Medicine 60, 27-36.

Mohamed F., Swafford S., Petrowski H., Bracht A., Schmit B., Fabian A., Pacheco J.M., Hartwig E., Berninger M., Carrillo C., Mayr G., Moran K., Kavanaugh D., Leibrecht H., White W., Metwally S., 2011. Foot-and-mouth disease in feral swine: susceptibility and transmission. Transboundary and Emerging Diseases 58, 358-371.

Mettenleiter T.C., Ehlers B., Müller T., Yoon K.-J., Teifke J.P., 2012. Herpesviruses. In: Zimmermann J.J., Karriker L.A., Ramirez A., Schwartz K.J., Stevenson G.W. (Editors). Diseases of Swine. Wiley-Blackwell, Chichester, West Sussex, United Kingdom, 1534-1625.

Miao L.-f., Zhang C.-f., Chen C.-m., Cui S.-j., 2009. Real-time PCR to detect and analyze virulent PPV loads in artificially challenged sows and their fetuses. Veterinary Microbiology 138, 145-149.

Moore C., 1992. Biosecurity and minimal disease herds. Food Animal Practice 8, 461-474.

12

Muñoz-González S., Ruggli N., Rosell R., Pérez L.J., Frías-Leuporeau M.T., Fraile L., Montoya M., Cordoba L., Domingo M., Ehrensperger F., Summerfield A., Ganges L., 2015. Postnatal persistent infection with classical swine fever virus and its immunological implications. PLoS One 10, e0125692.

Nathues H., Woeste H., Doehring S., Fahrion A.S., Doherr M.G., Grosse Beilage E., 2012. Detection of Mycoplasma hyopneumoniae in nasal swabs sampled from pig farmers. Veterinary Record 170, 623.

Neumann E.J., 2012. Disease transmission and biosecurity. In: Zimmerman J.J., Karriker L.A., Ramirez A., Schwartz K.J., Stevenson G.W. (editors), Diseases of Swine. 10th edition John Wiley & Sons Inc., Iowa, USA, 141-164.

Nicholson T.L., Brockmeier S.L., Loving C.L., Register K.B., Kehrli M.E., Stibitz S.E., Shore S.M., 2012. Phenotypic modulation of the virulent Bvg phase is not required for pathogenesis and transmission of Bordetella bronchiseptica in swine. Infection and Immunity 80, 1025-1036.

Olsen S.C., Garin-Bastuij B., Blasco J.M., Nicola A.M., Samartino L., 2012. Brucellosis. In: Zimmermann J.J., Karriker L.A., Ramirez A., Schwartz K.J., Stevenson G.W. (Editors). Diseases of Swine. Wiley-Blackwell, Chichester, West Sussex, United Kingdom, 2550-2594.

Opriessnig T., Patterson A.R., Meng X.-J., Halbur P.G., 2009. Porcine circovirus type 2 in muscle and bone marrow is infectious and transmissible to naïve pigs by oral consumption. Veterinary Microbiology 133, 54-64.

Opriessnig T. and Wood R.L., 2012. Erysipelas. In: Zimmermann J.J., Karriker L.A., Ramirez A., Schwartz K.J., Stevenson G.W. (Editors). Diseases of Swine. Wiley-Blackwell, Chichester, West Sussex, United Kingdom, 2746-2779.

Pacheco J.M., Tucker M., Hartwig E., Bishop E., Arzt J., Rodriguez L.L., 2012. Direct contact transmission of three different foot-and-mouth disease virus strains in swine demonstrates important strain-specific differences. Veterinary Journal 193, 456-463.

Pasick J., Berhane Y., Ojkic D., Maxie G., Embury-Hyatt C., Swekla K., Handel K., Fairles J., Alexandersen S., 2014. Investigation into the Role of Potentially Contaminated Feed as a Source of the First-Detected Outbreaks of Porcine Epidemic Diarrhea in Canada. Transboundary and Emerging Diseases 61, 397-410.

Patterson A.R., Ramamoorthy S., Madson D.M., Meng X.J., Halbur P.G., Opriessnig T., 2011. Shedding and infection dynamics of porcine circovirus type 2 (PCV2) after experimental infection. Veterinary Microbioly 149, 91-98.

Pearson H.E., Toribio J.A., Lapidge S.J., Hernández-Jover M., 2016. Evaluating the risk of pathogen transmission from wild animals to domestic pigs in Australia. Preventive Veterinary Medicine 123, 39-51.

Pinheiro A.L.B.C., Bulos L.H.S., Onofre T.S., de Paula Gabardo M., de Carvalho O.V., Fausto M.C., Guedes R.M.C., de Almeida M.R., Silva Júnior A., 2013. Verification of natural infection of peridomestic rodents by PCV2 on commercial swine farms. Research in Veterinary Science 94, 764-768.

Pointon A., Heap P., McCloud P., 1985. Enzootic pneumonia of pigs in South Australia—factors relating to incidence of disease. Australian Veterinary Journal 62, 98-100.

Postma M., Backhans A., Collineau L., Loesken S., Sjölund M., Belloc C., Emanuelson U., Grosse Beilage E., Stärk K.D.C., J., D., 2016. The biosecurity status and its associations with production and management characteristics in farrow-to-finish pig herds. Animal 10, 478-489.

Pritchard G., Dennis I., Waddilove J., 2005. Biosecurity: reducing disease risks to pig breeding herds. In Practice 27, 230-237.

Rajkowski K.T., Eblen S., Laubauch C., 1998. Efficacy of washing and sanitizing trailers used for swine transport in reduction of Salmonella and Escherichia coli. Journal of Food Protection 61, 31-35.

Reddy S., Montambault J., Masuda Y.J., Keenan E., Butler W., Fisher J.R.B., Asah S.T., Gneezy A., 2017. Advancing conservation by understanding and influencing human behavior. Conservation Letters 10, 248-256.

Register K.B., Brockmeier S.L., de Jong M.F., Pijoan C., 2012. Pasteurellosis. In: Zimmermann J.J., Karriker L.A., Ramirez A., Schwartz K.J., Stevenson G.W. (Editors). Diseases of Swine. Wiley-Blackwell, Chichester, West Sussex, United Kingdom, 2924-2975.

Ribbens S., Dewulf J., Koenen F., Maes D., De Kruif A., 2007. Evidence of indirect transmission of classical swine fever virus through contact with people. The Veterinary Record 160, 687-690.

Rojo-Gimeno C., Postma M., Dewulf J., Hogeveen H., Lauwers L., Wauters E., 2016. Farm-economic analysis of reducing antimicrobial use whilst adopting improved management strategies on farrow-to-finish pig farms. Preventive Veterinary Medicine. 129, 74-87.

Rose N. and Madec F., 2002. Occurrence of respiratory disease outbreaks in fattening pigs: Relation with the features of a densely and a sparsely populated pig area in France. Veterinary Research 33, 179-190.

Saif L.J., Pensaert M.B., Sestak K., Yeo S.-G., Jung K., 2012. Coronaviruses. In: Zimmermann J.J., Karriker L.A., Ramirez A., Schwartz K.J., Stevenson G.W. (Editors). Diseases of Swine. Wiley-Blackwell, Chichester, West Sussex, United Kingdom, 1821-1914.

Schembri N., Hernández-Jover M., Toribio J.A., Holyoake P.K., 2010. Feeding of prohibited substances (swill) to pigs in Australia. Australian Veterinary Journal 88, 294300.

Schijven J., Rijs G.B.J., De Roda Husman A.M., 2005. Quantitative risk assessment of FMD virus transmission via water. Risk Analysis 25, 13-21.

Scott A., McCluskey B., Brown-Reid M., Grear D., Pitcher P., Ramos G., Spencer D., Singrey A., 2016. Porcine epidemic diarrhoea virus introduction into the United States: root cause investigation. Preventive Veterinary Medicine 123, 192-201.

Segalés J., Allen G.M., Domingo M., 2012. Porcine circoviruses. In: Zimmermann J.J., Karriker L.A., Ramirez A., Schwartz K.J., Stevenson G.W. (Editors). Diseases of Swine. Wiley-Blackwell, Chichester, West Sussex, United Kingdom, 1470-1522.

Segalés J., Allan G.M., Domingo M., 2005. Porcine circovirus diseases. Animal Health Research Reviews 6, 119-142.

Sellers R.F., Donaldson A.I., Herniman K.A.J., 1970. Inhalation, persistence and dispersal of foot-and-mouth disease virus by man. Journal of Hygiene 68, 565-573.

Siekkinen K.M., Heikkilä J., Tammiranta N., Rosengren H., 2012. Measuring the costs of biosecurity on poultry farms: a case study in broiler production in Finland. Acta Veterinaria Scandinavica 54, 12.

Sliz I., Vlasakova M., Jackova A., Vilcek S., 2015. Characterization of porcine parvovirus type 3 and porcine circovirus type 2 in wild boars (sus scrofa) in Slovakia. Journal of Wildlife Diseases 51, 703-711.

12

Songer J.G., 2012. Clostridiosis. In: Zimmermann J.J., Karriker L.A., Ramirez A., Schwartz K.J., Stevenson G.W. (Editors). Diseases of Swine. Wiley-Blackwell, Chichester, West Sussex, United Kingdom, 2595-2648.

Stärk K., 2000. Epidemiological investigation of the influence of environmental risk factors on respiratory disease in swine. The Veterinary Journal 159, 37-56.

Thacker E. and Minion F.C., 2012. Mycoplasma hyopneumoniae. In: Zimmermann J.J., Karriker L.A., Ramirez A., Schwartz K.J., Stevenson G.W. (Editors). Diseases of Swine. Wiley-Blackwell, Chichester, West Sussex, United Kingdom, 2850-2923.

Thakur K.K., Sanchez J., Hurnik D., Poljak Z., Opps S., Revie C.W., 2015. Development of a network-based model to simulate the between-farm transmission of the porcine reproductive and respiratory syndrome virus. Veterinary Microbiology 180, 212-222.

Tobias T.J., Bouma A., van den Broek J., van Nes A., Daemen A.J.J.M., Wagenaar J.A., Stegeman J.A., Klinkenberg D., 2014. Transmission of Actinobacillus pleuropneumoniae among weaned piglets on endemically infected farms. Preventive Veterinary Medicine 117, 207-214.

Truyen U. and Streck, A.F., 2012. Porcine parvovirus. In: Zimmermann J.J., Karriker L.A., Ramirez A., Schwartz K.J., Stevenson G.W. (Editors). Diseases of Swine. Wiley-Blackwell, Chichester, West Sussex, United Kingdom, 1626-1657.

Vangroenweghe F., Ribbens S., Vandersmissen T., Beek J., Dewulf J., Maes D., Castryck F., 2009. Keeping Pigs Healthy (in Dutch). 1st editor F. Vangroenweghe, DCL Print & Signs, Zelzate, Belgium.

Van Reeth K., Brown I.H., Olsen C.W., 2012. Influenza virus. In: Zimmermann J.J., Karriker L.A. Ramirez, A., Schwartz K.J., Stevenson G.W. (Editors). Diseases of Swine. Wiley-Blackwell, Chichester, West Sussex, United Kingdom, 2036-2095.

Wentworth D.E., McGregor M.W., Macklin M.D., Neumann V., Hinshaw V.S., 1997. Transmission of swine influenza virus to humans after exposure to experimentally infected pigs. Journal of Infectious Diseases. 175, 7-15.

Windsor R.S. and Simmons J.R., 1981. Investigation into the spread of swine dysentery in 25 herds in East Anglia and assessment of its economic significance in five herds. The Veterinary Record 109, 482-484.

Woeste K., Grosse Beilage E., 2007. Transmission of agents of the porcine respiratory disease complex (PRDC) between swine herds: a review, Part 1 – diagnostics, pathogens transmission via pig movement. Berliner und Münchener Tierärztliche Wochenschrift 114, 324-337.

Wu N., Abril C., Thomann A., Grosclaude E., Doherr M.G., Boujon P., Ryser-Degiorgis M.-P., 2012. Risk factors for contact between wild boar and outdoor pigs in Switzerland and investigations into potential Brucella suis spill-over. BMC Veterinary Research 8, 116.

Zimmerman J.J., Benfield D.A., Dee S.A., Murtaugh M.P., Stadejek T., Stevenson G.W., Torremorell M., 2012. Porcine Reproductive and Respiratory Syndrome virus. In: Zimmermann J.J., Karriker L.A., Ramirez A., Schwartz K.J., Stevenson G.W. (editors), Diseases of Swine. Wiley-Blackwell, Chichester, West Sussex, United Kingdom, 1675-1777.

CHAPTER 13

TRANSMISSION OF POULTRY DISEASES AND BIOSECURITY IN POULTRY PRODUCTION

Hilde Van Meirhaeghe[1]

Anna Schwarz[3]

Jeroen Dewulf[2]

Filip Van Immerseel[3]

Bo Vanbeselaere[4]

Maarten De Gussem[1]

[1] Vetworks, 9880 Poeke, Belgium
[2] Faculty of Veterinary Medicine, Department of Obstetrics, Reproduction and Herd Health, Veterinary Epidemiology Unit, University of Ghent, 9820 Merelbeke, Belgium
[3] Faculty of Veterinary Medicine, Department of Obstetrics, Bacteriology and Avian Diseases, University of Ghent, 9820 Merelbeke, Belgium
[4] CID LINES NV, 8900 Ieper, Belgium

1 Introduction

1.1 Poultry production

In poultry production today disease control is mainly based on prevention. Prophylactic use of antibiotics should be limited because of the risk of antimicrobial resistance. The mainstays of disease prevention are vaccination programmes, good management and biosecurity (Butcher and Miles, 2012). Since the 1950s breeder companies have selected genetic lines to optimise meat and egg production (Anthony, 1998; Vaillancourt and Carver, 1998; Graham et al., 2008; Butcher and Miles, 2012). Genetic progress is very fast because females are able to produce many eggs and the generation interval is short. Only a few breeder companies operate globally and select pedigree birds. They produce lines of Great Grand Parents – GGP, these are mated to produce Grand Parents -GP, who produce Parent stock. These parent birds produce birds for production: broilers for meat and layers for egg production. This is called the poultry production pyramid (see Fig. 13.1) (Anthony, 1998; Pym, 2013; European Commission, 2016). The value of pedigree birds is easily 1000 times higher than that of parent stock and 10,000 times higher than that of broilers. The upper part of the pyramid from the pedigree birds to grandparents is generally occupied by breeder companies and contains very valuable animals, and as such disease prevention is a top priority; biosecurity rules are very strict in these farms. Parent stock, broilers and layers are mainly owned by integrations or private farmers. The implementation of biosecurity on these farms is not always adequate (Hiemstra and Napel, 2013). Other special features of poultry production include artificial incubation, usually in the hatchery, and intensive mass production in broiler and layer farms.

Fig. 13.1: Poultry production structure: Broilers (left) and Layers (right)
(adapted from Pym, 2013)

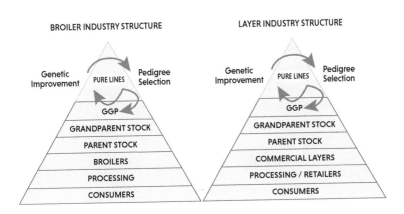

The poultry production process can be set up as an integrated system, or a non-integrated system. When choosing the integration approach the same company controls the whole production chain from parent stock, hatchery to production animals. The feed mills and processing plants also sometimes form part of the same company. In a non-integrated system farmers choose freely to work with different hatcheries, feed mills and slaughter houses. It is obvious that it is easier to impose biosecurity rules in integrated systems (Gillespie and Flanders, 2009; Hiemstra and Napel, 2013).

1.2 Disease transmission: horizontal and vertical

Most poultry diseases are transmitted horizontally from one infected bird to the other or, what is often more important, through mechanical carriers and people. Vertical transmission occurs when the pathogen infects the reproductive organs and is incorporated in the eggs and the embryo is born infected (Pattinson et al., 2008; Butcher and Miles, 2012; de Gussem et al., 2013). In commercial poultry operations eggs from different breeder flocks are hatched together, so horizontal spread of pathogens from vertically infected eggs may already start in the hatchery. Hatched chicks are often also transported over long distances bringing vertically transmitted pathogens to new farms. *Mycoplasma* and *Salmonella* are the most important examples of vertically transmitted pathogens and standard control programmes are implemented in breeders to protect the offspring (Hafez, 2007; Leon, 2015). In table 1 the most important poultry pathogens, their transmission route and persistence in the environment are listed.

Table 13.1: Transmission and persistence in the environment of the most important poultry diseases

Disease	Vertical transmission	Horizontal transmission	Horizontal spread	Persistence in the environment
Mycoplasma spp.	yes	yes	slow	low
Salmonella	yes	yes	fast	high
Avian influenza	?	yes	very fast	low
Newcastle disease	no	yes	fast	low
Infectious laryngotracheitis	no	yes	fast	low
Infectious bronchitis	no	yes	fast	low
Turkey rhinotracheitis	?	yes	medium	low
Fowl pox	no	yes	slow	high
Aspergillus	no	no	Environmental contamination	high
Pasteurellosis	no	yes	medium	low
Avibacterium paragallinarum	no	yes	fast	low
Ornithobacterium rhinotracheale	?	yes	fast	high
Escherichia coli	no	yes	fast	high
Gallibacterium anatis	no	yes	medium	low
Chlamidia psittaci	no	yes	medium	high
Gumboro	no	yes	fast	high
Marek disease	no	yes	medium	high
Coccidiosis	no	yes	fast	high
Worms	no	yes	medium	high
Clostridium Perfringens	no	yes	medium	high
Avian encephalomyelitis	yes	yes	fast	high

2 General biosecurity principles

The intensification of poultry production, with bigger farms and higher bird densities, has increased the level of infection pressure in poultry farms, resulting in higher risk of endemic and epidemic diseases with substantial economic consequences. Biosecurity in poultry production is the most effective and economic way to control poultry diseases (Butcher and Miles, 2012; Gelaude et al., 2014). Basic rules of biosecurity for any poultry unit include correct choice of geographical location of the farm, proper design of the buildings and positioning of equipment, well-planned operational protocols, focusing on potential sources of infection and the flow of people, materials, feed, eggs and flocks to and from the farm. When designing successful biosecurity programmes it is important to include education of all personnel involved in the operations of the unit.

2.1 Geographical location of the poultry farm

There are a few basic elements to take into consideration when setting up a poultry farm. First of all, it is essential to be aware of the location of all farming units in the planned area. The best strategy when building the new farm is to keep as far away from any other commercial (poultry) farming units and also processing plants as possible. This will limit natural transmission of pathogens. It is also essential to be aware of the prevailing wind currents (Nespeca et al., 1997; Graham et al., 2008; Vieira et al., 2009; Lister, 2008). This will help when designing an effective and economic ventilation programme, as many pathogens are air-borne and may be carried on the wind (Hartung and Schulz, 2007). Wild birds can be an important source of infection, and areas with a lot of forest or water, around lakes, rivers or moors should be avoided therefore (Kapperud et al., 1993; East, 2007; Charisis, 2008; Lister, 2008; Sims, 2008; Van Steenwinkel et al., 2011).

13

Fig. 13.2: Gates at the entrance of the farm where it is clearly marked that no access is allowed without permission. Guard dogs are only allowed if they are not permitted into the houses.

▼

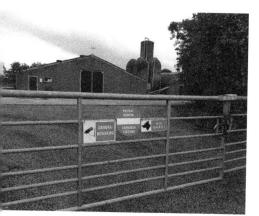

2.2 Structural layout of the poultry farm and buildings

Ideally, the buildings should be as far away as possible from roads, along which poultry, feed or litter are transported (De Gussem et al., 2013). The whole farm should be fenced off, access should only be via the gates (Fig. 13.2) where everything entering and leaving the farm is recorded and where all vehicles can be disinfected (Nespeca et al., 1997; Sims, 2008; Van Steenwinkel et al., 2011; De Gussem et al., 2013).

Within the unit, there should be a clear separation of the dirty (outside world) and the clean areas, where the animals are kept (Fig. 13.3 floor plan). The dirty route should be used by trucks to unload the feed or to pick up dead birds, without coming into the close vicinity of the broiler house (Al-Saffar et al., 2006; De Gussem et al., 2013; Ssematimba et al., 2013). The immediate area around the poultry house should be kept clean and free of any vegetation (Nespeca et al., 1997; Charisis, 2008; Lister, 2008; Anonymous, 2010; De Gussem et al., 2013).

Fig. 13.3: Floor plan of a broiler farm. The clean and dirty roads should be separated. Entry to the house should be via the clean road, while the gate of the poultry house for chick delivery and loading should be via the dirty road. Feed bins and fan-outlets should also be positioned along the dirty road.

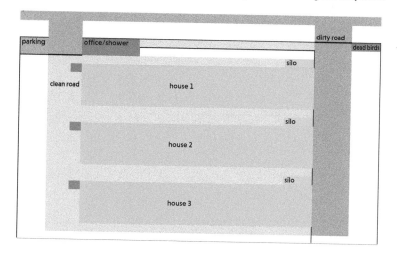

The buildings should be secure from wild birds, rodents and insects that may be carriers of *Salmonella*, *Mycoplasma* and other diseases (Lister, 2008; Gelaude et al., 2014). The entrance to the buildings should be made of solid and cleanable surfaces. Soil contains a lot of organic material, where pathogens can survive longer and can easily be carried inside the house. A 'hygiene lock' must be provided at the entrance of each building (Fig. 13.4), with a clear separation between clean and dirty section, a wash basin to wash and disinfect hands and clean clothes and footwear (Evans and Sayer, 2000; Bestman et al., 2012).

Litter and feed storage should be free of wild birds and vermin. Silos for feed storage must be clean and sealed (Nespeca et al., 1997; Charisis, 2008; Lister, 2008; Anonymous, 2010; Van Steenwinkel et al., 2011). The whole building and equipment should be conceived in order to allow for easy and efficient cleaning and disinfection. Floors and walls must be smooth and without cracks, the floor should ideally be covered with concrete. Feeding and water lines should be easy to disinfect.

An important biosecurity risk is having flocks of different ages on one site. The objective should be for single age and all-in all-out, but this is not always feasible. Older birds can be asymptomatic carriers of pathogens such as *Salmonella*, Gumboro, *Mycoplasma*, Newcastle and Infectious Bronchitis virus which can infect younger birds that have not yet developed a resistance to these germs (Nespeca et al., 1997; East et al., 2006; East, 2007; de Gussem et al., 2013). Bringing new birds from outside, for example in case of spiking (= introducing new males in a breeder flock) is associated with a high biosecurity risk (Jones, 2009; Woodger and Wirral, 2009; Ssematimba et al., 2013; De Gussem et al., 2013). During the sanitary void between flocks the houses should be cleaned, rinsed and disinfected, and this can only be done efficiently on farms if all houses are empty at the same time.

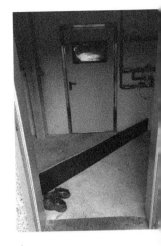

▲

Fig. 13.4: Example of a basic hygiene lock with a clear physical separation between the clean and the dirty sections. Ideally this hygiene lock should be a bit larger and the separation between clean and dirty areas should be made of material that is easy to clean and disinfect.

13

2.3 Potential sources of infection and operational flow on the farm

Identification of potential sources of infection and ensuring the proper control of all material and people entering and leaving the poultry unit are the fundamental aspects of biosecurity. A first rule is that diseases must be kept outside. The second important biosecurity rule is that diseases that have been brought inside, also should stay inside.

2.3.1 Introduction through humans

There are many ways in which micro-organisms can be introduced into farms. One of the potential vectors for the introduction of disease into farms are humans (Lister, 2008; Woodger and Wirral, 2009; Butcher and Miles, 2012). People can carry pathogens into farms and within farms between houses, on footwear and clothes. Hands can be contaminated with faeces or discharges when birds are examined. People may use and move equipment that is contaminated with dust, faeces or bird feathers (Lister, 2008; De Gussem et al., 2013). Some pathogens like *Mycoplasma* can survive for a few days on hair and clothing and can be transferred mechanically (Christensen et al., 1994). Workers on industrial poultry farms who keep back-yard poultry or pet birds at home can easily introduce disease into a commercial operation (Berndtson et al., 1996; Van Steenwinkel et al., 2011; Cormick, 2017a). Back-yard poultry are usually not well vaccinated compared to commercial flocks; they can also harbour diseases which have been eradicated in commercial poultry flocks such as CRD –Chronic Respiratory Disease (caused by *M. gallisepticum*). Contract work crews who perform vaccinations or other jobs like thinning, blood testing or moving birds to other locations, can also be an important source of infection. Such crews usually serve many poultry farms and travel from one farm to another within a short period of time. Sales and technical representatives and consultants may travel from one continent to another within a day or two and visit different poultry units with different infection pressure and problems, and also different levels of biosecurity protection. They should be especially careful to avoid introducing infections (Berndtson et al., 1996; Hald et al., 2000; Anonymous, 2010; De Gussem et al., 2013; Gelaude et al., 2014). In order to reduce the risk presented by humans, a general rule is to avoid unnecessary visitors at all times and to restrict access to the farm for any unauthorized people (Sims, 2008; Van Steenwinkel et al., 2011). If a visitor needs to enter the farm, he/she should be registered at the entrance, where the personal data, purpose of visit and the previous visit to the poultry unit is recorded. The visitors should be given clean clothing and boots; they should wash and disinfect their hands and if possible, take a shower. Farm personnel should also change clothes and footwear between houses (Nespeca et al., 1997; Lister, 2008; McDowell et al., 2008; Sims, 2008; Dorea et al., 2010a; Cormick, 2017a).

2.3.2 Introduction through equipment and vehicles

Equipment and delivery vehicles can also be important sources of infection. Trucks that transport poultry, eggs or feed must be cleaned, washed and disinfected each time before loading (Lister, 2008; Sims, 2008; Anonymous, 2010; Dorea et al., 2010a; Gelaude et al., 2014). The vehicles should be disinfected at the entrance of the farm. Vaccination instruments and other equipment should not be taken inside the house without first being cleaned and disinfected.

2.3.3 Feed

Another way that pathogens can be introduced into poultry farms is via feed. It can be contaminated with pathogens (e.g. *Salmonella*) through ingredients, during production, delivery or storage. A feed sample must be kept from each delivery batch until the end of the production cycle (Lister, 2008; Anonymous, 2010). Trucks transporting feed must be cleaned and disinfected on their return from the farms before they enter feed storage areas in order to avoid cross-contamination. The drivers should not be allowed to enter poultry houses and should wear clean clothes and footwear when they enter the feed storage area on the farm (Nespeca et al., 1997; Berndtson et al., 1996; Hald et al., 2000; McDowell et al., 2008; Sims, 2008; Anonymous, 2010; Dorea et al., 2010a; Gelaude et al., 2014).

13

2.3.4 Birds

Carrier birds can also contribute to the introduction and spread of pathogensin farms (Butcher and Miles, 2012; De Gussem et al., 2013). Multi-age farms harbour a serious risk of disease from both infected birds and recovered carriers. Layer pullets that have been reared on separate premises and exposed to infection can become carriers of some diseases not existing on the layer farms and introduce new pathogens to aproduction site. In some countries sick birds are put in a sick bay in the same house and can continue to infect the healthy chickens. Such birds should be euthanized and removed to stop continuous infection (Gelaude et al., 2014).

2.3.5 Disposal of dead birds and litter

Dead chickens are a perfect medium for bacterial growth. Chickens are curious and will pick on dead birds thus spreading more pathogens among the flock. Dead birds must be collected at least twice a day as carcasses remain a source of infection (Meroz and Samberg, 1995; Nespeca et al., 1997; Evans and Sayer, 2000; Anonymous, 2010; Bestman et al., 2012; De Gussem et al., 2013). If there is an acute infection with high mortality, dead birds must be collected more frequently. They must be stored in a container, preferably cooled and placed at the edge of the farm, far from live birds (Evans and Sayers, 2000; Gibbens et al., 2001; Anonymous, 2010). The storage location must be chosen so that trucks collecting dead birds do not need to enter the farm or at least not the clean area. After depopulation of the house, litter should be removed from the farm as soon as possible (Charisis, 2008; Lister, 2008; Anonymous, 2010). If needed storage should be far from the buildings so that insects cannot carry the infection back into the house.

2.3.6 Vermin

Mice and rats are important transmitters of poultry diseases including *Salmonella* and *Campylobacter* (Liljebjelke et al., 2005; Meerberg and Kijlstra, 2007; Lister, 2008; Backhans and Fellstrom, 2012; Robyn et al., 2015). Feed, manure and rubbish should never be kept outside the house (Nespeca et al., 1997; Charisis, 2008; Lister, 2008; Anonymous, 2010). Insects can also be an important source of infection. Flies and beetles and their larvae can spread pathogens (Bestman et al., 2012; De Gussem et al., 2013). An efficient and continuous control programme should be set up and continuously monitored (Nespeca et al., 1997; Evans and Sayer, 2000; Lister, 2008; Sims, 2008; Van Steenwinkel et al., 2011). More details on vermin and bird control can be found in chapters 10 and 11 of this book).

2.4 Cleaning and disinfection protocols for poultry

Once birds have left the house it should be cleaned and disinfected before new chicks arrive (Meroz et al., 1995; Tablante, 2008; De Gussem et al., 2013). The first stage is to eliminate the sources of infection. The house must be mechanically cleaned and measures be taken to deal with insects and rodents (Meroz and Samberg, 1995; De Gussem et al., 2013; Ledoux, 2017). The litter should be taken out of the house and ideally removed from the farm (Charisis, 2008; Lister, 2008; Anonymous, 2010; Ledoux, 2017). If this is not possible, the storage zone for litter must be as far from the poultry houses as possible. The surroundings of the building, the roof, outside walls, loading zones and personnel area, must be checked and cleaned to avoid recontamination of the house from outside (Studer et al., 1999; De Gussem et al., 2013). Air vents often get contaminated with manure and dust. *Salmonella* is often found in the dust and surface samples taken from vents. Special attention should be paid to the paved area in front of the entrance. It becomes heavily contaminated when loading birds and removing litter. The decontamination area or hygiene lock at the entrance of the house and electronic control system must also be cleaned. Inside the house the water lines must be flushed and treated to eliminate the biofilm (Watkins, 2006). Water and feed lines must be raised and feeder pans opened. All surfaces and equipment must be soaked with detergent for at least 20 minutes to remove all organic material. After soaking, the house must be rinsed down with water using high-pressure cleaning equipment.

Disinfectant should be applied by wet spray or foam application on dry surfaces but not later than 24 hours after cleaning. Optionally, a second disinfection by fog, mist or low-volume wet spray can be applied before birds are placed. Efficacy of the disinfection must be monitored visually and by taking samples for bacteriology as described in chapter 5 of this book (measuring efficacy of cleaning and disinfection). Sufficient time between flocks is needed in order to clean, disinfect and dry out poultry houses. Increasing the temperature helps to dry the house faster but in general, at least one week is recommended as a sanitary void between the flocks (Meroz et al., 1995).

2.5 Water quality in poultry houses

The main use for water in poultry farms is as drinking water for the birds. When a new flock of day-old chicks arrives on the farm, the temperature in the houses is very high, around 35°C. Because water consumption among small birds is very low the flow of the water in the drinking pipes is also very low. In these circumstances even a small amount of organic material in the drinking lines can promote bacterial growth and biofilm production (Sparks, 2009; de Gussem et al., 2013). It is important therefore, especially during the first week, to counteract these problems. The drinking lines should be flushed before arrival of the birds and at least once a day during the first week (De Gussem et al., 2013). The water should also be treated starting from the day of chick arrival, if possible. Water treatment is a common practice in poultry (Watkins, 2006; Jones, 2009). Tap water is very expensive, so most farms use ground or surface water. A lot of different techniques are possible: chlorine, chlorine dioxide, hydrogen peroxide, electrolysis, UV-treatment, heat treatment, ozone and reverse osmosis, but chlorine, chlorine dioxide and hydrogen peroxide are the ones that are used most frequently (Watkins, 2006; Sparks, 2009; De Gussem et al., 2013). Chlorine is dosed at 10ppm, while chlorine dioxide and hydrogen peroxide are dosed in a range of 150-250ppm when birds are present in the house. The correct dose however should be calculated according to the activity at the end of the drinking pipes. This evaluation can be carried out by ORP (Oxidative reduction potential)-measuring for chlorine or test-strips. Bacteriological analysis is also an important method for evaluating water quality and safety. When the water flow in the drinking pipes rises, doses of the products can be reduced. During vaccination it is important to stop the water treatment 1 day before the vaccination. Treatment can be resumed one day after vaccination (Sparks, 2009).

During the sanitary void and the cleaning and disinfection of the houses, the inside of the drinking lines should also be cleaned (Watkins, 2006; Sparks, 2009; De Gussem et al., 2013). This can be done first mechanically with a device that creates turbulence using a mix of air and water under high pressure. This will clear the majority of the organic material. Then a chemical, such as hydrogen peroxide or chlorine dioxide, should be used in high concentrations (500 ppm). The drinking lines should be filled with the product, leaving the end of the line open to evacuate the surplus gas created by the chemical reaction. After 15 minutes the drinking lines should be flushed with pure water to evacuate the last remaining waste and biofilm together with excess chemical product.

3 Biosecurity aspects that are specific to the different production systems

3.1 Breeders

Breeder birds occupy the upper part of the poultry production pyramid, so the level of biosecurity in breeder farms is generally higher than in production farms (Al-Saffar et al., 2006; Woodger and Willar, 2009; de Gussem et al., 2013). Breeder birds must come from healthy grandparents and are monitored for different pathogens, especially *Salmonella* and *Mycoplasma*. Extensive vaccination programmes in breeders are applied to protect the parent stock and to prevent vertical transmission of pathogens to the progeny, or to provide maternal antibodies in the chick for the first 3 weeks (Levisohn and Kleven, 2000; Kleven, 2008; Dorea et al., 2010b). The litter in the breeder house must be dry and of sufficient quantity. Eggs must be collected at least twice a day. Dirty, cracked or floor eggs must be separated from clean ones and ideally not incubated.

An important risk of pathogen introduction in breeder flocks is spiking of males (Jones, 2009; Woodger and Wirral, 2009; Ssematimba et al., 2013; De Gussem et al., 2013; van der Sluis, 2014). This usually occurs around 35 weeks, at which 20% of the older males are replaced by younger ones to compensate for the decline in fertility. It is important that spiking males come from a single source and that they are tested for disease (e.g. *Mycoplasma Gallisepticum, Salmonella*, Avian Influenza) before introduction.

Another biosecurity risk are chicks in one house coming from different breeder farms (Gelaude et al., 2014). In an ideal situation hatching eggs in a specific house on the production farm should come from a single breeder flock, with the same age and health status.

3.2 Production farms: broilers

Broilers grow very fast and there are usually 6-8 production cycles on a farm within a year. Most of the broilers are kept in all-in all-out production systems. This means that the houses are emptied of birds and litter and cleaned and disinfected after each cycle. One of the major biosecurity risks in broiler production units is thinning (Berndtson et al., 1996; Hald et al., 2000; Slader et al., 2002; Katsma et al., 2007; Allen et al., 2008; Lister, 2008; McDowell et al., 2008; Fraser et al., 2010; de Gussem et al., 2013; Koolman et al., 2014). To avoid excessively high density of broilers per m2 some birds can be taken out (thinned) in the third part of the grow-out period. As a general rule, 15-20% of the birds at 32-35 days old with body weight of 1700-1800 g are slaughtered. The remaining birds in the house are left to grow to the final slaughter weight. This procedure allows a maximum volume of meat per m2 at a lower cost, but it is also a substantial biosecurity risk (Katsma et al., 2007; Fraser et al., 2010). The catching teams and their equipment can easily introduce pathogens into the broiler house. Therefore they should wear clean overalls and footwear at least and wash and disinfect their hands before starting their work

(Berndtson et al., 1996; McDowell et al., 2008; Sims, 2008; Robyn et al., 2015). Transport crates and loaders must be clean (Slader et al., 2002). Before thinning, the whole house should be deprived of feed for a few hours in order to empty the intestines for slaughter. The feed withdrawal and distress during catching causes stress for the remaining birds. Stress has a negative impact on the immune responses of the birds making them more vulnerable to disease (Durant et al., 1999; Humphrey, 2006; Allen et al., 2008).

Slow-growing free-range broilers run a greater risk of picking up intestinal parasites. The free range area is difficult to clean and disinfect, so parasitic infection is able to build up (Permin et al., 1999).

3.3 Production farms: layers

Different housing systems exist for laying hens, with different biosecurity risks: cages, aviary or barn systems; with and without free range. Most of the layers worldwide are kept in cages. The cage system is the most efficient in terms of production and biosecurity (Lay et al., 2011; Bestman et al., 2012). It is easier to control disease spread in a closed house with a cage system as there is less contact between animals and there is minimal contact with the faeces. In general, in cage systems, layers are exposed to lower infection pressure and a lower variety of pathogens compared to floor and free-range systems. In the latter systems, birds are able to move around in- or outside the house and infection can spread faster than in cages. Free-running birds can easily carry pathogens throughout the whole building and there is more direct contact with other birds and their faeces. In the free-range system the birds move outside in the open air, posing a high biosecurity risk. Free-range chickens can come into contact with wild birds or their faeces and become infected with pathogens such as Avian Influenza, *Mycoplasma* or Newcastle disease virus. They can also pick up insects that carry pathogens. The free-range area can harbour different intestinal parasites, such as cestodes, nematodes and coccidosis (Permin et al., 1999; Miao et al., 2005; Bestman et al., 2012; Permin and Bisgaard, 2013). Earthworms are known to be intermediate hosts for *Ascaridia galli* and *Heterakis gallinarum*. The

13

free range area cannot be cleaned and disinfected and it attracts rodents and other vermin. *Dermanyssus gallinae* or red mites are blood-sucking parasites and are an important biosecurity issue in layer production farms. They can harbour bacteria and viruses and transfer them from one bird to another as they feed on them (De Luna et al., 2008). Red mites are difficult to eradicate and can survive many months in the environment. It is essential to prevent contamination of laying production farms with red mites that can derive from laying hen rearing farms. When entering production sites pullets should be free of *Dermanyssus* (Bestman et al., 2012). Another important biosecurity issue in layers is that these are often reared in multi-age farms (Wales et al., 2007). In general, layer birds are kept relatively long on the farm, for 70 up to almost 100 weeks of age. Older birds infected with for example *Mycoplasma* or *Salmonella* can spread the pathogens to flocks that contain younger birds, so that the pathogens persist on the farm. Farms rearing replacement pullets and production farms are not usually to be found at the same location, and pullets are transferred at around 17 weeks. Care should be taken not to introduce diseases to the production site. Monitoring for *Salmonella* and *Myco-plasma* is generally the rule before transfer, but internal and external parasites should also be looked for and if needed pullets should be treated before moving to the production farm. The crates and containers used for transfer should be cleaned and disinfected.

4 Biosecurity in hatcheries

4.1 Hatchery management from egg to chick

The hatchery has a central position in the poultry production chain in the spread of pathogens: eggs collected from different breeder farms are processed to deliver day-old chicks to different production farms (broiler or layer) (Thermote, 2006; Hill and van Roovert-Reijrink, 2010; Bestman et al., 2012; De Gussem et al., 2013). Good management in hatcheries should stop the spread of incoming infections and avoid cross-contamination (Thermote, 2006; Hafez, 2007; Lange, 2015; Leon, 2015; Bennett, 2017).

Biosecurity in hatcheries starts at the breeder farms producing the hatching eggs (Thermote, 2006; Ledoux, 2009; Woodger and Wirral, 2009; Bennet, 2017). Eggs received in hatcheries come from different breeder farms (De Lange, 2015). After storage (up to max 10 days) eggs are put into incubators from day 1 to 18, transferred to the hatcher, where they stay from days 19-21, after which the chicks are pulled (=removed from the hatcher) and prepared for transport to the production farm.

The production capacity in today's hatcheries has increased from 100.000 – 500.000 to up to 2 – 3 million chicks per week. Production rhythm has increased from 2 hatching days per week to up to 4 or even 6 days. As a consequence, the cleaning and disinfection of the different sections of the hatchery has become more complicated and there is more risk of cross-contamination, making increased biosecurity essential.

Previously incubation was carried out in a multi-stage setting, at which eggs of different ages and flock origin were incubated in the same machine and eggs were regularly removed and added (Almeida et al., 2008; Bennett, 2010). The major disadvantage of this system in terms of biosecurity is the higher risk of cross-contamination because of intermingling eggs from different origins (and quality) and because the machine is never empty to allow for thorough cleaning and disinfection (Thermote, 2006; Decuypere et al., 2007; De Lange, 2015). Modern hatcheries operate with single-stage incubation, where all eggs have the same embryonic age and ideally the same origin. This is an all-in/all-out procedure and allows good cleaning and disinfection every 18 days (Bennett, 2010; De Lange, 2015).

Hatchery routing can be divided into five steps: egg handling, incubation, transfer, hatching and chick handling. Each step involves biosecurity risks that need to be adequately controlled (Fig. 13.5).

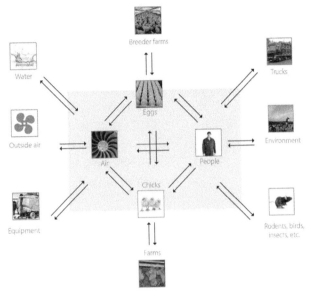

▲

Fig. 13.5: Biosecurity risks in hatcheries (from CID LINES NV)

13

4.2 Disease transmission in hatcheries

Diseases can be transmitted vertically or horizontally (Ledoux, 2003; Hafez, 2007; Pattinson et al., 2008; Butcher and Miles, 2012; de Gussem et al., 2013; Leon, 2015; Cormick, 2017a). With vertical transmission the embryo is infected during development and the infection originates from the breeder hen. External contamination of the eggs from the environment can occur and bacteria can migrate to the internal egg through pores or cracks in the egg shell. Horizontal transmission occurs through vectors: dust, insects, rodents, trays, transport equipment, people. Because eggs are hatched in the confinement of the hatcher, any infection that is present in one egg or chick can potentially spread to all other chicks in the same machine (Hafez, 2007; Leon, 2015; Cormick, 2017a). Special attention should be paid to controlling *Aspergillus* because climate conditions in hatcheries are ideal for the development of fungal growth (Oxley-Goody, 2008; Oxley-Goody, 2011; De Lange, 2015).

4.3 Hygiene and biosecurity in hatcheries

The aim of biosecurity in hatcheries is to prevent the introduction of contamination and to minimise the risk of spreading within the different hatchery compartments (Woodger and Wirral, 2009; De Lange, 2015; Bennett, 2017). The layout of the hatchery should therefore provide a good separation between 'clean' egg zone and 'dirty' chick zone (Ledoux, 2003; Thermote, 2006; Woodger and Wirral, 2009; Bennett, 2017) (See Fig. 13.6 below). It is important to create hygiene zones and work with uni-directional flow (Ledoux, 2003; Ledoux, 2009).

- Product flow: no crossing of eggs, chicks, offal
- People flow: from clean to dirty zone
- Airflow: incoming air should be filtered and the ventilation should create a positive pressure environment with single direction flows (from clean to dirty zones) with no air intake near a dirty zone exhaust
- Waste water flow: separate drains for clean and dirty zones

General hygiene rules apply to all personnel and visitors. Protocols for cleaning and disinfection should be established and controlled by regular monitoring, as applies to poultry houses.

Fig. 13.6: Layout hatchery with product flow (white arrows) (from CID LINES NV).

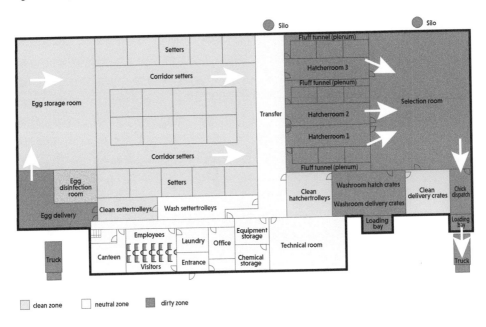

4.3.1 General hygiene measures for personnel and visitors

At the entrance everyone should change clothes and shoes used outside the hatchery after taking a shower, and change to clean disinfected clothes and shoes for inside the hatchery (Woodger and Wirral, 2009; Leon, 2015; Bennett, 2017). Before entering the premises visitors should register with their name, company and date of last contact with live poultry, and follow the hygiene instructions for personnel (Woodger and Wirral, 2009; Cormick, 2017a). There should be a clear barrier between dirty and clean zones. Hands should be washed or sanitised at all times after eating or using the toilet (Ledoux, 2003; Thermote, 2006; Woodger and Wirral, 2009; Bennett, 2017).

To prevent contamination spreading to the different compartments of the hatchery a one-way traffic system in line with the egg flow through the hatchery from 'clean' areas (i.e., egg rooms and incubators) to increasingly 'dirtier' areas (hatchery room, chick handling and hatch debris) should be installed (Ledoux, 2003; Thermote, 2006; Woodger and Wirral, 2009; Bennett, 2017; Cormick, 2017a). If possible personnel should be restricted to either 'clean' egg side or 'dirty' chick side, to avoid contamination of clean areas with chick fluff and debris. Using a designated colour for clothes and shoes per section can make this separation between areas more visual (Ledoux, 2003; Ledoux, 2009).

It is important to avoid air flow from dirty to clean rooms, so opening doors should be kept to a minimum and positive air pressure should be maintained in critical areas of the hatchery (Ledoux, 2003; Hafez, 2007; Ledoux, 2009; Bennett, 2017). Optimally, each area of the hatchery should be ventilated separately. If this is not possible, keep the incubation room under positive pressure (pushing air out of the room) to minimise potentially contaminated air from the dirty side of hatchery (Ledoux, 2003; Thermote, 2006; Oxley-Goody, 2008; Ledoux, 2009).

The perimeter of the hatchery facility should be fenced to avoid unauthorised people entering the premises. No poultry or other animals should be kept on the premises.

4.3.2 Egg handling

4.3.2.1 Storage and setting for incubation

Ideally eggs should be disinfected as soon as possible after collection from the breeder farm and again at the hatchery (Ledoux, 2003; Thermote, 2006; Hafez, 2007; Ledoux, 2009; Woodger and Wirral, 2009). Floor eggs should not be used as hatching eggs (Thermote, 2006; Hafez, 2007; De Lange, 2015). Washing eggs should be avoided. Ideally quality control at the farm should separate the non-hatching eggs, and if this is not carried out at the farm, it should be carried out upon receipt at the hatchery. Hatching eggs should be labelled and stored before incubation. During quality control, eggs that are unsuitable for hatching (misshapen, dirty or cracked) should be removed because they present a risk of contamination (Hafez, 2007; De Gussem et al., 2013; De Lange, 2015). Technical data of the parent flock should be recorded for each batch by the farm manager, and on receipt in the hatchery all trays should be labelled for traceability (Bennett, 2010; Hafez, 2007).

Conditions during storage and transport should avoid eggs 'sweating' because this provides the ideal conditions for pathogens to grow and penetrate inside the eggs. 'Sweating' is caused by condensation when cold eggs are exposed to higher temperatures (Thermote, 2006; Schulte-Drüggelte, 2011; Gradl et al., 2017). The storage room should be kept at 18°C and 70-80% relative humidity. If eggs are to be stored for more than 7 days, the temperature should be lowered (Cormick, 2017b). Before incubation, eggs should be placed in setter trays on setter trolleys and disinfected in the fumigation room. As mentioned above, care must be taken to avoid temperature changes and sweating. The fumigation room should be located between the egg traying room and the incubator room, and disinfection should be performed with registered disinfection products (Ledoux, 2003; Thermote, 2006; Hafez, 2007; Leon, 2015). The use of formaldehyde as an egg disinfectant is decreasing due to its negative effects on human health and on the environment. In some countries, moreover, use of this kind of disinfectant is already prohibited (De Lange, 2015). Trolleys should be moved in from the egg storage room and moved out onto the side of the setter room. It is important to ventilate after fumigation before moving the trolleys into the setter room. Setters should be washed and disinfected after each use (Ledoux, 2013; Thermote, 2006; De Lange, 2015).

4.3.2.2 Transfer to the hatcher

After 18 days of incubation eggs should be transferred to the hatcher in the transfer room. Before transfer, eggs can be candled to remove infertile eggs or dead embryos. Transfer should be completed in 30 minutes and the temperature in the room should be kept at 25°C. Eggs with different ID codes should be kept in differ-

13

ent hatcher baskets to ensure traceability. Hatcher baskets should be cleaned, disinfected and dried before transfer.

Recently, *in ovo* vaccination has become more popular and equipment more adequate and precise (Ricks et al., 1999; Williams, 2007; Williams and Villalobos, 2010). At transfer, eggs should be injected automatically with vaccines and the opening where the needle enters the egg should be disinfected after injection. If the procedure is executed correctly and equipment is well maintained this is a very efficient method of vaccination, causing less stress than injection at day 1.

Occasionally 'bangers' occur during transfer: these are eggs that explode with a loud bang and give off a very bad smell, due to gas producing bacteria, usually *Pseudomonas* spp.. Gas production causes pressure to build up inside the egg and small vibrations can trigger explosions. These exploders lead to heavy bacterial contamination in the hatcher that can lead to bad chick quality (Thermote, 2006; De Gussem et al., 2013; De Lange, 2015). Eggs from older flocks are more at risk because the shells are weaker and cracks occur more frequently.

Hatcher baskets get soiled by meconium, eggshells, fluff and should be cleaned and washed directly after hatching. This is usually done in a specially designed automatic washing machine.

4.3.2.3 Hatching and chick handling

After 3 days in the hatcher, and 21 days of incubation, chicks are pulled. The hygiene status of the environment has a direct impact on the quality of one-day old chicks and mortality in the first days. It is important to realize that at pipping – when the egg is opened by the chick, germ counts increase logarithmically in the confinement of the hatcher (Ledoux, 2003; Thermote, 2006; Ledoux, 2009). Just before pipping, a disinfecting fogging agent is used in the hatcher. The chick side is the 'dirty' zone of the hatchery: hatcher room, plenum, chick room, wash room are heavily contaminated with organic material and fluff, and high temperatures and humidity form ideal conditions for bacterial and fungal growth (Ledoux, 2003; Thermote, 2006; Ledoux, 2009; Woodger and Wirral, 2009; Bennett, 2017). Therefore it is important that air flow is controlled and exhausted, dirty air cannot be drawn back into the hatchery (Ledoux, 2003; Ledoux, 2009; Bennett, 2017). Cleaning and disinfection in this zone of the hatchery will be more challenging and very active products that can cope with organic material are needed.

The process from removing the chicks from the hatcher basket to dispatch in the transport crates is very much automated. All necessary equipment, including the hatcher basket destacker, transport belts, chick counter, automatic vaccinator and vaccine spray cabinet should be clean and well maintained. Waste removal from the hatchery should be carried out using a vacuum system and waste should be stored in a silo, or with offal containers (Thermote, 2006; Glatz et al., 2011). All this equipment should be regularly cleaned and disinfected.

4.3.2.4 Cleaning and disinfectant products in hatcheries

The hatchery is an ideal environment for pathogen multiplication (Thermote, 2006; De Lange, 2015). All essential components necessary for growth of micro-organisms are available here: nutrients, air, water and heat (Oxley-Goody, 2011; Thermote, 2006). Cleaning is very important and can remove at least 85% of micro-organisms, the rest should be removed by disinfection. Regular cleaning and keeping surfaces dry reduces the bacterial load. Surfaces should be smooth with no cracks or crevices. More detailed information on the cleaning and disinfection procedures can be found in chapter 6 of this book.

Monitoring the efficacy of cleaning and disinfection is essential: visual inspection is the first step, but it is essential to include monitoring using agar cultures for total bacterial loads (non-specific) and specific bacteria (*Salmonella, Mycoplasma*) and fungi (*Aspergillus)* (De Lange, 2015; Bennett, 2017). Special care should be taken to choose the correct sampling method and to sample the critical locations (plenum, washing machines, rubber equipment).

References

Allen V.M., Weaver H., Ridley A.M., Harris J. A., Sharma M., Emery J., Sparks N., Lewis M., Edge S., 2008. Sources and spread of thermophilic Campylobacter spp. during partial depopulation of broiler chicken flocks. Journal of food protection 71, 264-270.

Almeida J.G., Vieira S.L., Reis R.N., Berres J., Barros R.D., Ferreira A.K., Furtado F.V.F., 2008. Hatching distribution and embryo mortality of eggs laid by broiler breeders of different ages. Revista Brasileira de Ciência Avícola 10, 89-96.

Al-Saffar A., Al-Nasser A., Al-haddad A., Al-Bahouh M., Mashaly M., 2006. Principles of poultry biosecurity program. Kuwait Institute for Scientific Research, Safat, Kuwait, 1-67.

Anonymous, Australian Chicken Meat Federation, 2010. National farm biosecurity manual for chicken growers. ACMF, Sydney, 1-36.

Anthony N.B., 1998. A review of genetic practices in poultry: Efforts to improve meat quality. Journal of Muscle Foods 9, 25-33.

Backhans A. and Fellstrom C., 2012. Rodents on pig and chicken farms – a potential threat to human and animal health. Infection Ecology & Economy 2, 17093.

Bennett B., 2010. The advantage of single stage versus multi stage incubation. International Hatchery Practice 24, 7-9.

Bennett B., 2017. The importance of biosecurity in the modern day hatchery. International Hatchery Practice 31, 15-17.

Berndtson E., Emanuelson U., Engvall A., Danielsson-Tham L., 1996. A 1-year epidemiological study of Campylobacter in 18 Swedish chicken farms. Preventive Veterinary Medicine 26, 167-185.

Bestman M., Ruis M., Heijmans J., van Middelkoop K., 2012. Laying hens: a practical guide for layer focused management. Roodbont Publishers B.V., Zutphen, The Netherlands.

Butcher G.D. and Miles R.D., 2012. Disease prevention in commercial poultry (CR1079). University of Florida IFAS Extension http://edis.ifas.ufl.edu/pdffiles/VM/VM01100.pdf

Charisis N., 2008. Avian influenza biosecurity: a key for animal and human protection. Veterinaria Italiana 44, 657-669.

Christensen N.H., Yavari C.A., McBain A.J., Bradbury J.M., 1994. Investigations into the survival of Mycoplasma gallisepticum, Mycoplasma synoviae and Mycoplasma iowae on materials found in the poultry house environment. Avian Pathology 23, 127-143.

Cormick J., Petersime Hatchery Development Specialist – Petersime NV, 2017a. Bio-security: practical tips to minimize the human risk of contamination. Available at: http://www.petersime.com/hatchery-development-department/bio-security-practical-tips-to-minimize-the-human-risk-of-contamination/ (accessed October 2017).

Cormick J., Petersime Hatchery Development Specialist – Petersime NV, 2017b. Egg storage: good practices. Available at: http://www.petersime.com/hatchery-development-department/egg-storage/ (accessed October 2017).

Decuypere E., Tona K., Bruggeman V., Bamelis F., 2001. The day-old chick: a crucial hinge between breeders and broilers. World's Poultry Science Journal 57, 127-138.

de Gussem M., van Middelkoop K., van Mullem K., van 't Veer E., 2013. Broiler signals: a practical guide to broiler focused management. Roodbont Publishers B.V., Zutphen, The Netherlands.

De Lange G., 2015. Good hygiene: a must for the modern hatchery. International Hatchery Practice 29, 11-15.

De Luna C.J., Arkle S., Harrington D., George D. R., Guy J. H., Sparagano O.A., 2008. The Poultry Red Mite Dermanyssus gallinae as a Potential Carrier of Vector-borne Diseases. Annals of the New York Academy of Sciences 1149, 255-258.

Dorea F.C., Berghaus R., Hofacre C., Cole D.J., 2010a. Survey of biosecurity protocols and practices adopted by growers on commercial poultry farms in Georgia – USA. Avian Diseases 54, 1007-1015.

Dorea F.C., Cole D.J., Hofacre C., Zamperini K., Mathis D., Doyle M.P., Lee M.D., Maurer J.J., 2010b. Effect of Salmonella vaccination of breeder chickens on contamination of broiler chicken carcasses in integrated poultry operations. Applied and Environmental Microbiology 76, 7820-7825.

Durant J.A., Corrier D.E., Byrd J.A., Stanker L.H., Ricke S.C., 1999. Feed deprivation affects crop environment and modulates Salmonella enteritidis colonization and invasion of Leghorn hens. Applied and Environmental Microbiology 65, 1919-1923.

East I.J., Kite V., Daniels P., Garner G., 2006. A cross-sectional survey of Australian chicken farms to identify risk factors associated with seropositivity to Newcastle-disease virus. Preventive Veterinary Medicine 77, 199-214.

East I.J., 2007. Adoption of biosecurity practices in the Australian poultry industries. Australian Veterinary Journal 85, 107-112.

European Commission, 2016. Report from the Commission to the European Parliament and the Council. The impact of genetic selection on the welfare of chickens kept for meat production. http://eur-lex.europa.eu/legal-content/EN/TXT/?qid=1507288411148&uri=CELEX:52016DC0182

Evans S.J. and Sayer A.R., 2000. A longitudinal study of Campylobacter infection of broiler flock in Great Britain. Preventive Veterinary Medicine 46, 209-223.

Fraser R.W., Williams N.T., Powell L.F., Cook A.J.C., 2010. Reducing Campylobacter and Salmonella infection: two studies of the economic cost and attitude to adoption of on-farm biosecurity measures. Zoonoses Public Health 57, 109-115.

Gelaude P., Schlepers M., Verlinden M., Laanen M., Dewulf J., 2014. Biocheck.UGent: a quantitative tool to measure biosecurity at broiler farms and the relationship with technical performances and antimicrobial use. Poultry Science 93, 2740-2751.

Gibbens J.C., Pascoe S.J.S., Evans S.J., Davies R.H., Sayers A.R., 2001. A trial of biosecurity as a means to control Campylobacter infection of broiler chickens. Preventive Veterinary Medicine 48, 85-99.

Gillespie J.R. and Flanders F., 2009. Modern livestock & poultry production (8th edition), chapter 35: Selection of poultry. Cengage Learning, Clifton Park, USA.

Glatz P., Miao Z., Rodda B., 2011. Handling and treatment of poultry hatchery waste: a review. Sustainability 3, 216-237.

Gradl J.A., Curtis P. A., Jones D. R., Anderson K.E., 2017. Assessing the impact of egg sweating on Salmonella Enteritidis penetration into shell eggs. Poultry Science, pex011.

Graham J.P., Leibler J.H., Price L.B., Otte J.M., Pfeiffer D.U., Tiensin T., Silbergeld E.K., 2008. The animal – human interface and infectious disease in industrial food animal production: rethinking biosecurity and biocontainment. Public Health Reports 123, 282-299.

13

Hafez M.H., 2007. Breeder farms and hatchery as integrated operation. Lohmann Information 42, 29-34.

Hald B., Wedderkopp A., Madsen M., 2000. Thermophilic Campylobacter spp. in Danish broiler production: A cross-sectional survey and a retrospective analysis of risk factors for occurrence in broiler flocks. Avian Pathology 29, 123-131.

Hartung J. and Schulz J., 2007. Risks caused by bio-aerosols in poultry houses. International Conference: Poultry in the 21st century, avian influenza and beyond, Bangkok.

Hiemstra S.J. and Napel J.T., 2013. Study of the impact of genetic selection on the welfare of chickens bred and kept for meat production. Final Report Framework Contract No SANCO/2011/12254, IBF International Consulting.

Hill D., van Roovert-Reijrink I., 2010. Making innovations in hatchery hygiene by understanding the basics. International Hatchery Practice 24, 7-11.

Hoff J.C. and Akin E.W., 1986. Microbial resistance to disinfectants: mechanisms and significance. Environmental Health Perspectives 69, 7-13.

Humphrey T., 2006. Are happy chickens safer chickens? Poultry welfare and disease susceptibility. British Poultry Science 47, 379-391.

Iqbal, M., 2009. Controlling avian influenza infections: The challenge of the backyard poultry. Journal of molecular and genetic medicine: an international journal of biomedical research 3, 119.

Jones K.H., 2009. Health management of the modern broiler breeder male. Aviagen Brief, 1-9.

Kapperud G., Skjerve E., Vik E., Hauge K., Lysaker A., Aalmen I., Ostroff S.M., Potter M., 1993. Epidemiology investigation of risk factors for Campylobacter colonization in Norwegian broiler flocks. Epidemiology and Infection 111, 245-255.

Katsma W.E., De Koeijer A.A., Jacobs-Reitsma W.F., Mangen M.J.J., Wagenaar J.A., 2007. Assessing interventions to reduce the risk of Campylobacter prevalence in broilers. Risk Analysis 27, 863-876.

Kleven S.H., 2008. Control of avian mycoplasma infections in commercial poultry. Avian diseases 52, 367-374.

Koolman L., Whyte P., Bolton D.J., 2014. An investigation of broiler caecal Campylobacter counts at first and second thinning. Journal of applied microbiology 117, 876-881.

Lay Jr D.C., Fulton R.M., Hester P.Y., Karcher D.M., Kjaer J.B., Mench J.A., Mullens B.A., Newberry R.C., Nicol C.J., O'Sullivan N.P., Porter R.E., 2011. Hen welfare in different housing systems 1. Poultry Science 90, 278-294.

Ledoux L., 2003. Hatchery hygiene procedures and product choices. World Poultry 19, 20-21.

Ledoux L., 2009. Hatchery hygiene – getting the basics right for grade A chicks. International Hatchery Practice 23, 11-12.

Ledoux L., 2017. Effective use of disinfectants in disease prevention and control. International Hatchery Practice 31, 28-29.

Leon O., 2015. Taking steps towards a salmonella free hatchery. International Hatchery Practice 29, 12-13.

Levisohn S. and Kleven S.H., 2000. Avian mycoplasmosis (Mycoplasma gallisepticum). Revue scientifique et technique (International Office of Epizootics) 19, 425-442.

Liljebjelke K.A., Hofacre C.L., Liu T., White D.G., Ayers S., Young S., Maurere J.J., 2005. Vertical and horizontal transmission of salmonella within integrated broiler production system. Foodborne Pathogens and Disease 2, 90-102.

Lister S.A., 2008. Biosecurity in poultry management. M. Patisson, P. F. McMullin, J. M. Bradburry, Alexander D.J., ed. p. 48-65 in Poultry Diseases. 6th edition Saunders Elsevier, Beijing, China.

McDowell S.W.J., Menzies F.D., McBride S.H., Oza A.N., McKenna J.P., Gordon A.W., Neill S.D., 2008. Campylobacter spp. in conventional broiler flocks in Northern Ireland: Epidemiology and risk factors. Preventive Veterinary Medicine 84, 261-276.

McQuiston J.H., Garber L.P., Porter-Spalding B.A., Hahn F.W., Pierson S.H., Wainwright S.H., Senne D.A., Brignole T.J., Akey B.L., Holt T.J., 2005. Evaluation of risk factors for the spread of low pathogenicity H7N2 avian influenza virus among commercial poultry farms. Journal of the American Veterinary Medical Association 226, 767-772.

Meerburg B.G. and Kijlstra A., 2007. Role of rodents in transmission of Salmonella and Campylobacter. Journal of the Science of Food Agriculture 87, 2774-2781.

Meroz M. and Samberg Y., 1995. Disinfecting poultry production premises. Revue Scientifique et Technique (Office International des Epizooties) 14, 273-291.

Miao Z.H., Glatz P.C., Ru Y.J., 2005. Free-range poultry production-A review. Asian-Australian Journal of Animal Science 18, 113-132.

Nespeca R., Vaillancourt J.P., Morrow W.E.M., 1997. Validation of a poultry biosecurity survey. Preventive Veterinary Medicine 31, 73-86.

Oxley-Goody D., 2008. Effective Aspergillus control in the hatchery. International Hatchery Practice 23, 7-9.

Oxley-Goody D., 2011. Aspergillus in the hatchery. International Hatchery Practice 26, 7-9.

Patisson M. (Editor), McMullin P.F., Bradburry J.M., Alexander D.J., 2008. Poultry Diseases, 6th edition. Elsevier Health Sciences.

Permin A., Bisgaard M., Frandsen F., Pearman M., Kold J., Nansen P., 1999. Prevalence of gastrointestinal helminths in different poultry production systems. British poultry science 40, 439-443.

Permin A. and Bisgaard M., 2013. A general review on some important diseases in free-range chickens. INFPDE-CONFERENCE, 163.

Pym R., 2013. Poultry genetics and breeding in developing countries. Poultry Development Review FAO, 80-83.

Ricks C.A., Avakian A., Bryan T., Gildersleeve R., Haddad E., Ilich R., King S., Murray L., Phelps P., Poston R., Whitfill C., Williams C., 1999. In ovo vaccination technology. Advances in Veterinary Medicince – San Diego 41, 495-516.

Robyn J., Rasschaert G., Pasmans F., Heyndrickx M., 2015. Thermotolerant Campylobacter during broiler rearing: risk factors and intervention. Comprehensive Reviews in Food Science and Food Safety 14, 81-105.

Schulte-Drüggelte R., 2011. Recommendations for hatching, egg handling and storage. Lohmann Information 46, 56-60.

Sims L.D., 2008. Risks associated with poultry production systems. International conference: Poultry in the 21st century, 1-24.

13

Slader J., Domingue G., Jorgensen F., McAlphine K., Owen R.J., Bolton F.J., Humphrey T.J., 2002. Impact of transport crate reuse and of catching and processing on Campylobacter and Salmonella contamination of broiler chickens. Applied and Environmental Microbiology 68, 713-719.

Sparks N.H.C., 2009. The role of the water supply system in the infection and control of Campylobacter in chicken. World's Poultry Science Journal 65, 459-474.

Ssematimba A., Hagenaars T.J., de Wit J.J., Ruiterkamp F., Fabri T.H., Stegeman J.A., de Jong M.C.M., 2013. Avian influenza transmission risks: analysis of biosecurity measures and contact structure in Dutch poultry farming. Preventive Veterinary Medicine 109, 106-115.

Studer E., Luthy J., Hübner P., 1999. Study of the presence of Campylobacter jejuni and C. coli in sand samples from four Swiss chicken farms. Research in microbiology 111, 213-219.

Tablante N.L., 2008. Biosecurity: A vital key to poultry disease prevention. Poultry perspectives 8, 2-4.

Thermote L., 2006. Effective hygiene within the hatchery. International Hatchery Practice 20, 18-21.

Vaillancourt J.P. and Carver D.K., 1998. Biosecurity: Perception is not reality. Poultry Digest 57, 28-36.

Van der Sluis W., 2014. Spiking reduces fertility drop in older poultry flocks. World Poultry Magazine 30.

Vangroenweghe F., Ribbens S., Vandersmissen T., Beek J., Dewulf J., Maes D., Castryck F., 2009. Keeping Pigs Healthy (in Dutch). 1st editor F. Vangroenweghe, DCL Print & Signs, Zelzate, Belgium

Van Steenwinkel S., Ribbens S., Ducheyne E., Goossens E., Dewulf J., 2011. Assessing biosecurity practices, movements and densities of poultry sites across Belgium, resulting in different farm risk-groups for infectious disease introduction and spread. Preventive Veterinary Medicine 98, 259-270.

Vieira A.R., Hofacre C.L., Smith J.A., Cole D., 2009. Human contacts and potential pathways of disease introduction on Georgia poultry farms. Avian Diseases 53, 55-62.

Wales A., Breslin M., Carter B., Sayers R., Davies R., 2007. A longitudinal study of environmental Salmonella contamination in caged and free-range layer flocks. Avian Pathology 36, 187-197.

Watkins S., 2006. Clean water lines for flock health. Avian Advice 8, 3-5.

Williams C., 2007. In ovo vaccination for disease prevention. International Poultry Production 15, 7-8.

Williams C., Villalobos T., 2010. Critical success factor for in ovo vaccination. International Hatchery Practice 25, 7-9.

Woodger J. and Wirral, M., 2009. Effective biosecurity on the breeder farm and in the hatchery. International Hatchery Practice 23, 7-111.

Zenner L., Bon G., Chauve C., Nemoz C., Lubac S., 2009. Monitoring of Dermanyssus gallinae in free-range poultry farms. Experimental and Applied Acarology 48, 157-166.

CHAPTER 14

TRANSMISSION OF CATTLE DISEASES AND BIOSECURITY IN CATTLE FARMS

Steven Sarrazin[1]

Bert Damiaans[1]

Véronique Renault[2]

Claude Saegerman[2]

[1] Faculty of Veterinary Medicine, Department of Reproduction, Obstetrics and Herd Health, Veterinary Epidemiology Unit, University of Ghent, 9820 Merelbeke, Belgium
[2] Faculty of Veterinary Medicine, Department of Infectious and Parasitic Diseases, Research Unit in Epidemiology and Risk Analysis Applied to Veterinary Sciences, (UREAR-ULg), Fundamental and Applied Research for Animal and Health (FARAH) Center, University of Liege, 4000 Liege, Belgium

1 Introduction

In the first part of this chapter we provide a brief outline of the cattle industry. Since cattle production is a diverse sector, this outline will help readers to understand why the approach to biosecurity may sometimes differ between types of cattle farms. Although biosecurity does not necessarily focus on one particular infectious disease and aims at upgrading herd health in general, measures are based on the knowledge of the epidemiology of specific pathogens (Barrington et al., 2002). Therefore in the second part of this chapter on cattle biosecurity the transmission of endemic and epidemic cattle diseases is presented.

This outline is not meant to be exhaustive in terms of possible pathogens or diseases or the references of possible routes of transmission, but is based on recent work in the classification of cattle diseases of relevance to Belgium (Renault et al., 2017).

In the third part of this chapter we provide an overview of how biosecurity measures can be implemented in cattle farms. This overview is based on an elaborate review literature covering the risk factors for disease transmission as listed in the first part of this chapter. We will discuss the essential aspects of cattle biosecurity and specific practical biosecurity measures for dairy, beef and veal calf farms. Despite the fact that the overview of diseases is not exhaustive and that there are considerable epidemiologic differences between pathogens such as the reservoir, modes of transmission and incubation periods (Barrington et al., 2002; Villarroel et al., 2007), the basic principle of disease prevention is to reduce contact between disease agents and susceptible animals (Callan & Garry, 2002). Most biosecurity measures are not specific to a single infectious agent therefore (Barrington et al., 2002) and also apply to diseases that are not listed in the overview.

2 Outline of the cattle industry

Cattle production is a diverse sector as it comprises both dairy and beef production. Furthermore, the main focus of the highly integrated veal calf industry is rearing male dairy calves, a 'by-product' of the dairy sector.

In dairy farms the majority of female calves are kept as replacement heifers, while male calves and surplus female calves are sold at the age of 2 weeks. Young stock is usually inseminated at around the age of 15 months (more rarely fertilised by a bull) in order to have the first calf and start lactating at around the age of 2 years. After 60 days into lactation, cows are inseminated again to aim for a new birth 365 days after the previous calving. On average, 40 days before the second calving, a cow will be dried off and moved to a group of dry cows to prepare for the next lactation.

In beef farms cattle are reared for meat production and it is mainly specialised beef breeds that are used. Dual purpose breeds for both beef and dairy production are used but this is rarer. Calves born in beef herds are either immediately separated from the dam or are raised together with the dam as suckling calves. The majority of the calves are reared on the farm of origin, but some are sold to be reared until the age of slaughter on other beef farms or sold to the veal industry. Replacement heifers are inseminated or fertilised by a bull at the same age as dairy heifers.

Most of the veal production takes place in Europe, mainly in France, the Netherlands, Italy, Belgium and Germany (Pardon et al., 2014). The term veal is reserved for meat from bovines younger than eight months. White veal has white meat, rosé veal is a little more red and bobby veal originates from calves slaughtered within a week of birth. The production of white veal is highly integrated, while rosé veal is more privately owned. Calves are collected by salesmen from their farms of origin at the age of 2 weeks and pass through a sorting centre before entering the veal farm. Veal farms maintain an all-in all-out system and tend to be very closed. During the first eight weeks of age the calves are housed in separate boxes and then split up into groups of typically seven to eight animals.

14

3 Transmission of cattle diseases

The most important route of disease transmission is generally considered to be direct contact between live animals, but indirect transmission should not be ignored (Barrington et al., 2002; Callan and Garry, 2002; Brennan et al., 2008; Nöremark et al., 2013), this is especially true of pathogens that can survive for a long time in the environment (Saegerman et al., 2012). In addition to direct animal to animal contact, direct contact also includes transplacental and venereal transmission. The latter transmission pathway has become less important as artificial insemination is more frequently used instead of natural fertilisation by a breeding bull (Robertson & Rendel 1950, Salisbury & Vandemark 1961, Foote 2002). In this overview a distinction between several pathways of indirect disease transmission is made (Table 14.1, see p. 378-381). Disease is able to spread from cattle to cattle without direct contact through people, other animals besides cattle (e.g. cats, dogs, rodents), fomites (e.g. feeding utensils, syringes and needles), ingestion (water and feed, including colostrum), inhalation (droplets or aerosol), manure and vectors (either biological or mechanical). When the literature does not specify the specific pathway for a given disease, this is denoted in the overview as 'General'. Furthermore, this overview also indicates whether the diseases have a zoonotic aspect, i.e. the disease spreads naturally from vertebrate animals to humans and vice versa, which species are affected (including whether a wild life reservoir exists), and whether the disease spreads through asymptomatic carriers.

4 Biosecurity in cattle farms

The description of the biosecurity measures is subdivided into external and internal biosecurity, under which the most relevant subcategories of biosecurity in the prevention of cattle disease transmission on dairy, beef and veal calf farms are further discussed. Where necessary, the subcategories are split up in a paragraph on the prevention of direct and indirect contact.

4.1 External biosecurity

4.1.1 Purchase of animals

The introduction of new cattle through purchase is by far the most cited risk factor for introduction of disease pathogens in herds (Valle et al., 1999; Boelaert, 2005; Cuttance & Cuttance, 2014). Although the risk of introducing pathogens depends on the frequency of purchase and type of animals purchased (e.g. young stock, breeding bull, pregnant heifers, lactating cows), every introduction of new cattle is a risk of entering disease into a herd. Therefore the general advice is to avoid purchasing cattle as much as possible. However, it may be that cattle have to be purchased. For example a breeding bull may be needed when the conception rate through artificial insemination is too low, or when some female young stock are added as an exceptional to the herd when too many male calves have been born. Veal calf farms are a special case, since they typically purchase all their animals, which originate from many different farms. Whenever it is necessary to purchase cattle, measures to avoid disease transmission through direct and indirect contact should be implemented.

4.1.1.1 Direct contact

The risk of disease introduction can be reduced by purchasing cattle from farms with a sanitary status and health management that is equal to or higher than your own farm (Griffin et al., 2010; Sweiger & Nichols, 2010). If your farm has a specific pathogen-free (SPF) health status for a disease (e.g. infectious bovine rhinotracheïtis or bovine viral diarrhoea), it is advisable to purchase cattle from farms with the same or a higher status. Furthermore, farmers who pay attention to obtain an SPF status for some diseases are more likely to have good health management in general and consequently a lower occurrence of other diseases. Also, when purchasing sperm, embryos or colostrum attention should be paid to the health status of farms/institutions of origin.

Limiting the number of farms of origin where cattle are purchased can reduce the risk of disease introduction (Edwards, 2010; Mee

14

et al., 2012). This can pose a problem in particular for veal calves farms, since the animals originate from many different farms. In such cases calves could be divided in smaller risk groups, depending on one or more specific disease statuses (Pardon, 2012).

Even when cattle are purchased from farms with a sanitary status and health management that is equal to or higher than your own farm, the individual disease status of the purchased cattle should be checked by testing the animals, preferably at the farm of origin (Gorden & Plummer, 2010). In this way you avoid diseased animals entering the farm and whenever a test result is positive the purchase should be cancelled. It is important to remember that cattle may be carriers of other disease agents (e.g. Mortellaro disease, *Psoroptes ovis* mange, *Staphylococcus aureus* mastitis, Q fever) than the small number tested for. It is advisable to test milk samples of lactating cattle.

When cattle are transported to the farm, contact with cattle (or other animals) with an unknown disease status from other farms should be avoided (Mee et al., 2012). Ideally, only the cattle destined for your farm should be present in the transportation vehicle. When using your own transportation vehicle, you can also control the cleaning and disinfection status of the vehicle.

Once purchased cattle arrive on the farm they should be quarantined, i.e. the animals should be placed in isolation without contact with the farm's own herd for a sufficiently long period (Maunsell & Donovan, 2009; Gorden & Plummer, 2010; Raaperi et al., 2014). It should be pointed out that quarantining purchased cattle cannot be replaced by just testing these animals, since cattle can be carriers of other disease agents than the small number tested for (see above). Quarantine allows the newly introduced animals to adapt to the farm (e.g. feed, climate) and avoids the purchased cattle transmitting diseases to the herd. The recommended isolation duration of the quarantine varies, but for diseases with a short incubation period three to four weeks is recommended (Wells et al., 2002; Barrington et al., 2002; Callan & Garry, 2002; Villarroel et al., 2007; Maunsell & Donovan, 2008). An appropriate quarantine area is a space that prevents disease transmission through direct and indirect contact (e.g. aerosols). It should preferably be a separate building where no other cattle are present (Edwards,

2010). Farmers often argue that there is no space available on the farm to apply a good quarantine. However, a pasture or an old building can also serve as quarantine area.

Furthermore, one should also take into account that:
- a quarantine period of three to four weeks is insufficient for diseases with a long incubation period, e.g. paratuberculosis;
- when purchasing cattle in lactation, they should preferably be milked inside the quarantine area;
- when purchasing pregnant cattle, calving should preferably occur in the quarantine area and the new-born should be tested immediately after birth (before the intake of colostrum) and should be quarantined until test results are available;
- the all-in/all-out principle should be applied for animals in quarantine.

4.1.1.2 Indirect contact

Indirect disease transmission from cattle in quarantine is possible through people that enter the quarantine area, material that is used and through feed and water that are provided to the cattle. Specific clothing and boots (and/or a disinfection footbath) should be available at the entrance of the quarantine area and they should only be used for this purpose. Everyone who enters the quarantine area should make use of these facilities. Hands should preferably be washed when entering and leaving the quarantine area (Edwards, 2010). Moreover, farmers are advised to enter the quarantine area at the end of their daily work routine.
Specific material (e.g. feeding utensils) should be available in the quarantine area and must not be used in the farm's own herd. Feed that is present in the quarantine area should not be used to feed the farm's own herd (Edwards, 2010; Gorden & Plummer, 2010).

14

4.1.2 Animals that leave and return to the herd

Sometimes cattle leave the farm, but come back afterwards, e.g. a breeding bull shared with other farms or for auctions, contests, markets. Such animals should also preferably be quarantined when they return to the farm according to the same principles as mentioned above (Gorden & Plummer, 2010).

4.1.3 Pasture contact

Very often contact with cattle from other farms is possible on pastures shared with other farms in the same season or through an adjacent pasture. Furthermore, disease transmission between cattle from different farms is possible when they have access to the same surface water in the pastures. The general rule should therefore be to avoid pasture contact on the same or adjacent pastures (Fig. 14.1). In those instances when this is not possible, double fenced pastures can reduce the risk of disease transmission (Valle et al., 1999; Nafstad & Gronstol, 2001; Raaperi et al., 2014). However, for non-airborne diseases such as bovine viral diarrhoea, a distance of at least 3 meters is recommended (Laureyns et al., 2010). Another possibility is to pasture high-risk groups (i.e. where infection from those animals could have huge consequences, e.g. abortion of animals in gestation) on pastures with no adjacent pastures.

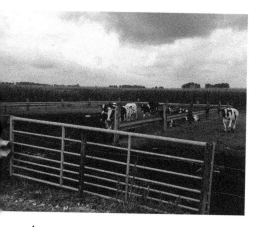

▲

Fig. 14.1.: These cattle are grazing on a pasture with no neighbouring pastures thus avoiding fence-line contact with cattle from other farms.

4.1.4 Removal of dead animals

For every dead animal the cause of death may be infectious and therefore dead animals should be removed from the farm as quickly as possible in order to avoid disease transmission through direct and indirect contact.

4.1.4.1 Direct contact

Until the carcasses are collected by the rendering company they should be stored in a separate storage space with at least a cemented floor (Smart et al., 1982). This storage space should preferably be located close to the public highway to avoid trucks of the rendering company having to enter the farm (Fig. 14.2).

4.1.4.2 Indirect contact

When handling carcasses it is recommendable to use disposable gloves and/or to clean and disinfect hands afterwards. It is also highly advisable to clean and disinfect the storage place after each use. To avoid disease transmission through rodents, cats and dogs the storage place should be sealed off. Ideally, waste water should be collected in a well.

4.1.5 Professional visitors and personnel

Cattle farms receive a lot of visits from professional visitors (Nöremark et al., 2013; Sarrazin et al., 2014). Professional visitors enter farms for work-related reasons and thus come into close contact with cattle. In addition to veterinarians, other professional visitors include artificial insemination (AI) technicians, cattle salesmen, feed suppliers, milk collectors, rendering companies, hoof trimmers and possibly also other caretakers (personnel).

Very often (professional) visitors can enter the farm and stables where cattle are housed freely (Sarrazin et al., 2014). Nevertheless, it is recommended that all visitors should only be able to enter the farm after notifying the farmer and the stables should only be entered together with the farmer. Fencing the farm and closing the entrance with a gate, making the phone number of the farmer visible and putting up restricted area signs (pictograms) are practical tips that make visitors aware that they should not enter the farm and stables freely (Fig. 14.3, see p. 306).

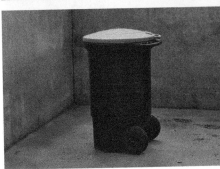

▲
Fig. 14.2: Until the carcasses are collected by the rendering company they should be stored in a separate storage space with at least a cemented floor. This storage space should preferably be close to the public highway to avoid trucks of the rendering company having to enter the farm.

14

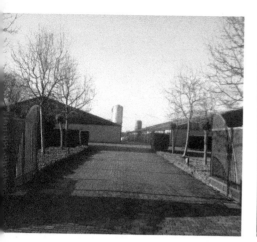
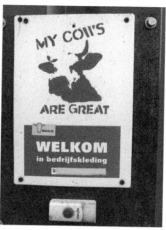

Fig. 14.3: Fencing the farm and closing the entrance with a gate, making the phone number of the farmer visible, a bell and putting up restricted area signs are practical tips that make visitors aware that they should not enter the farm and stables freely. (Translation: 'Welkom in bedrijfskleding' is 'Welcome when using herd-specific clothing')

Other adequate biosecurity measures for professional visitors are the use of herd-specific protective clothing and boots and/or well-maintained disinfection footbaths (Villarroel et al., 2007; Nöre-mark et al., 2013). These basic biosecurity measures should be easily accessible for the visitors, since it was noticed that although these measures were present in the majority of the cattle farms, they were rarely used (Sarrazin et al., 2014). Furthermore, we should also point out that it is not only veterinarians but every professional visitor that may represent a source of indirect trans-mission. A recent study revealed that biosecurity measures at entrances were not implemented by all visitors to the same extent: veterinarians used protective clothing and boots more often than AI technicians, followed by cattle salesmen (Sarrazin et al., 2014). A sanitary transition zone where visitors can change clothes and wash their hands should be located to ensure that a minimum amount of effort has to be made in order to access the sanitary transition zone before entering the stables (Fig. 14.4, see p. 307).

4.1.6 Vehicles and equipment

Although animal movements are generally considered as the major cause of disease spread, (professional) visitors and vehicles entering the farm should also be taken into consideration when establishing a biosecurity strategy for the farm (Alvarez et al., 2011). The risk of disease transmission depends among other things on the type of vehicle: for instance, rendering company trucks are considered to

BIOSECURITY IN ANIMAL PRODUCTION AND VETERINARY MEDICINE

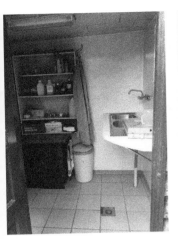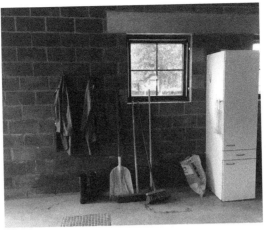

Fig. 14.4: This figure shows two examples of a sanitary transition zone where professional visitors can make use of the herd-specific clothing and boots and wash their hands before and after contact with the cattle.

be a higher biosecurity risk than feed trucks (Ribbens et al., 2009). Carcass storage space therefore should be located close to the public highway to avoid the truck of the rendering company having to enter the premises (see above). Although feed and milk collection trucks are rarely exposed to the animals on farms (Nöremark et al., 2013), these vehicles should be considered as a biosecurity risk as they visit several herds on the same day (Ribbens et al., 2009). Cattle stables should be designed in such a way that tractors can gain easy access to feed the animals and clean the pens. However, this means that vehicles from professional visitors can also enter the stables, and by so doing come close to the animals, and visitors will be less likely to pass through the sanitary transition zone. Therefore, it is recommended that vehicles should not enter the stables and that parking spaces should be provided close to the sanitary transition zone. Feed should be delivered and tank milk collected without the driver having to enter the stables.

When cattle leave the farm the animal transportation truck should preferably be empty, cleaned and disinfected on arrival at the farm (Crookshank et al., 1979). However, cattle from other farms are very often already present in the truck. It is advisable therefore that farmers do not enter the truck when animals are being loaded in order to avoid contact with cattle from other farms. and the transporter should not be allowed to enter the stables in order to avoid contact with the animals on the farm. Furthermore, cattle leaving the farm should be moved to a separate building or loading area to prevent contact with the herd. For example male dairy

14

calves that are sold at young age should be housed at a different location from the female calves remaining on the farm.

When equipment is shared with other farms, such as transportation vehicles or manure spreaders, attention should be paid to ensuring that the equipment is cleaned and disinfected when returned to the farm (Brennan et al., 2008).

4.1.7 Rodents, birds, dogs and cats

The presence of rodents, wild birds and cats is difficult to avoid on cattle farms. Domestic cats and dogs are also very often present. To avoid disease transmission through these animals (e.g. neosporosis, leptospirosis), access to the stables, manure storage facility and food storage facility should be limited as much as possible by closing or shielding doors, windows and gates (Synge et al., 2003; Fossler et al., 2005; Nielsen et al., 2007). Moreover, cats are not considered to be an effective good rodent control programme and traps and/or poison are recommended for controlling rodents (see chapter 11).

4.1.8 Feed and water quality

Contamination of feed by pathogens and or (myco)toxins can occur at all stages of feed production and storage. Crops can be contaminated with manure during fertilisation or even from fertilisation of neighbouring pastures. Therefore attention should be paid when manure from other farms used close to your own crops or pastures. Excretions and secretions of carrier animals may also contaminate feed (Maciorowski et al., 2007). All feeding utensils should be cleaned after each use to remove remnants that present a potential source of contamination. To avoid the growth of pathogens and/or production of myco(toxins) strict procedures for handling and storing feed should be observed, e.g. by adding products to improve the preservation of the silage pH.

Water contamination can occur at water sources, in reservoirs or pipes and at the outlets. It is therefore recommended to test the water quality at least once a year by carrying out bacteriological and chemical analysis at each of these places. Water troughs should also be checked and cleaned regularly to avoid contamination with faeces, urine and feed. For this reason, water troughs should be placed somewhat higher and at a distance from feeding troughs (Wright, 2007).

To avoid the contamination of feed and water by rodents, birds, dogs and cats, access to the food storage facility and water reservoirs should be limited as much as possible.

4.2 Internal biosecurity

4.2.1 Calving management

The period around calving is known to be a very critical period for dams that experience a temporary decrease in immunity as well as for the new-born calf that is born without any acquired immunity. A great deal of attention should be paid to the calving management therefore in order to avoid disease transmission through direct and indirect contact (Klein-Jöbstl et al., 2014).

4.2.1.1 Direct contact

Maternity pens are where dams are housed shortly before and after calving and should never be used to house sick animals. In the maternity pens there should be no contact with other cattle, although visible contact may be recommended to avoid stress (Svensson et al., 2003). Before and after each calving the maternity pens should be cleaned and disinfected (Gorden & Plummer, 2010). When calves cannot be born through natural calving a caesarean section has to be performed by the veterinarian. Similar biosecurity measures apply to this type of calving: a separate, clean and disinfected space without contact with other cattle and the use of herd-specific clothing by the veterinarian.

4.2.1.2 Indirect contact

It is recommended that the farmer is always present at the moment of calving. Hands, together with all obstetric material, should be cleaned and disinfected before and after each calving. Before a nat-

14

ural calving dams should be prepared by cleaning and disinfecting the udder and vulva (Meganck et al., 2015). After calving the foetal membranes and tissues should be removed from the calving area and the calf and attention must be paid to ensure that dogs in particular do not eat these membranes and tissues (Anderson et al., 2000; Wouda, 2000).

Immediately after birth the navel of the calf should be dipped into fresh disinfectant in a clean vessel. A disinfectant spray can also be used, but farmers have to be sure that the entire navel is sprayed and that it is only handled with clean and disinfected hands (Mee, 2008; Gorden & Plummer, 2010).

Since calves are born without acquired immunity, the ingestion of sufficient maternal antibodies through colostrum within the first hours of life is crucial (Harp & Goff, 1998; Mohammed, 1999). The administration of colostrum should fulfil the following requirements:

- A sufficient amount of colostrum has to be administered, i.e. 200 grams Ig G antibodies (Klein-Jöbstl et al., 2014). The concentration of IgG antibodies in the colostrum can be verified in several ways and depends among other things on the age and type of cattle. Given the amount of milk that dairy cattle produce, the concentration of maternal antibodies is lower and therefore more colostrum has to be given compared to beef cattle.

- The best quality colostrum is obtained from the first milking. Fresh colostrum is preferred over frozen colostrum. Frozen colostrum should never be thawed in a microwave oven – since antibodies are destroyed above 50 °C – but in warm water at 40-45 °C.

Using colostrum from other farms is not advised, given that the maternal antibodies in the colostrum of the dam or other cows present in the herd reflect the herd immunity better than colostrum from other farms and there is a potential for transmission of pathogens through colostrum (e.g. paratuberculosis).

- The absorption of antibodies through the gut quickly drops so the required amount of colostrum should be administered within 6 hours after birth (Gulliksen et al., 2009).

- Given the small capacity of the abomasum, colostrum should be administered *frequently* to avoid it flowing into the undeveloped rumen. The colostrum cannot be given all at once therefore, but should be spread over several feedings (Gorden & Plummer, 2010). Colostrum should not be left in the stable between feedings, but cooled in the refrigerator.

4.2.2 Disease management

4.2.2.1 Disease prevention

It is highly recommendable to have a register with animal health data in order to have an overview of the health and treatment status of individual and groups of animals (Edwards, 2010; Pardon et al., 2012). This type of register could contain the following information:

- Which animals are currently under treatment and which treatment are they receiving?
- Which animals are sick on a regular basis?
- What are the vaccination protocols for the different diseases and which (groups of) animals have to be vaccinated?
- When do cattle that go out to pasture: have to be rotated (every 2 to 6 weeks) or treated against endoparasites and ectoparasites?
- When do cows have to go through a disinfection footbath?
- What is the udder health status of lactating cows?

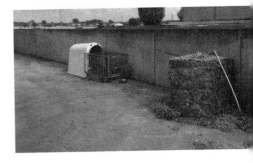

Fig. 14.5: This figure shows a diseased calf that is housed separately to avoid direct and indirect disease transmission. Specific material for use in this hospital pen only should be available.

14

▼

4.2.2.2 Direct contact

Hospital pens are where sick animals are housed to prevent disease transmission to other animals in the herd through direct and indirect contact (e.g. aerosols!) (Gorden & Plummer, 2010; Maunsell et al., 2011) (Fig. 14.5). Hospital pens should never be used as maternity pens and vice versa

(Fossler et al., 2005). Hospital pens should be cleaned and disinfected each time they are used (Edwards, 2010).

Cattle that have aborted should also be considered as sick animals and housed in hospital pens therefore until the reason for abortion has been determined.

When lactating cattle are diseased, it is advisable to milk them in the hospital pen or, if this is not possible, as last cow in the regular milking facility to avoid contact with the healthy animals (Hage et al., 2003; Fossler et al., 2005). If the latter option is chosen, special attention has to be paid to the cleaning and disinfection of milking material that is also used for healthy animals.

Chronically infected animals (e.g. paratuberculosis, bovine viral diarrhoea virus persistently infected animals, chronic subclinical mastitis, ...) are a continuous source of infection and perform in a suboptimal way and should therefore be removed from the farm. Such animals are often kept in the herd or in isolation until the moment of slaughter, but this practice should be discouraged because of the risk of disease transmission through direct and indirect contact.

4.2.2.3 Indirect contact

In the same way as when entering the quarantine area at the end of the daily working routine, diseased animals should be taken care of after the healthy animals (Maunsell et al., 2011).

Similar biosecurity measures to avoid indirect disease transmission as those adopted in the quarantine area also apply in hospital pens: the use of specific clothing, washing hands before and after contact with diseased animals and use of specific material only in the hospital pen, are strongly recommended.

4.2.3 Age groups and specific material

Except for suckling calves, new-born calves should be removed from the dam within one hour of the birth (Maunsell et al., 2011; Gorden & Plummer, 2010). They should preferably be housed in individual calf boxes or hutches during the first weeks of their life

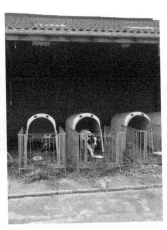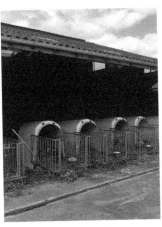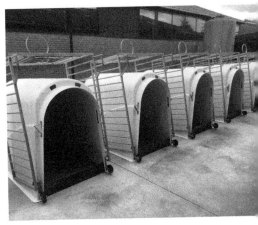

Fig. 14.6: Calves should preferably be housed in individual calf boxes or hutches during the first weeks of their life without physical, but with visible contact with other calves Hutches should be draught-free and placed on a paved/cemented and easy to clean surface Attention should be paid to ensure that urine and faeces cannot spread from one hutch to another. Calves should receive milk in their own and always the same bucket. After each feeding the buckets should be cleaned and placed upside down until the next use to avoid the introduction of dust, water, flies, etc.

without physical, but with visible contact with other calves (Klein-Jöbstl et al., 2014) (Fig. 14.6). Hutches should be draught-free and placed on a paved/cemented and easy-to-clean surface (Lundborg et al., 2005). Attention must be paid to ensuring that urine and faeces cannot spread from one hutch to another.

Calves should receive milk in their own and always the same bucket. This can be done very easily by numbering the boxes/hutches and buckets. After each feeding the buckets should be cleaned and placed upside down until the next use to avoid the introduction of dust, water, flies, etc. (Lassen et al., 2009; Meganck et al., 2015).

When calves leave their individual housing, it is advisable to split them up into group pens of calves that are the same age (Fig. 14.7). Initially this means that a variation in age of one week is allowed,

Fig. 14.7: This figure shows a stable with beef cattle; the young stock are housed in groups of the same age. The youngest animals are housed at the end of the stable at the left and move up towards the front of the stable when they grow older. To avoid stress and lesions, they are grouped per sex. The position of the different age groups in the stable depends on the direction in the airflow in the stable: air flows from the younger calves to the older animals.

◀

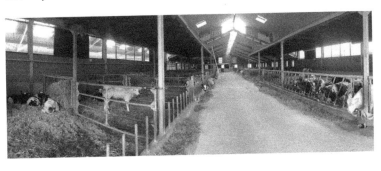

for older calves variation in age of about eight weeks is allowed (Gulliksen et al., 2009). Calves that do not grow well should not be put back in a younger age group, but should be examined for the presence of a disease and should be isolated to avoid them acting as a continuous source of infection. Calves and young stock should preferably be housed in different stable from the adult cattle, or at least well separated (i.e. no physical contact and a distance of minimum three meters between the boxes) to avoid disease transmission through direct and indirect contact, including aerosols and air transmission (Maunsell et al., 2011).

To avoid stress and lesions, beef cattle can be grouped by sex (Sanderson et al., 2008).

Disease transmission through aerosol is very important for calves. The position of the different age groups in the stable is important therefore. If there is a specific direction in the airflow in the stable, and if the stable houses different age groups, attention should be paid to ensuring that air flows from the younger calves to the older animals. If necessary the climate (temperature, humidity, etc.) should be controlled in the stables (Daugschies et al., 2005; Gorden & Plummer, 2010).

4.2.4 Working lines

It was already mentioned that sick animals and quarantined animals should be taken care of at the end of the daily routine. It is furthermore advisable to work *from young to old* in the daily working schedule, i.e. farm-specific working lines (Maunsell & Donovan, 2009; Gorden & Plummer, 2010; Maunsell, 2011). Farmers often argue that this young-to-old scheme is difficult to apply, since lactating cows first have to be milked in order to give this milk to the calves. This issue can be solved by feeding the calves with tank milk or by having different people milk the cows and feed the calves. Furthermore, feeding calves with milk from cows under antimicrobial treatment is strongly discouraged (Virtala et al., 1999).

It is recommendable to use age-specific material for each age group and feeding utensils should only be used for feed, i.e. no double use for removing manure. Distinction between age-specific material or feeding-specific utensils can easily be made by labelling the material. Feeding utensils should preferable cleaned and disinfected after each use.

Ideally a sanitary transition zone (changing clothes, washing hands) should be provided for each age group of animals and it should be used correctly. The application of these biosecurity measures together with the use of age-specific material can be encouraged by providing physical barriers between the age groups. This may be a different stable, or a bench or door which has to be passed in order to go to the next age group.

4.2.5 Milking management

Optimal milking management starts with well-functioning milking equipment. A yearly maintenance and audit of the milking equipment should be carried out in a static (without milking cows) and dynamic (while milking cows) test. A dynamic test evaluates the milking process by the machine and the farmer and only by carrying out a dynamic test is it possible to obtain a complete overview of the functioning of the milking process. The frequency of replacing teat cup liners depends on the type: rubber and silicone teat cup liners should be replaced after 2500 and 6000 milkings, respectively.

An optimal milking technique is a next crucial factor in the milking management (Fig. 14.8). The following recommendations apply more specifically to manual milking, but they also apply generally to robot milking:

- The farmer should wash, clean and disinfect his/her hands before milking and/or use gloves;
- Teats should be dry cleaned before milking with a clean cloth. If teats are also disinfected before milking, they should be dried after disinfection;
- Foremilk should be examined visually;

Fig. 14.8: Optimal milking management includes clean milking equipment and parlour.

▼

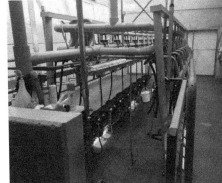

- Teats should be disinfected after removing the teat cups;
- The milking equipment and parlour should be cleaned after milking.

Cows should be milked in the best possible conditions by ensuring optimal comfort and hygiene:

- The flanks and udders should be clipped;
- To avoid stress the hierarchical order amongst cow should be respected, but keeping in mind that sick cows in lactation (e.g. mastitis) should preferably be milked as last;
- After milking, the teats remain open for about 30 to 60 minutes. It is advisable therefore to keep the cows standing for at least 30 minutes after milking. This can be facilitated by providing fresh feed at the feeding fence.
- If cows are housed in stables with slatted floors, rubber mats or an equivalent surface should be present in the resting spaces to avoid cows lying down on the slatted floors.

As mentioned above, cows with chronic subclinical mastitis should be removed from the herd.

Table 14.1: Overview of transmission pathways for epidemic and endemic cattle diseases of relevance to Belgium (references see pp. 382-405) ▶

| Disease | Species affected and asymptomatic carriers | | | | Direct contact | | | | |
	Zoonotic	Other reservoirs	Asymptomatic	Wildlife reservoir	Animal to animal	Transplacental	Venereal	General	People
Anaplasmosis		Mammals, birds	X	X		X		X	
Anthrax	X	Mammals, birds	X		X			X	
Aujeszky's Disease		Pigs, sheep, dogs, cats, rodents,....	X	X	X	X	X	X	
Babesiosis (bovine)	X	Buffaloes, deer	X	X					
Bluetongue		Ruminants, carnivores	X	X	X	X	X	X	
Botulism	X	Most animals	X	X	X			X	X
Bovine enzootic leucosis			X		X	X		X	
Bovine herpesvirus 4		Ruminants	X				X		
Bovine respiratory disease [a]		Ruminants	X	X	X			X	X
Bovine Spongiform Encephalopathy	X	Sheep, goats	X	X		X			
Bovine Viral Diarrhoea			X		X	X	X	X	X
Brucellosis	X	Ruminants, pigs, dogs, rodents, ...	X	X	X	X	X		
Campylobacteriosis	X	Vertebrates	X	X	X		X	X	
Coccidiosis			X		X			X	X
Cryptosporidiosis	X	Mammals	X	X	X			X	X
Cysticercosis	X		X	X					
Dermatophytosis	X	Mammals, birds	X	X	X			X	
Diarrhoea / enteritis (coronavirus, rotavirus, E. coli)	X	Mammals	X	X	X			X	X
Distomatosis	X	Ruminants	X	X					
E. Coli (verotoxic)	X	Mammals			X			X	X
Echinococcosis	X	Mammals, birds	X	X					

a The bovine respiratory disease complex includes the bovine respiratory syncytial virus, parainfluenza virus 3 (PI3), Mannheimia haemolytica, Pasteurella multocida, Histophilus somni, Mycoplasma bovis.

Animals	Rodents	Fomites	Syringes/needles	Feed	Water	General	Droplet	Aerosol	Soil / Manure	Vector	References
			X							X	[1-4]
		X		X	X	X			X	X	[5, 6]
		X			X	X		X	X		[4, 7]
										X	[4]
			X							X	[4, 7, 8]
X	X	X	X	X	X	X		X	X		[9-19]
			X							X	[20-23]
				X	X	X					[24]
X	X	X		X	X	X	X	X			[25-123]
				X							[4, 7, 124, 125]
X	X	X		X		X		X	X		[48, 65, 126-137]
				X	X	X			X		[4, 7, 138-144]
		X		X	X				X		[4, 8]
	X	X		X	X				X		[145-160]
X	X	X		X	X				X		[148, 150, 161-176]
				X	X						[4, 177, 178]
		X								X	[4, 179]
X	X	X		X	X				X		[56, 59, 66, 67, 161, 165, 167, 170, 176, 180-199]
				X							[21, 200, 201]
X	X	X		X	X				X		[202-212]
				X	X						[4, 213, 214]

Indirect contact

14

Disease	Zoonotic	Other reservoirs	Asymptomatic	Wildlife reservoir	Animal to animal	Transplacental	Venereal	General	People
		Species affected and asymptomatic carriers			Direct contact				
Enterotoxemia (*Clostridium* spp.)		Humans	X	X	X			X	X
Foot-and-mouth Disease		Cloven-hooved livestock, wildlife	X	X	X			X	X
Giardiasis	X	Mammals	X	X	X			X	X
Infectious Bovine Keratoconjunctivitis			X		X			X	X
Infectious Bovine Rhinotracheitis (IBR)			X		X	X	X	X	X
(Inter)digital infections		All			X			X	
Intestinal parasites	X	Ruminants	X	X				X	X
Leptospirosis	X	Mammals			X		X	X	
Lice and ectoparasites	X				X			X	
Listeriosis	X	Mammals, birds	X	X	X	X		X	X
(Sub)clinical mastitis	X		X		X			X	X
Metritis: trichomoniasis (T) + chlamydiosis(C)					T		T+C	T	
Necrobacillosis (laryngitis)			X		X			X	
Neosporosis	X	Mammals	X			X			
Papillomatosis			X		X	X		X	
Paratuberculosis		Mammals	X	X		X	X		
Q Fever / Coxiellosis	X	Vertebrates	X	X	X	X	X	X	
Rabies	X	Mammals		X	X			X	
Salmonellosis	X		X	X	X			X	X
Scabies					X			X	
Schmallenberg disease		Ruminants	X	X		X	X		
Tuberculosis (bovine)	X	Mammals	X	X		X		X	

Animals	Rodents	Fomites	Syringes/needles	Feed	Water	General	Droplet	Aerosol	Soil / Manure	Vector	References
				Ingestion		**Inhalation**					
X	X	X		X	X				X		[215-225]
X	X	X	X	X		X		X			[4, 226-323]
X	X	X		X	X				X		[168, 173, 233]
X		X								X	[234-244]
		X				X		X			[48, 65, 68, 120, 245-268]
									X		[21]
X		X		X	X				X		[269-291]
		X		X	X	X			X		[4, 292]
X	X	X									[293-308]
X	X	X		X							[309-333]
		X				X		X	X		[21, 334-338]
				C	C	C					[8, 339-342]
		X									[343-361]
				X	X						[362-366]
		X								X	[8, 21, 367-369]
		X		X	X						[4, 370-374]
		X		X	X	X			X		[4, 375-377]
X		X	X	X	X						[378-393]
X	X	X		X	X	X		X	X		[161, 394-410]
		X									[411-425]
										X	[8, 426-430]
		X		X	X	X	X		X		[4, 431, 432]

Table 14.1: References

1. Aiello, S. E., & Moses, M. A. (2016). The Merck Veterinary Manual.
2. Aubry, P., & Geale, D. (2011). A review of bovine anaplasmosis. *Transboundary and Emerging Diseases 58*(1), 1-30.
3. Kocan, K. M., Step, D., Blouin, E., Coetzee, J., Simpson, K., Genova, S., et al. (2010). Current challenges of the management and epidemiology of bovine anaplasmosis. *Bovine Practitioner 44*(2), 93-102.
4. Technology, I. S. U. o. S. a. Bovine Diseases and Resources. 2016, from Bovine Diseases and Resources
5. AR, S. Animal disease information. 2016, from http://www.cfsph.iastate.edu/DiseaseInfo/index.php.
6. Organization, W. H., & Epizootics, I. O. o. (2008). Anthrax in humans and animals: World Health Organization.
7. FAVV/AFSCA. 2016, from http://www.favv-afsca.be/santeanimale/aujeszky/
8. Francoz, D., Buczinski, S., Bélanger, A., Forté, G., Labrecque, O., Tremblay, D., et al. (2015). Respiratory pathogens in Québec dairy calves and their relationship with clinical status, lung consolidation, and average daily gain. *Journal of Veterinary Internal Medicine 29*(1), 381-387.
9. Critchley, E. (1991). A comparison of human and animal botulism: a review. *Journal of the Royal Society of Medicine 84*(5), 295-298.
10. Galey, F., Terra, R., Walker, R., Adaska, J., Etchebarne, M., Puschner, B., et al. (2000). Type C botulism in dairy cattle from feed contaminated with a dead cat. *Journal of Veterinary Diagnostic Investigation 12*(3), 204-209.
11. Gilbert, R. (1974). Staphylococcal food poisoning and botulism. *Postgraduate Medical Journal 50*(588), 603-611.
12. Heider, L. C., McClure, J., & Leger, E. R. (2001). Presumptive diagnosis of Clostridium botulinum type D intoxication in a herd of feedlot cattle. *The Canadian Veterinary Journal 42*(3), 210.
13. Lindström, M., Myllykoski, J., Sivelä, S., & Korkeala, H. (2010). Clostridium botulinum in cattle and dairy products. *Critical Reviews in Food Science and Nutrition 50*(4), 281-304.
14. Meyer, K. (1956). The status of botulism as a world health problem. *Bulletin of the World Health Organization 15*(1-2), 281.
15. Rodloff, A. C., & Krüger, M. (2012). Chronic Clostridium botulinum infections in farmers. *Anaerobe 18*(2), 226-228.
16. Seeliger, H. (1960). Food-borne infections and intoxications in Europe. *Bulletin of the World Health Organization 22*(5), 469.
17. Shapiro, R. L., Hatheway, C., & Swerdlow, D. L. (1998). Botulism in the United States: a clinical and epidemiologic review. *Annals of Internal Medicine 129*(3), 221-228.
18. Smart, J., Jones, T., Clegg, F., & McMurtry, M. (1987). Poultry waste associated type C botulism in cattle. *Epidemiology and Infection 98*(01), 73-79.
19. Sobel, J. (2005). Botulism. *Clinical Infectious Diseases 41*(8), 1167-1173.
20. Hopkins, S. G., & DiGiacomo, R. F. (1997). Natural transmission of bovine leukemia virus in dairy and beef cattle. *Veterinary Clinics of North America: Food Animal Practice 13*(1), 107-128.
21. L'ÉLEVAGE, I. D. (2000.). Maladies des bovins, Manuel pratique. Paris.
22. Nagy, D. W., Tyler, J. W., & Kleiboeker, S. B. (2007). Decreased Periparturient Transmission of Bovine Leukosis Virus in Colostrum-Fed Calves. *Journal of Veterinary Internal Medicine 21*(5), 1104-1107.

23. Rodríguez, S. M., Florins, A., Gillet, N., De Brogniez, A., Sánchez-Alcaraz, M. T., Boxus, M., et al. (2011). Preventive and therapeutic strategies for bovine leukemia virus: lessons for HTLV. *Viruses 3*(7), 1210-1248.

24. Markine-Goriaynoff, N., Minner, F., De Fays, K., Gillet, L., Thiry, E., Pastoret, P.-P., et al. (2003). L'herpèsvirus bovin 4. *Annales de Médecine Vétérinaire 147*, 215-247.

25. Assie, S., Seegers, H., Makoschey, B., Desire-Bousquie, L., & Bareille, N. (2009). Exposure to pathogens and incidence of respiratory disease in young bulls on their arrival at fattening operations in France. *The Veterinary Record 165*(7), 195-199.

26. Brscic, M., Leruste, H., Heutinck, L., Bokkers, E., Wolthuis-Fillerup, M., Stockhofe, N., et al. (2012). Prevalence of respiratory disorders in veal calves and potential risk factors. *Journal of Dairy Science 95*(5), 2753-2764.

27. Bureau, F., Detilleux, J., Dorts, T., Uystepruyst, C., Coghe, J., Leroy, P., et al. (2001). Spirometric performance in Belgian Blue calves: I. Effects on economic losses due to the bovine respiratory disease complex. *Journal of Animal Science 79*(5), 1301-1304.

28. Bureau, F., Michaux, C., Coghe, J., Uystepruyst, C., Leroy, P., & Lekeux, P. (2001). Spirometric performance in Belgian Blue calves: II. Analysis of environmental factors and estimation of genetic parameters. *Journal of Animal Science 79*(5), 1162-1165.

29. Cusack, P., McMeniman, N., & Lean, I. (2003). The medicine and epidemiology of bovine respiratory disease in feedlots. *Australian Veterinary Journal 81*(8), 480-487.

30. Edwards, T. (2010). Control methods for bovine respiratory disease for feedlot cattle. *Veterinary Clinics of North America: Food Animal Practice 26*(2), 273-284.

31. Francoz, D., & Couture, Y. (2014). Manuel de médecine des bovins. Editions MED'COM, 37-49.

32. Fulton, R. W. (2009). Bovine respiratory disease research (1983-2009). *Animal Health Research Reviews 10*(02), 131-139.

33. Gay, E., & Barnouin, J. (2009). A nation-wide epidemiological study of acute bovine respiratory disease in France. *Preventive Veterinary Medicine 89*(3), 265-271.

34. Gorden, P. J., & Plummer, P. (2010). Control, management, and prevention of bovine respiratory disease in dairy calves and cows. *Veterinary Clinics of North America: Food Animal Practice 26*(2), 243-259.

35. Griffin, D., Chengappa, M. M., Kuszak, J., & McVey, D. S. (2010). Bacterial pathogens of the bovine respiratory disease complex. *Veterinary Clinics of North America: Food Animal Practice 26*(2), 381-394.

36. Gulliksen, S. M., Lie, K. I., Løken, T., & Østerås, O. (2009). Calf mortality in Norwegian dairy herds. *Journal of Dairy Science 92*(6), 2782-2795.

37. Gulliksen, S. M., Jor, E., Lie, K. I., Løken, T., Åkerstedt, J., & Østerås, O. (2009). Respiratory infections in Norwegian dairy calves. *Journal of Dairy Science 92*(10), 5139-5146.

38. Gulliksen, S. M., Lie, K. I., & Østerås, O. (2009). Calf health monitoring in Norwegian dairy herds. *Journal of Dairy Science 92*(4), 1660-1669.

39. Hägglund, S., Svensson, C., Emanuelson, U., Valarcher, J., & Alenius, S. (2006). Dynamics of virus infections involved in the bovine respiratory disease complex in Swedish dairy herds. *The Veterinary Journal 172*(2), 320-328.

40. Hilton, W. M. (2014). BRD in 2014: where have we been, where are we now, and where do we want to go? *Animal Health Research Reviews 15*(02), 120-122.

41. Klem, T., Gulliksen, S., Lie, K.-I., Løken, T., Østerås, O., & Stokstad, M. (2013). Bovine respiratory syncytial virus: infection dynamics within and between herds. *Veterinary Record 173*, 476.

42. Lundborg, G., Svensson, E., & Oltenacu, P. (2005). Herd-level risk factors for infectious diseases in Swedish dairy calves aged 0-90 days. *Preventive Veterinary Medicine 68*(2), 123-143.

14

43. Lundborg, G., Oltenacu, P., Maizon, D., Svensson, E., & Liberg, P. (2003). Dam-related effects on heart girth at birth, morbidity and growth rate from birth to 90 days of age in Swedish dairy calves. *Preventive Veterinary Medicine* 60(2), 175-190.

44. Mosier, D. (2014). Review of BRD pathogenesis: the old and the new. *Animal Health Research Reviews* 15(02), 166-168.

45. Norström, M., Skjerve, E., & Jarp, J. (2000). Risk factors for epidemic respiratory disease in Norwegian cattle herds. *Preventive Veterinary Medicine* 44(1), 87-96.

46. Pardon, B., De Bleecker, K., Dewulf, J., Callens, J., Boyen, F., Catry, B., et al. (2011). Prevalence of respiratory pathogens in diseased, non-vaccinated, routinely medicated veal calves. *Veterinary Record-English Edition* 169(11), 278.

47. Pardon, B. (2012). Morbidity, mortality and drug use in white veal calves with emphasis on respiratory disease. Ghent University.

48. Roshtkhari, F., Mohammadi, G., & Mayameei, A. (2012). Serological evaluation of relationship between viral pathogens (BHV-1, BVDV, BRSV, PI-3V, and Adeno3) and dairy calf pneumonia by indirect ELISA. *Tropical Animal Health and Production* 44(5), 1105-1110.

49. Sanderson, M. W., Dargatz, D. A., & Wagner, B. A. (2008). Risk factors for initial respiratory disease in United States' feedlots based on producer-collected daily morbidity counts. *Canadian Veterinary Journal* 49(4), 373-378.

50. Stokka, G. L. (2010). Prevention of respiratory disease in cow/calf operations. *Veterinary Clinics of North America: Food Animal Practice* 26(2), 229-241.

51. Stott, E., Thomas, L., Collins, A., Crouch, S., Jebbett, J., Smith, G., et al. (1980). A survey of virus infections of the respiratory tract of cattle and their association with disease. *Journal of Hygiene* 85(02), 257-270.

52. Svensson, C., Lundborg, K., Emanuelson, U., & Olsson, S.-O. (2003). Morbidity in Swedish dairy calves from birth to 90 days of age and individual calf-level risk factors for infectious diseases. *Preventive Veterinary Medicine* 58(3), 179-197.

53. Svensson, C., & Jensen, M. B. (2007). Short communication: Identification of diseased calves by use of data from automatic milk feeders. *Journal of Dairy Science* 90(2), 994-997.

54. Sweiger, S. H., & Nichols, M. D. (2010). Control methods for bovine respiratory disease in stocker cattle. *Veterinary Clinics of North America: Food Animal Practice* 26(2), 261-271.

55. Taylor, J. D., Fulton, R. W., Lehenbauer, T. W., Step, D. L., & Confer, A. W. (2010). The epidemiology of bovine respiratory disease: What is the evidence for predisposing factors? *Canadian Veterinary Journal* 51(10), 1095-1102.

56. Torsein, M., Lindberg, A., Sandgren, C. H., Waller, K. P., Törnquist, M., & Svensson, C. (2011). Risk factors for calf mortality in large Swedish dairy herds. *Preventive Veterinary Medicine* 99(2), 136-147.

57. Van Donkersgoed, J., Janzen, E. D., Potter, A. A., & Harland, R. J. (1994). The occurrence of Haemophilus somnus in feedlot calves and its control by postarrival prophylactic mass medication. *The Canadian Veterinary Journal* 35(9), 573.

58. Virtala, A.-M., Gröhn, Y., Mechor, G., & Erb, H. (1999). The effect of maternally derived immunoglobulin G on the risk of respiratory disease in heifers during the first 3 months of life. *Preventive Veterinary Medicine* 39(1), 25-37.

59. Windeyer, M., Leslie, K., Godden, S., Hodgins, D., Lissemore, K., & LeBlanc, S. (2014). Factors associated with morbidity, mortality, and growth of dairy heifer calves up to 3 months of age. *Preventive Veterinary Medicine* 113(2), 231-240.

60. Woolums, A. R., Berghaus, R. D., Smith, D. R., White, B. J., Engelken, T. J., Irsik, M. B., et al. (2013). Producer survey of herd-level risk factors for nursing beef calf respiratory disease. *Journal of the American Veterinary Medical Association* 243(4), 538-547.

61. Almeida, R., Domingues, H., Spilki, F., Larsen, L. E., Hagglund, S., Belak, S., et al. (2006). Circulation of bovine respiratory syncytial virus in Brazil. *Veterinary Record* *158*(18), 632.

62. Brodersen, B. W. (2010). Bovine respiratory syncytial virus. *Veterinary Clinics of North America: Food Animal Practice 26*(2), 323-333.

63. Figueroa-Chávez, D., Segura-Correa, J. C., García-Márquez, L. J., Pescador-Rubio, A., & Valdivia-Flores, A. G. (2012). Detection of antibodies and risk factors for infection with bovine respiratory syncytial virus and parainfluenza virus 3 in dual-purpose farms in Colima, Mexico. *Tropical Animal Health and Production 44*(7), 1417-1421.

64. Luzzago, C., Bronzo, V., Salvetti, S., Frigerio, M., & Ferrari, N. (2010). Bovine respiratory syncytial virus seroprevalence and risk factors in endemic dairy cattle herds. *Veterinary Research Communications 34*(1), 19-24.

65. Mars, M., Bruschke, C., & Van Oirschot, J. (1999). Airborne transmission of BHV1, BRSV, and BVDV among cattle is possible under experimental conditions. *Veterinary Microbiology 66*(3), 197-207.

66. Oevermann, A., Zurbriggen, A., & Vandevelde, M. (2010). Rhombencephalitis caused by listeria monocytogenes in humans and ruminants: A zoonosis on the rise? *Interdisciplinary Perspectives on Infectious Diseases 2010.*

67. Ohlson, A., Alenius, S., Tråvén, M., & Emanuelson, U. (2013). A longitudinal study of the dynamics of bovine corona virus and respiratory syncytial virus infections in dairy herds. *The Veterinary Journal 197*(2), 395-400.

68. Raaperi, K., Bougeard, S., Aleksejev, A., Orro, T., & Viltrop, A. (2012). Association of herd BHV-1 seroprevalence with respiratory disease in youngstock in Estonian dairy cattle. *Research in Veterinary Science 93*(2), 641-648.

69. Saa, L. R., Perea, A., Jara, D. V., Arenas, A. J., Garcia-Bocanegra, I., Borge, C., et al. (2012). Prevalence of and risk factors for bovine respiratory syncytial virus (BRSV) infection in non-vaccinated dairy and dual-purpose cattle herds in Ecuador. *Tropical Animal Health and Production 44*(7), 1423-1427.

70. Sacco, R. E., McGill, J., Pillatzki, A. E., Palmer, M., & Ackermann, M. R. (2014). Respiratory syncytial virus infection in cattle. *Veterinary Pathology 51*(2), 427-436.

71. Sarmiento-Silva, R. E., Nakamura-Lopez, Y., & Vaughan, G. (2012). Epidemiology, molecular epidemiology and evolution of bovine respiratory syncytial virus. *Viruses 4*(12), 3452-3467.

72. Solís-Calderón, J., Segura-Correa, J., Aguilar-Romero, F., & Segura-Correa, V. (2007). Detection of antibodies and risk factors for infection with bovine respiratory syncytial virus and parainfluenza virus-3 in beef cattle of Yucatan, Mexico. *Preventive Veterinary Medicine 82*(1), 102-110.

73. Valarcher, J.-F., & Taylor, G. (2007). Bovine respiratory syncytial virus infection. *Veterinary Research 38*(2), 153-180.

74. Valarcher, J.-F., Bourhy, H., Lavenu, A., Bourges-Abella, N., Roth, M., Andreoletti, O., et al. (2001). Persistent infection of B lymphocytes by bovine respiratory syncytial virus. *Virology 291*(1) 55-67.

75. Van der Poel, W., Brand, A., Kramps, J., & Van Oirschot, J. (1994). Respiratory syncytial virus infections in human beings and in cattle. *Journal of Infection 29*(2), 215-228.

76. Allen, J., Viel, L., Bateman, K., Rosendal, S., Shewen, P., & Physick-Sheard, P. (1991). The microbial flora of the respiratory tract in feedlot calves: associations between nasopharyngeal and bronchoalveolar lavage cultures. *Canadian Journal of Veterinary Research 55*(4), 341.

77. Catry, B., Haesebrouck, F., Vliegher, S. D., Feyen, B., Vanrobaeys, M., Opsomer, G., et al. (2005). Variability in acquired resistance of Pasteurella and Mannheimia iso-

14

lates from the nasopharynx of calves, with particular reference to different herd types. *Microbial Drug Resistance 11*(4), 387-394.

78. Dewey, K., & Little, P. (1984). Environmental survival of Haemophilus somnus and influence of secretions and excretions. *Canadian Journal of Comparative Medicine 48*(1), 23.

79. Griffin, D., Chengappa, M., Kuszak, J., & McVey, D. S. (2010). Bacterial pathogens of the bovine respiratory disease complex. *Veterinary Clinics of North America: Food Animal Practice 26*(2), 381-394.

80. Harris, F. W., & Janzen, E. D. (1989). The Haemophilus somnus disease complex (Hemophilosis): A review. *The Canadian Veterinary Journal 30*(10), 816.

81. Headley, S., Alfieri, A., Oliveira, V., Beuttemmüller, E., & Alfieri, A. (2014). Histophilus somni is a potential threat to beef cattle feedlots in Brazil. *The Veterinary Record 175*(10), 249.

82. Highlander, S. K. (2001). Molecular genetic analysis of virulence in Mannheimia (Pasteurella) haemolytica. *Frontiers in Bioscience 6*(September), D1128-D1150.

83. Jánosi, K., Stipkovits, L., Glávits, R., Molnár, T., Makrai, L., Gyuranecz, M., et al. (2009). Aerosol infection of calves with Histophilus somni. *Acta Veterinaria Hungarica 57*(3), 347-356.

84. Martin, S., Harland, R., Bateman, K., & Nagy, E. (1998). The association of titers to Haemophilus somnus, and other putative pathogens, with the occurrence of bovine respiratory disease and weight gain in feedlot calves. *Canadian Journal of Veterinary Research 62*(4), 262.

85. O'Reilly, L. M., & Daborn, C. (1995). The epidemiology of Mycobacterium bovis infections in animals and man: a review. *Tubercle and Lung disease 76*, 1-46.

86. O'Connor, A., Shen, H., Wang, C., & Opriessnig, T. (2012). Descriptive epidemiology of Moraxella bovis, Moraxella bovoculi and Moraxella bovis in beef calves with naturally occurring infectious bovine keratoconjunctivitis (Pinkeye). *Veterinary Microbiology 155*(2), 374-380.

87. Portis, E., Lindeman, C., Johansen, L., & Stoltman, G. (2012). A ten-year (2000-2009) study of antimicrobial susceptibility of bacteria that cause bovine respiratory disease complex—Mannheimia haemolytica, Pasteurella multocida, and Histophilus somni—in the United States and Canada. *Journal of Veterinary Diagnostic Investigation 24*(5), 932-944.

88. Sandal, I., & Inzana, T. J. (2010). A genomic window into the virulence of Histophilus somni. *Trends in Microbiology 18*(2), 90-99.

89. Sanfacon, D., & Higgins, R. (1983). Epidemiology of Haemophilus somnus infection in dairy cattle in Quebec. *Canadian Journal of Comparative Medicine 47*(4), 456.

90. Saunders, J., Thiessen, W., & Janzen, E. (1980). Haemophilus somnus infections I. A ten year (1969-1978) retrospective study of losses in cattle herds in Western Canada. *The Canadian Veterinary Journal 21*(4), 119.

91. Van Donkersgoed, J., Ribble, C. S., Boyer, L., & Townsend, H. (1993). Epidemiological study of enzootic pneumonia in dairy calves in Saskatchewan. *Canadian Journal of Veterinary Research 57*(4), 247.

92. Jaramillo-Arango, C., Hernández-Castro, R., Suárez-Güemes, F., Martínez-Maya, J., Aguilar-Romero, F., Jaramillo-Meza, L., et al. (2008). Characterisation of Mannheimia spp. strains isolated from bovine nasal exudate and factors associated to isolates, in dairy farms in the Central Valley of Mexico. *Research in Veterinary Science 84*(1), 7-13.

93. Katsuda, K., Kamiyama, M., Kohmoto, M., Kawashima, K., Tsunemitsu, H., & Eguchi, M. (2008). Serotyping of Mannheimia haemolytica isolates from bovine pneumonia: 1987-2006. *The Veterinary Journal 178*(1), 146-148.

94. Noyes, N., Benedict, K., Gow, S., Booker, C., Hannon, S., McAllister, T., et al. (2015). Mannheimia haemolytica in feedlot cattle: prevalence of recovery and associations with antimicrobial use, resistance, and health outcomes. *Journal of Veterinary Internal Medicine 29*(2), 705-713.

95. Rice, J., Carrasco-Medina, L., Hodgins, D., & Shewen, P. (2007). Mannheimia haemolytica and bovine respiratory disease. *Animal Health Research Reviews 8*(02), 117-128.

96. Taylor, J., Holland, B., Step, D., Payton, M., & Confer, A. (2015). Nasal isolation of Mannheimia haemolytica and Pasteurella multocida as predictors of respiratory disease in shipped calves. *Research in Veterinary Science 99*, 41-45.

97. Timsit, E., Arcangioli, M.-A., Bareille, N., Seegers, H., & Assié, S. (2012). Transmission dynamics of Mycoplasma bovis in newly received beef bulls at fattening operations. *Journal of Veterinary Diagnostic Investigation 24*(6), 1172-1176.

98. Arcangioli, M.-A., Duet, A., Meyer, G., Dernburg, A., Bézille, P., Poumarat, F., et al. (2008). The role of Mycoplasma bovis in bovine respiratory disease outbreaks in veal calf feedlots. *The Veterinary Journal 177*(1), 89-93.

99. Ayling, R., Bashiruddin, S., & Nicholas, R. (2004). Mycoplasma species and related organisms isolated from ruminants in Britain between 1990 and 2000. *The Veterinary Record 155*(14), 413-416.

100. Caswell, J. L., & Archambault, M. (2007). Mycoplasma bovis pneumonia in cattle. *Animal Health Research Reviews 8*(02), 161-186.

101. Caswell, J. L., Bateman, K. G., Cai, H. Y., & Castillo-Alcala, F. (2010). Mycoplasma bovis in respiratory disease of feedlot cattle. *Veterinary Clinics of North America: Food Animal Practice 26*(2), 365-379.

102. Gagea, M. I., Bateman, K. G., Shanahan, R. A., van Dreumel, T., McEwen, B. J., Carman, S., et al. (2006). Naturally Occurring Mycoplasma Bovis—Associated Pneumonia and Polyarthritis in Feedlot Beef Calves. *Journal of Veterinary Diagnostic Investigation 18*(1), 29-40.

103. Giovannini, S., Zanoni, M., Salogni, C., Cinotti, S., & Alborali, G. (2013). Mycoplasma bovis infection in respiratory disease of dairy calves less than one month old. *Research in Veterinary Science 95*(2), 576-579.

104. Horwood, P., Schibrowski, M., Fowler, E., Gibson, J., Barnes, T., & Mahony, T. (2014). Is Mycoplasma bovis a missing component of the bovine respiratory disease complex in Australia? *Australian Veterinary Journal 92*(6), 185-191.

105. Howard, C. (1983). Mycoplasmas and bovine respiratory disease: studies related to pathogenicity and the immune response--a selective review. *The Yale Journal of Biology and Medicine 56*(5-6), 789.

106. Jasper, D. (1982). The role of Mycoplasma in bovine mastitis. *Journal of the American Veterinary Medical Association 181*(2), 158-162.

107. Knudtson, W., Reed, D., & Daniels, G. (1986). Identification of mycoplasmatales in pneumonic calf lungs. *Veterinary Microbiology 11*(1-2), 79-91.

108. Lamm, C. G., Munson, L., Thurmond, M. C., Barr, B. C., & George, L. W. (2004). Mycoplasma otitis in California calves. *Journal of Veterinary Diagnostic Investigation 16*(5), 397-402.

109. Maunsell, F., Woolums, A., Francoz, D., Rosenbusch, R., Step, D., Wilson, D. J., et al. (2011). Mycoplasma bovis infections in cattle. *Journal of Veterinary Internal Medicine 25*(4), 772-783.

110. Maunsell, F. P., & Donovan, G. A. (2009). Mycoplasma bovis infections in young calves. *Veterinary Clinics of North America: Food Animal Practice 25*(1), 139-177.

111. Nicholas, R., & Ayling, R. (2003). Mycoplasma bovis: disease, diagnosis, and control. *Research in Veterinary Science 74*(2), 105-112.

14

112. Soehnlen, M., Aydin, A., Murthy, K., Lengerich, E., Hattel, A., Houser, B., et al. (2012). Epidemiology of Mycoplasma bovis in Pennsylvania veal calves. *Journal of Dairy Science 95*(1), 247-254.

113. Timsit, E., Christensen, H., Bareille, N., Seegers, H., Bisgaard, M., & Assié, S. (2013). Transmission dynamics of Mannheimia haemolytica in newly-received beef bulls at fattening operations. *Veterinary Microbiology 161*(3), 295-304.

114. schopp, R., Bonnemain, P., Nicolet, J., & Burnens, A. (2001). Epidemiological study of risk factors for Mycoplasma bovis infections in fattening calves. *Schweizer Archiv fur Tierheilkunde 143*(9), 461-467.

115. Wilson, D. J., Justice-Allen, A., Goodell, G., Baldwin, T. J., Skirpstunas, R. T., & Cavender, K. (2011). Risk of Mycoplasma bovis transmission from contaminated sand bedding to naive dairy calves. *Journal of Dairy Science 94*(3), 1318-1324.

116. Dabo, S. M., Confer, A., Montelongo, M., York, P., & Wyckoff, J. H. (2008). Vaccination with Pasteurella multocida recombinant OmpA induces strong but non-protective and deleterious Th2-type immune response in mice. *Vaccine 26*(34), 4345-4351.

117. Hotchkiss, E., Hodgson, J., Schmitt-Van De Leemput, E., Dagleish, M., & Zadoks, R. (2011). Molecular epidemiology of Pasteurella multocida in dairy and beef calves. *Veterinary Microbiology 151*(3), 329-335.

118. Hotchkiss, E., Dagleish, M., Willoughby, K., Finlayson, J., Zadoks, R., Newsome, E., et al. (2010). Prevalence of Pasteurella multocida and other respiratory pathogens in the nasal tract of Scottish calves. *The Veterinary Record 167*(15), 555.

119. Hunt, M. L., Adler, B., & Townsend, K. M. (2000). The molecular biology of Pasteurella multocida. *Veterinary Microbiology 72*(1), 3-25.

120. Yates, W. (1982). A review of infectious bovine rhinotracheitis, shipping fever pneumonia and viral-bacterial synergism in respiratory disease of cattle. *Canadian Journal of Comparative Medicine 46*(3), 225.

121. Elazhary, M., & Derbyshire, J. (1979a). Aerosol stability of bovine parainfluenza type 3 virus. *Canadian Journal of Comparative Medicine 43*(3), 295.

122. Ellis, J. A. (2010). Bovine parainfluenza-3 virus. *Veterinary Clinics of North America: Food Animal Practice 26*(3), 575-593.

123. Frank, G., & Marshall, R. (1971). Relationship of serum and nasal secretion--neutralizing antibodies in protection of calves against parainfluenza-3 virus. *American Journal of Veterinary Research 32*(11), 1707-1713.

124. Doherr, M. G. (2007). Brief review on the epidemiology of transmissible spongiform encephalopathies (TSE). *Vaccine 25*(30), 5619-5624.

125. Ducrot, C., Arnold, M., De Koeijer, A., Heim, D., & Calavas, D. (2008). Review on the epidemiology and dynamics of BSE epidemics. *Veterinary Research 39*(4), 1-18.

126. Cuttance, W., & Cuttance, E. (2014). Analysis of individual farm investigations into bovine viral diarrhoea in beef herds in the North Island of New Zealand. *New Zealand Veterinary Journal 62*(6), 338-342.

127. Fredriksen, B., Press, C. M., Løken, T., & Ødegaard, S. (1999). Distribution of viral antigen in uterus, placenta and foetus of cattle persistently infected with bovine virus diarrhoea virus. *Veterinary Microbiology 64*(2), 109-122.

128. Gates, M., Humphry, R., & Gunn, G. (2013). Associations between bovine viral diarrhoea virus (BVDV) seropositivity and performance indicators in beef suckler and dairy herds. *The Veterinary Journal 198*(3), 631-637.

129. Humphry, R., Brlisauer, F., McKendrick, I., Nettleton, P., & Gunn, G. (2012). Prevalence of antibodies to bovine viral diarrhoea virus in bulk tank milk and associated risk factors in Scottish dairy herds. *Veterinary Record-English Edition 171*(18), 445.

130. Lanyon, S. R., Hill, F. I., Reichel, M. P., & Brownlie, J. (2014). Bovine viral diarrhoea: pathogenesis and diagnosis. *The Veterinary Journal 199*(2), 201-209.

131. Meyling, A., Houe, H., & Jensen, A. (1990). Epidemiology of bovine viral diarrhoea virus. *Revue scientifique et technique (International Office of Epizootics) 9*(1), 75-93.

132. Negrón, M., Raizman, E. A., Pogranichniy, R., Hilton, W. M., & Lévy, M. (2011). Survey on management practices related to the prevention and control of bovine viral diarrhea virus on dairy farms in Indiana, United States. *Preventive Veterinary Medicine 99*(2), 130-135.

133. Ridpath, J. F., Falkenberg, S. M., Bauermann, F. V., VanderLey, B. L., Do, Y., Flores, E. F., et al. (2013). Comparison of acute infection of calves exposed to a high-virulence or low-virulence bovine viral diarrhea virus or a HoBi-like virus. *American Journal of Veterinary Research 74*(3), 438-442.

134. Sarrazin, S., Veldhuis, A., Méroc, E., Vangeel, I., Laureyns, J., Dewulf, J., et al. (2013). Serological and virological BVDV prevalence and risk factor analysis for herds to be BVDV seropositive in Belgian cattle herds. *Preventive Veterinary Medicine 108*(1), 28-37.

135. Smith, D. R., & Grotelueschen, D. M. (2004). Biosecurity and biocontainment of bovine viral diarrhea virus. *Veterinary Clinics of North America: Food Animal Practice 20*(1), 131-149.

136. Valle, P., Martin, S., Tremblay, R., & Bateman, K. (1999). Factors associated with being a bovine-virus diarrhoea (BVD) seropositive dairy herd in the Møre and Romsdal County of Norway. *Preventive Veterinary Medicine 40*(3), 165-177.

137. Villarroel, A., Dargatz, D. A., Lane, V. M., McCluskey, B. J., & Salman, M. D. (2007). Suggested outline of potential critical control points for biosecurity and biocontainment on large dairy farms. *Journal of the American Veterinary Medical Association 230*(6), 808-819.

138. Aparicio, E. D. (2013). Epidemiology of brucellosis in domestic animals caused by Brucella melitensis, Brucella suis and Brucella abortus. *Revue scientifique et technique (International Office of Epizootics) 32*(1), 53-60.

139. Gwida, M., Al Dahouk, S., Melzer, F., Rösler, U., Neubauer, H., & Tomaso, H. (2010). Brucellosis – regionally emerging zoonotic disease? *Croatian Medical Journal 51*(4), 289-295.

140. Mailles, A., Rautureau, S., Le Horgne, J., Poignet-Leroux, B., d'Arnoux, C., Dennetière, G., et al. (2012). Re-emergence of brucellosis in cattle in France and risk for human health. *Eurosurveillance 17*(30), 20227.

141. Mukhtar, F. (2010). Brucellosis in a high-risk occupational group: seroprevalence and analysis of risk factors. *Journal of the Pakistan Medical Association 60*(12), 1031.

142. Nicoletti, P. (1980). The epidemiology of bovine brucellosis. *Advances in Veterinary Science and Comparative Medicine 24*, 69.

143. Plommet, M., Renoux, G., Philippon, A., Gestin, J., & Fensterbank, R. (1971). Congenital transmission of bovine brucellosis from one generation to another. *Bulletin de l'Academie vétérinaire de France 44*(1), 53-59.

144. Ron-Román, J., Ron-Garrido, L., Abatih, E., Celi-Erazo, M., Vizcaino-Ordonez, L., Calva-Pacheco, J., et al. (2014). Human brucellosis in northwest Ecuador: typifying Brucella spp., seroprevalence, and associated risk factors. *Vector-Borne and Zoonotic Diseases 14*(2), 124-133.

145. Abebe, R., Wossene, A., & Kumsa, B. (2008). Epidemiology of Eimeria infections in calves in Addis Ababa and Debre Zeit dairy farms, Ethiopia. *International Journal of Applied Research in Veterinary Medicine 6*(1), 24-30.

146. Daugschies, A., & Najdrowski, M. (2005). Eimeriosis in cattle: current understanding. *Journal of Veterinary Medicine, Series B 52*(10), 417-427.

147. Faber, J.-E., Kollmann, D., Heise, A., Bauer, C., Failing, K., Bürger, H.-J., et al. (2002). Eimeria infections in cows in the periparturient phase and their calves: oocyst

excretion and levels of specific serum and colostrum antibodies. *Veterinary Parasitology* 104(1), 1-17.

148. Fayer, R., Morgan, U., & Upton, S. J. (2000). Epidemiology of Cryptosporidium: transmission, detection and identification. *International Journal for Parasitology* 30(12), 1305-1322.

149. Jolley, W. R., & Bardsley, K. D. (2006). Ruminant coccidiosis. *Veterinary Clinics of North America: Food Animal Practice* 22(3), 613-621.

150. Lassen, B., Viltrop, A., Raaperi, K., & Järvis, T. (2009). Eimeria and Cryptosporidium in Estonian dairy farms in regard to age, species, and diarrhoea. *Veterinary Parasitology* 166(3), 212-219.

151. Lentze, T., Hofer, D., Gottstein, B., Gaillard, C., & Busato, A. (1999). Prevalence and importance of endoparasites in calves raised in Swiss cow-calf farms. DTW. *Deutsche Tierärztliche Wochenschrift* 106(7), 275-281.

152. Lucas, A. S., Swecker, W. S., Lindsay, D. S., Scaglia, G., Elvinger, F. C., & Zajac, A. M. (2007). The effect of weaning method on coccidial infections in beef calves. *Veterinary Parasitology* 145(3), 228-233.

153. Manya, P., Sinha, S., Sinha, S., Verma, S., Sharma, S., & Mandal, K. (2008). Prevalence of bovine coccidiosis at Patna. *Journal of Veterinary Parasitology* 22(2), 73-76.

154. Mitchell, E., Smith, R., & Ellis-Iversen, J. (2012). Husbandry risk factors associated with subclinical coccidiosis in young cattle. *The Veterinary Journal* 193(1), 119-123.

155. Radostits, O., & Stockdale, P. (1980). A brief review of bovine coccidiosis in western Canada. *The Canadian Veterinary Journal* 21(8), 227.

156. Rehman, T. U., Khan, M. N., Sajid, M. S., Abbas, R. Z., Arshad, M., Iqbal, Z., et al. (2011). Epidemiology of Eimeria and associated risk factors in cattle of the Toba Tek Singh District, Pakistan. *Parasitology Research* 108(5), 1171-1177.

157. Sánchez, R., Romero, J., & Founroge, R. (2008). Dynamics of Eimeria oocyst excretion in dairy calves in the Province of Buenos Aires (Argentina), during their first 2 months of age. *Veterinary Parasitology* 151(2), 133-138.

158. Step, D., Streeter, R., & Kirkpatrick, J. (2002). Bovine Coccidiosis – A Review. *Bovine Practitioner* 36(2), 126-135.

159. von Samson-Himmelstjerna, G., Epe, C., Wirtherle, N., Von der Heyden, V., Welz, C., Radeloff, I., et al. (2006). Clinical and epidemiological characteristics of Eimeria infections in first-year grazing cattle. *Veterinary Parasitology* 136(3), 215-221.

160. Waruiru, R., Kyvsgaard, N., Thamsborg, S., Nansen, P., Bøgh, H., Munyua, W., et al. (2000). The prevalence and intensity of helminth and coccidial infections in dairy cattle in central Kenya. *Veterinary Research Communications* 24(1), 39-53.

161. Andrews, A. H., Blowey, R. W., Boyd, H., & Eddy, R. G. (2008a). Bovine medicine: diseases and husbandry of cattle, Chapter 14: John Wiley & Sons.

162. Bartels, C. J., Holzhauer, M., Jorritsma, R., Swart, W. A., & Lam, T. J. (2010). Prevalence, prediction and risk factors of enteropathogens in normal and non-normal faeces of young Dutch dairy calves. *Preventive Veterinary Medicine* 93(2), 162-169.

163. Delafosse, A., Chartier, C., Dupuy, M., Dumoulin, M., Pors, I., & Paraud, C. (2015). Cryptosporidium parvum infection and associated risk factors in dairy calves in western France. *Preventive Veterinary Medicine* 118(4), 406-412.

164. Fayer, R., Trout, J., Graczyk, T., & Lewis, E. (2000). Prevalence of Cryptosporidium, Giardia and Eimeria infections in post-weaned and adult cattle on three Maryland farms. *Veterinary Parasitology* 93(2), 103-112.

165. Frank, N. A., & Kaneene, J. B. (1993). Management risk factors associated with calf diarrhea in Michigan dairy herds. *Journal of Dairy Science* 76(5), 1313-1323.

166. Garber, L., Salman, M., Hurd, H., Keefe, T., & Schlater, J. (1994). Potential risk factors for Cryptosporidium infection in dairy calves. *Journal of American Veterinary Medical Association* 205(1), 86-86.

167. Harp, J., & Goff, J. (1998). Strategies for the Control of Cryptosporidium parvum Infection in Calves. *Journal of Dairy Science 81*(1), 289-294.

168. Hunter, P. R. and Thompson, R. A. (2005). The zoonotic transmission of Giardia and Cryptosporidium. *International Journal for Parasitology 35*(11), 1181-1190.

169. Maldonado-Camargo, S., Atwill, E., Saltijeral-Oaxaca, J., & Herrera-Alonso, L. (1998). Prevalence of and risk factors for shedding of Cryptosporidium parvum in Holstein Friesian dairy calves in central Mexico. *Preventive Veterinary Medicine 36*(2), 95-107.

170. Mohammed, H., Wade, S., Schaaf, S. (1999). Risk factors associated with Cryptosporidium parvum infection in dairy cattle in southeastern New York State. *Veterinary Parasitology 83*(1), 1-13.

171. Naciri, M., Lefay, M. P., Mancassola, R., Poirier, P., Chermette, R. (1999). Role of Cryptosporidium parvum as a pathogen in neonatal diarrhoea complex in suckling and dairy calves in France. *Veterinary Parasitology 85*(4), 245-257.

172. Sischo, W., Atwill, E. R., Lanyon, L., George, J. (2000). Cryptosporidia on dairy farms and the role these farms may have in contaminating surface water supplies in the northeastern United States. *Preventive Veterinary Medicine 43*(4), 253-267.

173. Thompson, R. A. (2000). Giardiasis as a re-emerging infectious disease and its zoonotic potential. *International Journal for Parasitology 30*(12), 1259-1267.

174. Trotz-Williams, L. A., Martin, S. W., Leslie, K. E., Duffield, T., Nydam, D. V., & Peregrine, A. S. (2008). Association between management practices and within-herd prevalence of Cryptosporidium parvum shedding on dairy farms in southern Ontario. *Preventive Veterinary Medicine 83*(1), 11-23.

175. Trotz-Williams, L. A., Martin, S. W., Leslie, K. E., Duffield, T., Nydam, D. V., & Peregrine, A. S. (2007). Calf-level risk factors for neonatal diarrhea and shedding of Cryptosporidium parvum in Ontario dairy calves. *Preventive Veterinary Medicine 82*(1), 12-28.

176. Waltner-Toews, D., Martin, S., & Meek, A. (1986). Dairy calf management, morbidity and mortality in Ontario Holstein herds. II. Age and seasonal patterns. *Preventive Veterinary Medicine 4*(2), 125-135.

177. CDC. (2013). CDC – Taeniasis – Biology. Retrieved May 30, 2016, from http://www.cdc.gov/parasites/taeniasis/biology.html

178. Dorny, P., Devleesschauwer, B., Stoliaroff, V., Sothy, M., Chea, R., Chea, B., et al. (2015). Prevalence and associated risk factors of toxocara vitulorum infections in buffalo and cattle calves in three provinces of central Cambodia. *Korean Journal of Parasitology 53*(2), 197-200.

179. Bond, R. (2010). Superficial veterinary mycoses. *Clinics in Dermatology 28*(2), 226-236.

180. Bartels, C. J., Holzhauer, M., Jorritsma, R., Swart, W. A., Lam, T. J. (2010). Prevalence, prediction and risk factors of enteropathogens in normal and non-normal faeces of young Dutch dairy calves. *Preventive Veterinary Medicine 93*(2-3), 162-169.

181. Garcıa, A., Ruiz-Santa-Quiteria, J., Orden, J., Cid, D., Sanz, R., Gómez-Bautista, M., et al. (2000). Rotavirus and concurrent infections with other enteropathogens in neonatal diarrheic dairy calves in Spain. *Comparative Immunology, Microbiology and Infectious Diseases 23*(3), 175-183.

182. Ijaz, M., Sattar, S., Alkarmi, T., Dar, F., Bhatti, A., & Elhag, K. (1994). Studies on the survival of aerosolized bovine rotavirus (UK) and a murine rotavirus. *Comparative Immunology, Microbiology and Infectious Diseases 17*(2), 91-98.

183. Ijaz, M. K., Sattar, S. A., Johnson-Lussenburg, C. M., & Springthorpe, V. (1985). Comparison of the airborne survival of calf rotavirus and poliovirus type 1 (Sabin) aerosolized as a mixture. *Applied and Environmental Microbiology 49*(2), 289-293.

184. Kahrs, R. F. (2002). Viral Diseases of Cattle (2nd ed.).

14

185. Sattar, S. A., Ijaz, M. K., Johnson-Lussenburg, C. M., & Springthorpe, V. (1984). Effect of relative humidity on the airborne survival of rotavirus SA11. *Applied and Environmental Microbiology* 47(4), 879-881.

186. Berry, E. D., Wells, J. E., Bono, J. L., Woodbury, B. L., Kalchayanand, N., Norman, K. N., et al. (2015). Effect of proximity to a cattle feedlot on Escherichia coli O157: H7 contamination of leafy greens and evaluation of the potential for airborne transmission. *Applied and Environmental Microbiology* 81(3), 1101-1110.

187. Kolenda, R., Burdukiewicz, M., & Schierack, P. (2015). A systematic review and meta-analysis of the epidemiology of pathogenic Escherichia coli of calves and the role of calves as reservoirs for human pathogenic E. coli. *Frontiers in Cellular and Infection Microbiology* 5, 23.

188. Meganck, V., Hoflack, G., Piepers, S., & Opsomer, G. (2015). Evaluation of a protocol to reduce the incidence of neonatal calf diarrhoea on dairy herds. *Preventive Veterinary Medicine* 118(1), 64-70.

189. Sanz, M., Viñas, M., & Parma, A. (1998). Prevalence of bovine verotoxin-producing Escherichia coli in Argentina. *European Journal of Epidemiology* 14(4), 399-403.

190. Younis, E. E., Ahmed, A. M., El-Khodery, S. A., Osman, S. A., & El-Naker, Y. F. (2009). Molecular screening and risk factors of enterotoxigenic Escherichia coli and Salmonella spp. in diarrheic neonatal calves in Egypt. *Research in Veterinary Science* 87(3), 373-379.

191. Autio, T., Pohjanvirta, T., Holopainen, R., Rikula, U., Pentikäinen, J., Huovilainen, A., et al. (2007). Etiology of respiratory disease in non-vaccinated, non-medicated calves in rearing herds. *Veterinary Microbiology* 119(2), 256-265.

192. Bidokhti, M. R., Tråvén, M., Fall, N., Emanuelson, U., & Alenius, S. (2009). Reduced likelihood of bovine coronavirus and bovine respiratory syncytial virus infection on organic compared to conventional dairy farms. *The Veterinary Journal* 182(3), 436-440.

193. Saif, L. J. (2010). Bovine respiratory coronavirus. *Veterinary Clinics of North America: Food Animal Practice* 26(2), 349-364.

194. Vijgen, L., Keyaerts, E., Moës, E., Thoelen, I., Wollants, E., Lemey, P., et al. (2005). Complete genomic sequence of human coronavirus OC43: molecular clock analysis suggests a relatively recent zoonotic coronavirus transmission event. *Journal of Virology* 79(3), 1595-1604.

195. Al Mawly, J., Grinberg, A., Prattley, D., Moffat, J., Marshall, J., & French, N. (2015). Risk factors for neonatal calf diarrhoea and enteropathogen shedding in New Zealand dairy farms. *The Veterinary Journal* 203(2), 155-160.

196. Curtis, C. R., Scarlett, J. M., Erb, H. N., & White, M. E. (1988). Path model of individual-calf risk factors for calfhood morbidity and mortality in New York Holstein herds. *Preventive Veterinary Medicine* 6(1), 43-62.

197. Klein-Jöbstl, D., Iwersen, M., & Drillich, M. (2014). Farm characteristics and calf management practices on dairy farms with and without diarrhea: a case-control study to investigate risk factors for calf diarrhea. *Journal of Dairy Science* 97(8), 5110-5119.

198. Lievaart, J., Charman, N., Scrivener, C., Morton, A., & Allworth, M. (2013). Incidence of calf scours and associated risk factors in southern New South Wales beef herds. *Australian Veterinary Journal* 91(11), 464-468.

199. Murray, C., Fick, L., Pajor, E., Barkema, H., Jelinski, M., & Windeyer, M. (2016). Calf management practices and associations with herd-level morbidity and mortality on beef cow-calf operations. *Animal* 10(03), 468-477.

200. Cwiklinski, K., O'Neill, S., Donnelly, S., & Dalton, J. (2016). A prospective view of animal and human Fasciolosis. *Parasite Immunology* 38(9), 558-568.

201. Mitchell, G. B. (2003). Treatment and Control of liver fluke in sheep and cattle: Scottish Agricultural Colleges.
202. Berends, I., Graat, E., Swart, W., Weber, M., Van de Giessen, A., Lam, T., et al. (2008). Prevalence of VTEC O157 in dairy and veal herds and risk factors for veal herds. *Preventive Veterinary Medicine 87*(3), 301-310.
203. Cernicchiaro, N., Pearl, D., McEwen, S., Harpster, L., Homan, H., Linz, G., et al. (2012). Association of wild bird density and farm management factors with the prevalence of E. coli O157 in dairy herds in Ohio (2007-2009). *Zoonoses and Public Health 59*(5), 320-329.
204. Cernicchiaro, N., Pearl, D., Ghimire, S., Gyles, C., Johnson, R., LeJeune, J., et al. (2009). Risk factors associated with Escherichia coli O157: H7 in Ontario beef cow—calf operations. *Preventive Veterinary Medicine 92*(1), 106-115.
205. Cho, S., Fossler, C. P., Diez-Gonzalez, F., Wells, S. J., Hedberg, C. W., Kaneene, J. B., et al. (2009). Cattle-level risk factors associated with fecal shedding of Shiga toxin-encoding bacteria on dairy farms, Minnesota, USA. *Canadian Journal of Veterinary Research 73*(2), 151-156.
206. Cho, S., Fossler, C. P., Diez-Gonzalez, F., Wells, S. J., Hedberg, C. W., Kaneene, J. B., et al. (2013). Herd-level risk factors associated with fecal shedding of Shiga toxin-encoding bacteria on dairy farms in Minnesota, USA. *The Canadian Veterinary Journal 54*(7), 693.
207. Eriksson, E., Aspan, A., Gunnarsson, A., & Vågsholm, I. (2005). Prevalence of vero-toxin-producing Escherichia coli (VTEC) O157 in Swedish dairy herds. *Epidemiology and Infection 133*(02), 349-358.
208. Jackson, S., Goodbrand, R., Johnson, R., Odorico, V., Alves, D., Rahn, K., et al. (1998). Escherichia coli O157 [ratio] H7 diarrhoea associated with well water and infected cattle on an Ontario farm. *Epidemiology and Infection 120*(01), 17-20.
209. Nielsen, E. M., Tegtmeier, C., Andersen, H. J., Grønbæk, C., & Andersen, J. S. (2002). Influence of age, sex and herd characteristics on the occurrence of verocyto-toxin-producing Escherichia coli O157 in Danish dairy farms. *Veterinary Microbiology 88*(3), 245-257.
210. Pennington, H. (2010). Escherichia coli O157. *The Lancet 376*(9750), 1428-1435.
211. Schouten, J., Graat, E., Frankena, K., Van De Giessen, A., Van Der Zwaluw, W., & De Jong, M. (2005). A longitudinal study of Escherichia coli O157 in cattle of a Dutch dairy farm and in the farm environment. *Veterinary Microbiology 107*(3), 193-204.
212. Widgren, S., Eriksson, E., Aspan, A., Emanuelson, U., Alenius, S., & Lindberg, A. (2013). Environmental sampling for evaluating verotoxigenic Escherichia coli O157: H7 status in dairy cattle herds. *Journal of Veterinary Diagnostic Investigation 25*(2), 189-198.
213. Craig, P. S., McManus, D. P., Lightowlers, M. W., Chabalgoity, J. A., Garcia, H. H., Gavidia, C. M., et al. (2007). Prevention and control of cystic echinococcosis. *The Lancet Infectious Diseases 7*(6), 385-394.
214. Lightowlers, M. (2012). Cysticercosis and echinococcosis. *Current Topics in Microbiology and Immunology 365*, 315-335.
215. Abutarbush, S. M., & Radostits, O. M. (2005). Jejunal hemorrhage syndrome in dairy and beef cattle: 11 cases (2001 to 2003). *The Canadian Veterinary Journal 46*(8), 711.
216. Charlebois, A., Jacques, M., & Archambault, M. (2014). Biofilm formation of Clostridium perfringens and its exposure to low-dose antimicrobials. *Frontiers in Microbiology 5*, 183.

14

217. Manteca, C., Daube, G., Jauniaux, T., Linden, A., Pirson, V., Detilleux, J., et al. (2002). A role for the Clostridium perfringens ß2 toxin in bovine enterotoxaemia? *Veterinary Microbiology 86*(3), 191-202.

218. Manteca, C., Daube, G., Pirson, V., Limbourg, B., Kaeckenbeeck, A., & Mainil, J. (2001). Bacterial intestinal flora associated with enterotoxaemia in Belgian Blue calves. *Veterinary Microbiology 81*(1), 21-32.

219. Niilo, L. (1980). Clostridium perfringens in animal disease: a review of current knowledge. *The Canadian Veterinary Journal 21*(5), 141.

220. Niilo, L. (1988). Clostridium perfringens type C enterotoxemia. *The Canadian Veterinary Journal 29*(8), 658.

221. Uzal, F. A., Freedman, J. C., Shrestha, A., Theoret, J. R., Garcia, J., Awad, M. M., et al. (2014). Towards an understanding of the role of Clostridium perfringens toxins in human and animal disease. *Future Microbiology 9*(3), 361-377.

222. Valgaeren, B., Pardon, B., Goossens, E., Verherstraeten, S., Schauvliege, S., Timbermont, L., et al. (2013). Lesion development in a new intestinal loop model indicates the involvement of a shared Clostridium perfringens virulence factor in haemorrhagic enteritis in calves. *Journal of Comparative Pathology 149*(1), 103-112.

223. Valgaeren, B. R., Pardon, B., Goossens, E., Verherstraeten, S., Roelandt, S., Timbermont, L., et al. (2015). Veal calves produce less antibodies against C. Perfringens alpha toxin compared to beef calves. *Toxins 7*(7), 2586-2597.

224. van Asten, A. J., Nikolaou, G. N., & Gröne, A. (2010). The occurrence of cpb2-toxigenic Clostridium perfringens and the possible role of the ß2-toxin in enteric disease of domestic animals, wild animals and humans. *The Veterinary Journal 183*(2), 135-140.

225. Verherstraeten, S., Goossens, E., Valgaeren, B., Pardon, B., Timbermont, L., Vermeulen, K., et al. (2013). The synergistic necrohemorrhagic action of Clostridium perfringens perfringolysin and alpha toxin in the bovine intestine and against bovine endothelial cells. *Veterinary Research 44*(1), 45.

226. Arzt, J., Juleff, N., Zhang, Z., & Rodriguez, L. (2011). The Pathogenesis of Foot-and-Mouth Disease I: Viral Pathways in Cattle. *Transboundary and Emerging Diseases 58*(4), 291-304.

227. Bartley, L., Donnelly, C., & Anderson, R. (2002). Review of foot-and-mouth disease virus survival in animal excretions and on fomites. *Veterinary Record 151*(22), 667-669.

228. Dekker, A., Vernooij, H., Bouma, A., & Stegeman, A. (2008). Rate of Foot-and-Mouth Disease Virus Transmission by Carriers Quantified from Experimental Data. *Risk Analysis 28*(2), 303-309.

229. Jamal, S. M., & Belsham, G. J. (2013). Foot-and-mouth disease: past, present and future. *Veterinary Research 44*(1), 116.

230. Kitching, R. P., Hutber, A., & Thrusfield, M. (2005). A review of foot-and-mouth disease with special consideration for the clinical and epidemiological factors relevant to predictive modelling of the disease. *The Veterinary Journal 169*(2), 197-209.

231. Moutou, F. (2002). Epidemiological basis useful for the control of foot-and-mouth disease. *Comparative Immunology, Microbiology and Infectious Diseases 25*(5), 321-330.

232. Sutmoller, P., Barteling, S. S., Olascoaga, R. C., & Sumption, K. J. (2003). Control and eradication of foot-and-mouth disease. *Virus Research 91*(1), 101-144.

233. Thompson, R. A., Palmer, C. S., & O'Handley, R. (2008). The public health and clinical significance of Giardia and Cryptosporidium in domestic animals. *The Veterinary Journal 177*(1), 18-25.

234. Angelos, J. A. (2015). Infectious bovine keratoconjunctivitis (pinkeye). *Veterinary Clinics of North America: Food Animal Practice 31*(1), 61-79.

235. Angelos, J. A., Hess, J. F., & George, L. W. (2004). Prevention of naturally occurring infectious bovine keratoconjunctivitis with a recombinant Moraxella bovis cyto-toxin-ISCOM matrix adjuvanted vaccine. *Vaccine 23*(4), 537-545.

236. Brown, M. H., Brightman, A. H., Fenwick, B. W., & Rider, M. A. (1998). Infectious bovine keratoconjunctivitis: a review. *Journal of Veterinary Internal Medicine 12*(4), 259-266.

237. O'Connor, A., Martin, S. W., Harland, R., Shewen, P., & Menzies, P. (2001). The relationship between the occurrence of undifferentiated bovine respiratory disease and titer changes to Haemophilus somnus and Mannheimia haemolytica at 3 Ontario feedlots. *Canadian Journal of Veterinary Research 65*(3), 143.

238. Postma, G. C., Carfagnini, J. C., & Minatel, L. (2008). Moraxella bovis pathogenicity: an update. *Comparative Immunology, Microbiology and Infectious Diseases 31*(6), 449-458.

239. Pugh Jr, G., McDonald, T., Kopecky, K., & Kvasnicka, W. (1986). Infectious bovine keratoconjunctivitis: comparison of infection, signs of disease and weight gain in vaccinated versus nonvaccinated purebred Hereford heifer calves. *Canadian Journal of Veterinary Research 50*(2), 259.

240. Snowder, G., Van Vleck, L. D., Cundiff, L., & Bennett, G. (2005). Genetic and environmental factors associated with incidence of infectious bovine keratoconjunctivitis in preweaned beef calves. *Journal of Animal Science 83*(3), 507-518.

241. Takele, G., & Zerihun, A. (2000). Epidemiology of Infectious Keratoconjunctivitis in Cattle in Southeast Ethiopia. *Journal of Veterinary Medicine Series A 47*(3), 169-173.

242. Tarry, D. (1985). Cattle fly control using controlled-release insecticides. *Veterinary Parasitology 18*(3), 229-234.

243. Weech, G. M., & Renshaw, H. W. (1983). Infectious bovine keratoconjunctivitis: bacteriologic, immunologic, and clinical responses of cattle to experimental exposure with Moraxella bovis. *Comparative Immunology, Microbiology and Infectious Diseases 6*(1), 81-94.

244. Zbrun, M., Zielinski, G., Piscitelli, H., Descarga, C., & Urbani, L. (2011). Dynamics of Moraxella bovis infection and humoral immune response to bovine herpes virus type 1 during a natural outbreak of infectious bovine keratoconjunctivitis in beef calves. *Journal of Veterinary Science 12*(4), 347-352.

245. Bielanski, A., Algire, J., Lalonde, A., & Garceac, A. (2013). Prevention of bovine herpesvirus-1 transmission by the transfer of embryos disinfected with recombinant bovine trypsin. *Theriogenology 80*(9), 1104-1108.

246. Boelaert, F., Biront, P., Soumare, B., Dispas, M., Vanopdenbosch, E., Vermeersch, J., et al. (2000). Prevalence of bovine herpesvirus-1 in the Belgian cattle population. *Preventive Veterinary Medicine 45*(3), 285-295.

247. Boelaert, F., Speybroeck, N., de Kruif, A., Aerts, M., Burzykowski, T., Molenberghs, G., et al. (2005). Risk factors for bovine herpesvirus-1 seropositivity. *Preventive Veterinary Medicine 69*(3), 285-295.

248. Carbonero, A., Saa, L., Jara, D., García-Bocanegra, I., Arenas, A., Borge, C., et al. (2011). Seroprevalence and risk factors associated to Bovine Herpesvirus 1 (BHV-1) infection in non-vaccinated dairy and dual purpose cattle herds in Ecuador. *Preventive Veterinary Medicine 100*(1), 84-88.

249. Dias, J., Alfieri, A., Ferreira-Neto, J., Gonçalves, V., & Muller, E. (2013). Seroprevalence and risk factors of bovine herpesvirus 1 infection in cattle herds in the state of Paraná, Brazil. *Transboundary and Emerging Diseases 60*(1), 39-47.

250. Elazhary, M., & Derbyshire, J. (1979b). Effect of temperature, relative humidity and medium on the aerosol stability of infectious bovine rhinotracheitis virus. *Canadian Journal of Comparative Medicine 43*(2), 158.

14

251. Hage, J., Schukken, Y., Schols, H., Maris-Veldhuis, M., Rijsewijk, F., & Klaassen, C. (2003). Transmission of bovine herpesvirus 1 within and between herds on an island with a BHV1 control programme. *Epidemiology and infection 130*(03), 541-552.

252. Jones, C., & Chowdhury, S. (2007). A review of the biology of bovine herpesvirus type 1 (BHV-1), its role as a cofactor in the bovine respiratory disease complex and development of improved vaccines. *Animal Health Research Reviews 8*(02), 187-205.

253. Jones, C., & Chowdhury, S. (2010). Bovine herpesvirus type 1 (BHV-1) is an important cofactor in the bovine respiratory disease complex. *Veterinary Clinics of North America: Food Animal Practice 26*(2), 303-321.

254. Mars, M., De Jong, M., Van Maanen, C., Hage, J., & Van Oirschot, J. (2000). Airborne transmission of bovine herpesvirus 1 infections in calves under field conditions. *Veterinary Microbiology 76*(1), 1-13.

255. Mollema, L., Koene, P., & de Jong, M. (2006). Quantification of the contact structure in a feral cattle population and its hypothetical effect on the transmission of bovine herpesvirus 1. *Preventive Veterinary Medicine 77*(3), 161-179.

256. Muylkens, B., Thiry, J., Kirten, P., Schynts, F., & Thiry, E. (2007). Bovine herpesvirus 1 infection and infectious bovine rhinotracheitis. *Veterinary Research 38*(2), 181-209.

257. Nandi, S., Kumar, M., Manohar, M., & Chauhan, R. (2009). Bovine herpes virus infections in cattle. *Animal Health Research Reviews 10*(01), 85-98.

258. Pardon, B., De Bleecker, K., Hostens, M., Callens, J., Dewulf, J., & Deprez, P. (2012). Longitudinal study on morbidity and mortality in white veal calves in Belgium. *BMC Veterinary Research 8*(1), 26.

259. Raaperi, K., Bougeard, S., Aleksejev, A., Orro, T., & Viltrop, A. (2012). Association of herd BRSV and BHV-1 seroprevalence with respiratory disease and reproductive performance in adult dairy cattle. *Acta Veterinaria Scandinavica 54*(1), 4.

260. Raaperi, K., Aleksejev, A., Orro, T., & Viltrop, A. (2012). Dynamics of bovine herpesvirus type 1 infection in Estonian dairy herds with and without a control programme. *The Veterinary Record 171*(4), 99-99.

261. Raaperi, K., Nurmoja, I., Orro, T., & Viltrop, A. (2010). Seroepidemiology of bovine herpesvirus 1 (BHV1) infection among Estonian dairy herds and risk factors for the spread within herds. *Preventive Veterinary Medicine 96*(1), 74-81.

262. Raaperi, K., Orro, T., & Viltrop, A. (2014). Epidemiology and control of bovine herpesvirus 1 infection in Europe. *The Veterinary Journal 201*(3), 249-256.

263. Solis-Calderon, J., Segura-Correa, V., Segura-Correa, J., & Alvarado-Islas, A. (2003). Seroprevalence of and risk factors for infectious bovine rhinotracheitis in beef cattle herds of Yucatan, Mexico. *Preventive Veterinary Medicine 57*(4), 199-208.

264. Straub, O. C. (1991). BHV1 infections: relevance and spread in Europe. *Comparative Immunology, Microbiology and Infectious Diseases 14*(2), 175-186.

265. Van Engelenburg, F., Van Schie, F. W., Rijsewijk, F., & Van Oirschot, J. (1995). Excretion of bovine herpesvirus 1 in semen is detected much longer by PCR than by virus isolation. *Journal of Clinical Microbiology 33*(2), 308-312.

266. Van Schaik, G., Schukken, Y., Nielen, M., Dijkhuizen, A., & Huirne, R. (1999). Application of survival analysis to identify management factors related to the rate of BHV1 seroconversions in a retrospective study of Dutch dairy farms. *Livestock Production Science 60*(2), 371-382.

267. van Schaik, G., Dijkhuizen, A. A., Huirne, R. B., Schukken, Y. H., Nielen, M., & Hage, H. J. (1998). Risk factors for existence of Bovine Herpes Virus 1 antibodies on nonvaccinating Dutch dairy farms. *Preventive Veterinary Medicine 34*(2), 125-136.

268. Williams, D., & Winden, S. (2014). Risk factors associated with high bulk milk antibody levels to common pathogens in UK dairies. *Veterinary Record 174*(23), 580-580.

269. Adams, V. J., Markus, M. B., Adams, J. F. A., Jordaan, E., Curtis, B., Dhansay, M. A., et al. (2005). Paradoxical helminthiasis and giardiasis in Cape Town, South Africa: Epidemiology and control. *African Health Sciences 5*(2), 131-136.

270. Barger, I. (1997). Control by management. *Veterinary Parasitology 72*(3-4), 493-506.

271. Beck, M. A., Colwell, D. D., Goater, C. P., & Kienzle, S. W. (2015). Where's the risk? Landscape epidemiology of gastrointestinal parasitism in Alberta beef cattle. *Parasites & Vectors 8*(1), 434-434.

272. Borgsteede, F. H. M., Sol, J., Van Uum, A., De Haan, N., Huyben, R., & Sampimon, O. (1998). Management practices and use of anthelmintics on dairy cattle farms in The Netherlands: Results of a questionnaire survey. *Veterinary Parasitology 78*(1), 23-26.

273. Brooker, S., Bethony, J., & Hotez, P. J. (2008). Europe PMC Funders Group Human Hookworm Infection in the 21st Century. *International Journal of Tropical Medicine* (04), 1-59.

274. Craig, T. M. (2006). Anthelmintic Resistance and Alternative Control Methods. *Veterinary Clinics of North America – Food Animal Practice 22*(3), 567-581.

275. Dorny, P., & Praet, N. (2007). Taenia saginata in Europe. *Veterinary Parasitology 149*(1), 22-24.

276. Ekong, P. S., Juryit, R., Dika, N. M., Nguku, P., & Musenero, M. (2012). Prevalence and risk factors for zoonotic helminth infection among humans and animals – Jos, Nigeria, 2005-2009. *The Pan African Medical Journal 12*, 6-6.

277. Keyyu, J. D., Kyvsgaard, N. C., Monrad, J., & Kassuku, A. A. (2005). Epidemiology of gastrointestinal nematodes in cattle on traditional, small-scale dairy and large-scale dairy farms in Iringa district, Tanzania. *Veterinary Parasitology 127*(3-4), 285-294.

278. Keyyu, J. D., Kyvsgaard, N. C., Kassuku, A. A., & Willingham, A. L. (2003). Worm control practices and anthelmintic usage in traditional and dairy cattle farms in the southern highlands of Tanzania. *Veterinary Parasitology 114*(1), 51-61.

279. Kumar, N., Rao, T. K. S., Varghese, A., & Rathor, V. S. (2013). Internal parasite management in grazing livestock. *Journal of Parasitic Diseases 37*(2), 151-157.

280. Larsen, M. (1999). Biological control of helminths. *International Journal for Parasitology 29*(1), 139-146.

281. Le Jambre, L. F. (2006). Eradication of targeted species of internal parasites. *Veterinary Parasitology 139*(4), 360-370.

282. Manuscript, A., Beane, W. S., Morokuma, J., Adams, D. S., Levin, M., & Monitoring, R.-t. (2013). *NIH Public Access 2014*(1), 70-76.

283. Niezen, J. H., Charleston, W. A. G., Hodgson, J., Mackay, A. D., & Leathwick, D. M. (1996). Controlling internal parasites in grazing ruminants without recourse to anthelmintics: Approaches, experiences and prospects. *International Journal for Parasitology 26*(8-9), 983-992.

284. Power, P.-s. D. A. (1926). (Zomparative flemtcine.

285. Schunn, A. M., Conraths, F. J., Staubach, C., Fröhlich, A., Forbes, A., Schnieder, T., et al. (2013). Lungworm Infections in German Dairy Cattle Herds – Seroprevalence and GIS-Supported Risk Factor Analysis. *PLoS ONE 8*(9).

286. Slocombe, J. O. D. (1973). Gastrointestinal parasites in cattle in Ontario. *Canadian Veterinary Journal 14*(4), 91-95.

287. Smith, H. J., & Archibald, R. M. (1968). The Effects of Age and Previous Infection on the Development of Gastrointestinal Parasitism in Cattle. *Canadian Journal of Comparative Medicine 32*(4), 511-517.

14

288. Thamsborg, S. M., Roepstorff, A., & Larsen, M. (1999). Integrated and biological control of parasites in organic and conventional production systems. *Veterinary Parasitology 84*(3-4), 169-186.

289. van Wyk, J. A., Hoste, H., Kaplan, R. M., & Besier, R. B. (2006). Targeted selective treatment for worm management – How do we sell rational programs to farmers? *Veterinary Parasitology 139*(4), 336-346.

290. Walker, J. G., & Morgan, E. R. (2014). Generalists at the interface: Nematode transmission between wild and domestic ungulates. International Journal for Parasitology: *Parasites and Wildlife 3*(3), 242-250.

291. Waller, P. J. (2006). Sustainable nematode parasite control strategies for ruminant livestock by grazing management and biological control. *Animal Feed Science and Technology 126*(3-4), 277-289.

292. Ellis, W. A. (2015). Animal leptospirosis, Leptospira and Leptospirosis (pp. 99-137): Springer.

293. Andrews, J. M. (1950). Advancing Frontiers in Insect Vector Control. *American Journal of Public Health and the Nation's Health 40*(4), 409-416.

294. Athrey, G., Hodges, T. K., Reddy, M. R., Overgaard, H. J., Matias, A., Ridl, F. C., et al. (2012). The Effective Population Size of Malaria Mosquitoes: Large Impact of Vector Control. *PLoS Genetics 8*(12).

295. Cabezas-Cruz, A., & Valdés, J. J. (2014). Are ticks venomous animals? *Frontiers in Zoology 11*, 47-47.

296. Chanda, E., Ameneshewa, B., Angula, H. A., Iitula, I., Uusiku, P., Trune, D., et al. (2015). Strengthening tactical planning and operational frameworks for vector control: the roadmap for malaria elimination in Namibia. *Malaria Journal 14*(1), 302-302.

297. Elsener, J., Villeneuve, A., & DesCôteaux, L. (2001). Evaluation of a strategic deworming program in dairy heifers in Quebec based on the use of moxidectin, an endectocide with a long persistency. *Canadian Veterinary Journal 42*(1), 38-44.

298. Holdsworth, P. A., Vercruysse, J., Rehbein, S., Peter, R. J., Bruin, C. D., Letonja, T., et al. (2006). World Association for the Advancement of Veterinary Parasitology (W.A.A.V.P.) guidelines for evaluating the efficacy of ectoparasiticides against myiasis causing parasites on ruminants. *Veterinary Parasitology 136*(1 SPEC. ISS.), 15-28.

299. Jabbar, A., Abbas, T., Sandhu, Z.-U.-D. U., Saddiqi, H. A., Qamar, M. F., & Gasser, R. B. (2015). Tick-borne diseases of bovines in Pakistan: major scope for future research and improved control. *Parasites & Vectors 8*, 283-283.

300. Jaenson, T. G. T., Hjertqvist, M., Bergström, T., & Lundkvist, A. (2012). Why is tick-borne encephalitis increasing? A review of the key factors causing the increasing incidence of human TBE in Sweden. *Parasites & Vectors 5*(1), 184-196.

301. Killeen, G. F., Kiware, S. S., Seyoum, A., Gimnig, J. E., Corliss, G. F., Stevenson, J., et al. (2014). Comparative assessment of diverse strategies for malaria vector population control based on measured rates at which mosquitoes utilize targeted resource subsets. *Malaria Journal 13*, 338-338.

302. Lyimo, I. N., Ng'Habi, K. R., Mpingwa, M. W., Daraja, A. A., Mwasheshe, D. D., Nchimbi, N. S., et al. (2012). Does cattle milieu provide a potential point to target wild exophilic anopheles arabiensis (Diptera: Culicidae) with entomopathogenic fungus? A bioinsecticide zooprophylaxis strategy for vector control. *Journal of Parasitology Research 2012*.

303. Lyimo, I. N., Haydon, D., Russell, T. L., Mbina, K. F., Daraja, A. A., Mbehela, E. M., et al. (2013). The impact of host species and vector control measures on the fitness of African malaria vectors. Proceedings of the Royal Society B: *Biological Sciences 280*(1754), 20122823-20122823.

304. Mathison, B. A., & Pritt, B. S. (2014). Laboratory identification of arthropod ectoparasites. *Clinical Microbiology Reviews 27*(1), 48-67.

305. Matthews, K. R. (2011). Controlling and Coordinating Development in Vector-Transmitted Parasites. *Science 331*(6021), 1149-1153.

306. Nafstad, O., & Grønstøl, H. (2001). Eradication of lice in cattle. *Acta Veterinaria Scandinavica 42*(1), 81-89.

307. Slocombe, J. D. (1973). Parasitisms in domesticated animals in Ontario. I. Ontario Veterinary College Record 1965-70. *Canadian Veterinary Journal 14*(2), 36-42.

308. To, D. C. (1934). And communicable diseases common to man and animals. III(580).

309. Barkallah, M., Gharbi, Y., Hassena, A. B., Slima, A. B., Mallek, Z., Gautier, M., et al. (2014). Survey of infectious etiologies of bovine abortion during mid- to late gestation in dairy herds. *PLoS ONE 9*(3).

310. Bäumler, A., & Fang, F. C. (2013). Host specificity of bacterial pathogens. *Cold Spring Harbor Perspectives in Medicine 3*(12), a010041-a010041.

311. Boerlin, P., Boerlin-Petzold, F., & Jemmi, T. (2003). Use of Listeriolyson O and Internalin A in a Seroepidemiological Study of Listeriosis in Seiss Dairy Cows. *Journal of Clinical Microbiology 41*(3), 1055-1061.

312. Doyle, M. P., Glass, K. A., Beery, J. T., Garcia, G. A., Pollard, D. J., & Schultz, R. D. (1987). Survival of Listeria monocytogenes in milk during high-temperature, short-time pasteurization. *Applied and Environmental Microbiology 53*(7), 1433-1438.

313. Esteban, J. I., Oporto, B., Aduriz, G., Juste, R. A., & Hurtado, A. (2009). Faecal shedding and strain diversity of Listeria monocytogenes in healthy ruminants and swine in Northern Spain. *BMC Veterinary Research 5*, 2-2.

314. Farber, J. M., & Losos, J. Z. (1988). Listeria monocytogenes: a foodborne pathogen. *Canadian Medical Association Journal 138*(5), 413-418.

315. Farber, J. M., & Peterkin, P. I. (1991). Listeria monocytogenes, a food-borne pathogen. *Microbiological Reviews 55*(3), 476-511.

316. Fedio, W. M., Schoonderwoerd, M., Shute, R. H., & Jackson, H. (1990). A case of bovine mastitis caused by Listeria monocytogenes. *Canadian Veterinary Journal 31*(November), 773-775.

317. Galbraith, S. (1990). The epidemiology of foodborne disease in England and Wales. *British Journal of General Practice 40*(335), 221-223.

318. Gray, M. L., & Killinger, A. H. (1966). Listeria monocytogenes and listeric infections. *Bacteriological Reviews 30*(2), 309-382.

319. Hayes, P. S., Feeley, J. C., Graves, L. M., Ajello, G. W., & Fleming, D. W. (1986). Isolation of Listeria monocytogenes from raw milk. *Applied and Environmental Microbiology 51*(2), 438-440.

320. Headrick, M. L., Korangy, S., Bean, N. H., Angulo, F. J., Altekruse, S. F., Potter, M. E., et al. (1998). The epidemiology of raw milk-associated foodborne disease outbreaks reported in the United States, 1973 through 1992. *American Journal of Public Health 88*(8), 1219-1221.

321. Hoelzer, K., Pouillot, R. g., & Dennis, S. (2012). Animal models of listeriosis: A comparative review of the current state of the art and lessons learned. *Veterinary Research 43*(1), 18-18.

322. Konosonoka, I. H., Jemeljanovs, A., Osmane, B., Ikauniece, D., & Gulbe, G. (2012). Incidence of Listeria spp. in Dairy Cows Feed and Raw Milk in Latvia. *ISRN Veterinary Science 2012*, 1-5.

323. Lund, B. M., & O 'Brien, S. J. (2011). The Occurrence and Prevention of Foodborne Disease in Vulnerable People 8(9).

324. Nightingale, K. K., Schukken, Y. H., Nightingale, C. R., Fortes, E. D., Ho, A. J., Her, Z., et al. (2004). *Ecology and Transmission of. Society 70*(8), 4458-4467.

14

325. Odugbo, M. O., Ogunjumo, S. O., Chukwukere, S. C., Kumbish, P. R., Musa, A., Ekundayo, S. O., et al. (2009). The first report of Histophilus somni pneumonia in Nigerian dairy cattle. *The Veterinary Journal 181*(3), 340-342.

326. Robertson, M. H. (1977). *Listeriosis* (October), 618-622.

327. Salamina, G., Dalle Donne, E., Niccolini, A., Poda, G., Cesaroni, D., Bucci, M., et al. (1996). A foodborne outbreak of gastroenteritis involving Listeria monocytogenes. *Epidemiology and Infection 117*(3), 429-436.

328. Sharp, J. C. (1987). Infections associated with milk and dairy products in Europe and North America, 1980-85. *Bulletin of the World Health Organization 65*(3), 397-406.

329. Strawn, L. K., Gröhn, Y. T., Warchocki, S., Worobo, R. W., Bihn, E. A., & Wiedmann, M. (2013). Risk factors associated with Salmonella and Listeria monocytogenes Contamination of Produce Fields. *Applied and Environmental Microbiology 79*(24), 7618-7627.

330. Vivant, A.-L., Garmyn, D., & Piveteau, P. (2013). Listeria monocytogenes, a down-to-earth pathogen. *Frontiers in Cellular and Infection Microbiology 3*(November), 87-87.

331. Welshimer, H. J. (1960). Survival of Listeria monocytogenes in soil. *Journal of Bacteriology 80*(3), 316-320.

332. Who. (1988). Foodborne listeriosis. WHO Working Group. *Bulletin of the World Health Organization 66*(4), 421-428.

333. Wieczorek, K., Dmowska, K., & Osek, J. (2012). Prevalence, characterization, and antimicrobial resistance of Listeria monocytogenes isolates from bovine hides and carcasses. *Applied and Environmental Microbiology 78*(6), 2043-2045.

334. Barkema, H., Green, M., Bradley, A., & Zadoks, R. (2009). Invited review: The role of contagious disease in udder health. *Journal of Dairy Science 92*(10), 4717-4729.

335. Bradley, A. J. (2002). Bovine mastitis: an evolving disease. *The Veterinary Journal 164*(2), 116-128.

336. Erskine, R. J. Mastitis in cattle. 2016, from http://www.merckvetmanual.com/mvm/reproductive_system/mastitis_in_large_animals/mastitis_in_cattle.html

337. Fox, L., Chester, S., Hallberg, J., Nickerson, S., Pankey, J., & Weaver, L. (1995). Survey of Intramammary Infections in Dairy Heifers at Breeding Age and First Parturition1. *Journal of Dairy Science 78*(7), 1619-1628.

338. Nickerson, S., Owens, W., & Boddie, R. (1995). Mastitis in Dairy Heifers: Initial Studies on Prevalence and Control1. *Journal of Dairy Science 78*(7), 1607-1618.

339. Kemmerling, K., Müller, U., Mielenz, M., & Sauerwein, H. (2009). Chlamydophila species in dairy farms: polymerase chain reaction prevalence, disease association, and risk factors identified in a cross-sectional study in western Germany. *Journal of Dairy Science 92*(9), 4347-4354.

340. Michi, A. N., Favetto, P. H., Kastelic, J., & Cobo, E. R. (2016). A review of sexually transmitted bovine trichomoniasis and campylobacteriosis affecting cattle reproductive health. *Theriogenology 85*(5), 781-791.

341. Reinhold, P., Jaeger, J., Liebler-Tenorio, E., Berndt, A., Bachmann, R., Schubert, E., et al. (2008). Impact of latent infections with Chlamydophila species in young cattle. *The Veterinary Journal 175*(2), 202-211.

342. Walker, E., Lee, E. J., Timms, P., & Polkinghorne, A. (2015). Chlamydia pecorum infections in sheep and cattle: A common and under-recognised infectious disease with significant impact on animal health. *The Veterinary Journal 206*(3), 252-260.

343. Anderson, D. E., & St. Jean, G. (2008). Surgery of the Upper Respiratory System. *Veterinary Clinics of North America – Food Animal Practice 24*(2), 319-334.

344. Antiabong, J. F., Boardman, W., Adetutu, E. M., Brown, M. H., & Ball, A. S. (2013). Does anaerobic bacterial antibiosis decrease fungal diversity in oral necrobacillosis disease? *Research in Veterinary Science* 95(3), 1012-1020.

345. Bennett, G., Hickford, J., Sedcole, R., & Zhou, H. (2009). Dichelobacter nodosus, Fusobacterium necrophorum and the epidemiology of footrot. *Anaerobe* 15(4), 173-176.

346. Bicalho, M. L. S., Machado, V. S., Oikonomou, G., Gilbert, R. O., & Bicalho, R. C. (2012). Association between virulence factors of Escherichia coli, Fusobacterium necrophorum, and Arcanobacterium pyogenes and uterine diseases of dairy cows. *Veterinary Microbiology* 157(1-2), 125-131.

347. Blowey, R. W., & Weaver, a. D. (2003). Neonatal disorders. *Color Atlas of Diseases and Disorders of Cattle* (33), 11-22.

348. Checkley, S. L., Janzen, E. D., Campbell, J. R., & McKinnon, J. J. (2005). Efficacy of vaccination against Fusobacterium necrophorum infection for control of liver abscesses and footrot in feedlot cattle in western Canada. *Canadian Veterinary Journal* 46(11), 1002-1007.

349. Darling, M. J., Bryant, S. D., Kunz, A. N., & Weisse, M. E. (2010). Necrobacillosis: A case report of complicated Fusobacterium necrophorum septicemia. Anaerobe, 16(2), 171-173.

350. Härtel, H., Nikunen, S., Neuvonen, E., Tanskanen, R., Kivelä, S. L., Aho, P., et al. (2004). Viral and Bacterial Pathogens in Bovine Respiratory Disease in Finland. *Acta Veterinaria Scandinavia*, 45(4), 193-200.

351. Heppelmann, M., Rehage, J., & Starke, A. (2007). Diphtheroid necrotic laryngitis in three calves – Diagnostic procedure, therapy and post-operative development. *Journal of Veterinary Medicine Series A: Physiology Pathology Clinical Medicine 54(7)*, 390-392.

352. Kumar, A., Gart, E., Nagaraja, T. G., & Narayanan, S. (2013). Adhesion of Fusobacterium necrophorum to bovine endothelial cells is mediated by outer membrane proteins. *Veterinary Microbiology* 162(2-4), 813-818.

353. Langworth, B. F. (1977). Fusobacterium necrophorum: its characteristics and role as an animal pathogen. *Bacteriological Reviews* 41(2), 373-390.

354. Machado, V. S., De Souza Bicalho, M. L., De Souza Meira, E. B., Rossi, R., Ribeiro, B. L., Lima, S., et al. (2014). Subcutaneous immunization with inactivated bacterial components and purified protein of Escherichia coli, Fusobacterium necrophorumand Trueperella pyogenes prevents puerperal metritis in Holstein dairy cows. *PLoS ONE 9(3)*.

355. Martens, A., & Sobiraj, A. (2004). Summary: Einleitung W IEDERKÄUER Operative Behandlung der Necrobacillosis laryngis beim Kalb Material und Methoden. 32, 7-12.

356. Miesner, M. D., & Anderson, D. E. (2015). Surgical Management of Common Disorders of Feedlot Calves. *Veterinary Clinics of North America – Food Animal Practice 31(3)*, 407-424.

357. Nagaraja, T. G., Narayanan, S. K., Stewart, G. C., & Chengappa, M. M. (2005). Fusobacterium necrophorum infections in animals: Pathogenesis and pathogenic mechanisms. *Anaerobe 11(4)*, 239-246.

358. Nichols, S., & Anderson, D. E. (2009). Subtotal or partial unilateral arytenoidectomy for treatment of arytenoid chondritis in five calves. *Journal of the American Veterinary Medical Association 235(4)*, 420-425.

359. Summary, E. (2004). Otolaryngology – Head and Neck Surgery. *Health (San Francisco) 130*(January), 1-45.

360. Tadepalli, S., Narayanan, S. K., Stewart, G. C., Chengappa, M. M., & Nagaraja, T. G. (2009). Fusobacterium necrophorum: A ruminal bacterium that invades liver to cause abscesses in cattle. *Anaerobe 15*(1-2), 36-43.

361. West, H. J. (1997). Tracheolaryngostomy as a treatment for laryngeal obstruction in cattle. *Veterinary Journal 153*(1), 81-86.

362. Anderson, M. L., Reynolds, J. P., Rowe, J. D., Sverlow, K. W., Packham, A. E., Barr, B. C., et al. (1997). Evidence of vertical transmission of Neospora sp infection in dairy cattle. *Journal of the American Veterinary Medical Association 210*(8), 1169-1172.

363. Dijkstra, T. (2002). Horizontal and vertical transmission of Neospora caninum: Utrecht Univ.

364. Dubey, J., & Lindsay, D. (1996). A review of Neospora caninum and neosporosis. *Veterinary Parasitology 67*(1-2), 1-59.

365. Gay, J. M. (2006). Neosporosis in dairy cattle: An update from an epidemiological perspective. *Theriogenology 66*(3), 629-632.

366. Gondim, L. F. P., Gao, L., & McAllister, M. (2002). Improved production of Neospora caninum oocysts, cyclical oral transmission between dogs and cattle, and in vitro isolation from oocysts. *Journal of Parasitology 88*(6), 1159-1163.

367. Bocaneti, F., Altamura, G., Corteggio, A., Velescu, E., Roperto, F., & Borzacchiello, G. (2016). Bovine papillomavirus: new insights into an old disease. *Transboundary and Emerging Diseases 63*(1), 14-23.

368. Finlay, M., Yuan, Z., Burden, F., Trawford, A., Morgan, I. M., Campo, M. S., et al. (2009). The detection of Bovine Papillomavirus type 1 DNA in flies. *Virus Research 144*(1), 315-317.

369. Yaguiu, A., Dagli, M. L. Z., Birgel Jr, E., Alves Reis, B., Ferraz, O., Pituco, E. M., et al. (2008). Simultaneous presence of bovine papillomavirus and bovine leukemia virus in different bovine tissues: in situ hybridization and cytogenetic analysis. *Genetics and Molecular Research 7*(2), 487-497.

370. Cocito, C., Gilot, P., Coene, M., de Kesel, M., Poupart, P., & Vannuffel, P. (1994). Paratuberculosis. *Clinical Microbiology Reviews 7*(3), 328-345.

371. Kopecky, K., Larsen, A., & Merkal, R. (1967). Uterine infection in bovine paratuberculosis. *American Journal of Veterinary Research, 28*(125), 1043.

372. Larsen, A., Stalheim, O., Hughes, D., Appell, L., Richards, W., & Himes, E. (1981). Mycobacterium paratuberculosis in the semen and genital organs of a semen-donor bull. *Journal of the American Veterinary Medical Association 179*(2), 169-171.

373. Streeter, R. N., Hoffsis, G., Bech-Nielsen, S., Shulaw, W., & Rings, D. (1995). Isolation of Mycobacterium paratuberculosis from colostrum and milk of subclinically infected cows. *American Journal of Veterinary Research 56*(10), 1322-1324.

374. Whittington, R. J., & Windsor, P. A. (2009). In utero infection of cattle with Mycobacterium avium subsp. paratuberculosis: a critical review and meta-analysis. *The Veterinary Journal 179*(1), 60-69.

375. Agerholm, J. S. (2013). Coxiella burnetii associated reproductive disorders in domestic animals – a critical review. *Acta Veterinaria Scandinavica 55*(1), 13.

376. Angelakis, E., & Raoult, D. (2010). Q fever. *Veterinary Microbiology 140*(3), 297-309.

377. Kruszewska, D., & Tylewska-Wierzbanowska, S. (1997). Isolation of Coxiella burnetii from bull semen. *Research in Veterinary Science 62*(3), 299-300.

378. Andriamandimby, S. F., Héraud, J. M., Ramiandrasoa, R., Ratsitorahina, M., Rasambainarivo, J. H., Dacheux, L., et al. (2013). Surveillance and control of rabies in La Reunion, Mayotte, and Madagascar. *Veterinary Research 44*(1), 1-9.

379. Barasona, J. A., Latham, M. C., Acevedo, P., Armenteros, J. A., Latham, A. D. M., Gortazar, C., et al. (2014). Spatiotemporal interactions between wild boar and cattle: Implications for cross-species disease transmission. *Veterinary Research* 45(1), 1-11.

380. Causes, S. (1995). Original Articles. 126, 22-24.

381. Finnegan, C. J., Brookes, S. M., Johnson, N., Smith, J., Mansfield, K. L., Keene, V. L., et al. (2002). Rabies in North America and Europe. *Journal of the Royal Society of Medicine 95*, 9-13.

382. Hueffer, K., Parkinson, A. J., Gerlach, R., & Berner, J. (2013). Zoonotic infections in Alaska: Disease prevalence, potential impact of climate change and recommended actions for earlier disease detection, research, prevention and control. *International Journal of Circumpolar Health 72*(1), 1-11.

383. Lee, D. N., Pape, M., & van Den Bussche, R. A. (2012). Present and potential future distribution of common Vampire bats in the Americas and the associated risk to cattle. *PLoS ONE 7*(8), 1-9.

384. Mackey, T. K., Liang, B. A., Cuomo, R., Hafen, R., Brouwer, K. C., & Lee, D. E. (2014). Emerging and reemerging neglected tropical diseases: A review of key characteristics, Risk factors, and the policy and innovation environment. *Clinical Microbiology Reviews 27*(4), 949-979.

385. McDaniel, C. J., Cardwell, D. M., Moeller, R. B., & Gray, G. C. (2014). Humans and Cattle: A Review of Bovine Zoonoses. *Vector-Borne and Zoonotic Diseases 14*(1), 1-19.

386. Walker, V. (1969). Rabies today – man and animal. *Canadian Veterinary Journal 10*(1), 11-17.

387. More, S. J., Radunz, B., & Glanville, R. J. (2015). Lessons learned during the successful eradication of bovine tuberculosis from Australia. *The Veterinary Record 177*(9), 224-232.

388. Nöremark, M., & Sternberg-Lewerin, S. (2014). On-farm biosecurity as perceived by professionals visiting Swedish farms. *Acta veterinaria Scandinavica 56*, 28-28.

389. Saegerman, C., Berkvens, D., Claes, L., Dewaele, A., Coignoul, F., Ducatelle, R., et al. (2005). Population-level retrospective study of neurologically expressed disorders in ruminants before the onset of Bovine Spongiform Encephalopathy (BSE) in Belgium, a BSE risk III country. *Journal of Clinical Microbiology 43*(2), 862-869.

390. Takahashi-Omoe, H., Omoe, K., & Okabe, N. (2008). Regulatory systems for prevention and control of rabies, Japan. *Emerging Infectious Diseases 14*(9), 1368-1374.

391. Thiptara, A., Atwill, E. R., Kongkaew, W., & Chomel, B. B. (2011). Epidemiologic trends of rabies in domestic animals in southern Thailand, 1994-2008. *American Journal of Tropical Medicine and Hygiene 85*(1), 138-145.

392. Thumbi, S. M., Bronsvoort, B. M. D. C., Poole, E. J., Kiara, H., Toye, P. G., Mbole-Kariuki, M. N., et al. (2014). Parasite co-infections and their impact on survival of indigenous cattle. *PLoS ONE 9*(2).

393. West, S. G. (2007). The nervous system.

394. Andrews, A. H., Blowey, R. W., Boyd, H., & Eddy, R. G. (2008b). Bovine medicine: diseases and husbandry of cattle, Chapter 15: John Wiley & Sons.

395. Berge, A. C. B., Moore, D. A., & Sischo, W. M. (2006). Prevalence and antimicrobial resistance patterns of Salmonella enterica in preweaned calves from dairies and calf ranches. American Journal of Veterinary Research 67(9), 1580-1588.

396. Boqvist, S., & Vågsholm, I. (2005). Risk factors for hazard of release from Salmonella-control restriction on Swedish cattle farms from 1993 to 2002. *Preventive Veterinary Medicine 71*(1), 35-44.

397. Davison, H., Sayers, A., Smith, R., Pascoe, S., Davies, R., Weaver, J., et al. (2006). Risk factors associated with the Salmonella status of dairy farms in England and Wales. *The Veterinary Record 159*, 871-880.

14

398. Fossler, C., Wells, S., Kaneene, J., Ruegg, P., Warnick, L., Bender, J., et al. (2005). Herd-level factors associated with isolation of Salmonella in a multi-state study of conventional and organic dairy farms: I. Salmonella shedding in cows. *Preventive Veterinary Medicine 70(3), 257-277.*

399. Fossler, C. P., Wells, S. J., Kaneene, J. B., Ruegg, P. L., Warnick, L. D., Bender, J. B., et al. (2005). Herd-level factors associated with isolation of Salmonella in a multi-state study of conventional and organic dairy farms. II. Salmonella shedding in calves. *Preventive Veterinary Medicine 70(3-4), 279-291.*

400. Hermesch, D. R., Thomson, D. U., Loneragan, G. H., Renter, D. R., & White, B. J. (2008). Effects of a commercially available vaccine against Salmonella enterica serotype Newport on milk production, somatic cell count, and shedding of Salmonella organisms in female dairy cattle with no clinical signs of salmonellosis. *American Journal of Veterinary Research 69(9), 1229-1234.*

401. Huston, C. L., Wittum, T. E., Love, B. C., & Keen, J. E. (2002). Prevalence of fecal shedding of Salmonella spp in dairy herds. *Journal of the American Veterinary Medical Association 220(5), 645-649.*

402. Jones, F. (2011). A review of practical Salmonella control measures in animal feed. *The Journal of Applied Poultry Research 20(1), 102-113.*

403. Lomborg, S. R., Agerholm, J. S., Jensen, A. L., & Nielsen, L. R. (2007). Effects of experimental immunosuppression in cattle with persistently high antibody levels to Salmonella Dublin lipopolysaccharide O-antigens. *BMC Veterinary Research 3(1),* 17.

404. Nielsen, L. R., Baggesen, D. L., Aabo, S., Moos, M., & Rattenborg, E. (2011). Prevalence and risk factors for Salmonella in veal calves at Danish cattle abattoirs. *Epidemiology and Infection 139(7), 1075.*

405. Nielsen, L. R., Warnick, L., & Greiner, M. (2007). Risk factors for changing test classification in the Danish surveillance program for Salmonella in dairy herds. *Journal of Dairy Science 90(6), 2815-2825.*

406. Svensson, C., Hultgren, J., & Oltenacu, P. (2006). Morbidity in 3-7-month-old dairy calves in south-western Sweden, and risk factors for diarrhoea and respiratory disease. *Preventive Veterinary Medicine 74(2), 162-179.*

407. Tarazi, Y. H., & Abo-Shehada, M. N. (2015). Herd- and individual-level prevalence of and risk factors for Salmonella spp. fecal shedding in dairy farms in Al-Dhulail Valley, Jordan. *Tropical Animal Health and Production 47(7), 1241-1248.*

408. Vanselow, B., Hornitzky, M., Walker, K., Eamens, G., Bailey, G., Gill, P., et al. (2007). Salmonella and on-farm risk factors in healthy slaughterage cattle and sheep in eastern Australia. *Australian Veterinary Journal 85(12), 498-502.*

409. Wathes, C., Zaidan, W., Pearson, G., Hinton, M., & Todd, N. (1988). Aerosol infection of calves and mice with Salmonella typhimurium. *The Veterinary Record 123(23), 590-594.*

410. Younis, E. E., Ahmed, A. M., El-Khodery, S. A., Osman, S. A., & El-Naker, Y. F. I. (2009). Molecular screening and risk factors of enterotoxigenic Escherichia coli and Salmonella spp. in diarrheic neonatal calves in Egypt. *Research in Veterinary Science 87(3), 373-379.*

411. Amer, S., El Wahab, T. A., El Naby Metwaly, A., Feng, Y., & Xiao, L. (2015). Morphologic and genotypic characterization of Psoroptes mites from water buffaloes in Egypt. *PLoS ONE 10(10), 1-11.*

412. Cameron, T. W. M., Ph., D., & Sc, D. Parasites of Animals and the Public Health in North America *. 46-50.

413. Domínguez-Peñafiel, G., Giménez-Pardo, C., Gegúndez, M., & Lledó, L. (2011). Prevalence of ectoparasitic arthropods on wild animals and cattle in the Las Merindades area (Burgos, Spain). *Parasite (Paris, France) 18, 251-260.*

414. Field, J., Millar, H. D., & Guillain-barre, T. (1967). Problem of Cholestasis. (April).

415. Gakuya, F., Ombui, J., Heukelbach, J., Maingi, N., Muchemi, G., Ogara, W., et al. (2012). Knowledge of mange among Masai pastoralists in Kenya. *PLoS ONE* 7(8), 1-7.

416. Giadinis, N. D., Farmaki, R., Papaioannou, N., Papadopoulos, E., Karatzias, H., & Koutinas, A. F. (2011). Moxidectin efficacy in a goat herd with chronic and generalized sarcoptic mange. Veterinary Medicine International, 2011, 476348-476348.

417. Munang'andu, H. M., Siamudaala, V. M., Matandiko, W., Munyeme, M., Chembensofu, M., & Mwase, E. (2010). Sarcoptes mite epidemiology and treatment in African buffalo (Syncerus caffer) calves captured for translocation from the Kafue game management area to game ranches. *BMC Veterinary Research* 6, 29-29.

418. Sarre, C., González-Hernández, A., Van Coppernolle, S., Grit, R., Grauwet, K., Van Meulder, F., et al. (2015). Comparative immune responses against Psoroptes ovis in two cattle breeds with different susceptibility to mange. *Veterinary Research* 46(1), 1-10.

419. Scabies, O. F. (1941). Of scabies.

420. Suh, G. H., Hur, T. Y., Lim, S., Shin, S. M., Kwon, J., Cho, S. H., et al. (2008). The first outbreak of Chorioptes texanus (Acari: Psoroptidae) infestation in a cattle farm in Korea. *Korean Journal of Parasitology* 46(4), 273-278.

421. Thompson, R. C. A., Kutz, S. J., & Smith, A. (2009). Parasite zoonoses and wildlife: Emerging issues. *International Journal of Environmental Research and Public Health* 6(2), 678-693.

422. Vercruysse, J., Rehbein, S., Holdsworth, P. A., Letonja, T., & Peter, R. J. (2006). World Association for the Advancement of Veterinary Parasitology (W.A.A.V.P.) guidelines for evaluating the efficacy of acaricides against (mange and itch) mites on ruminants. *Veterinary Parasitology* 136(1 SPEC. ISS.), 55-66.

423. Walton, S. F., & Currie, B. J. (2007). Problems in diagnosing scabies, a global disease in human and animal populations. *Clinical Microbiology Reviews* 20(2), 268-279.

424. Youn, H. (2009). Review of zoonotic parasites in medical and veterinary fields in the Republic of Korea. *Korean Journal of Parasitology* 47(SUPPL.), 133-142.

425. Youssef, A. I., & Uga, S. (2014). Review of parasitic zoonoses in Egypt. *Tropical Medicine and Health* 42(1), 3-14.

426. Garigliany, M.-M., Bayrou, C., Kleijnen, D., Cassart, D., & Desmecht, D. (2012). Schmallenberg virus in domestic cattle, Belgium, 2012. *Emerging Infectious Diseases* 18(9), 1512.

427. Hoffmann, B., Schulz, C., & Beer, M. (2013). First detection of Schmallenberg virus RNA in bovine semen, Germany, 2012. *Veterinary microbiology* 167(3), 289-295.

428. Ohlson, A., Heuer, C., Lockhart, C., Tråvén, M., Emanuelson, U., & Alenius, S. (2010). Risk factors for seropositivity to bovine coronavirus and bovine respiratory syncytial virus in dairy herds. *Veterinary Record* 167(6), 201-206.

429. Ponsart, C., Pozzi, N., Bréard, E., Catinot, V., Viard, G., Sailleau, C., et al. (2014). Evidence of excretion of Schmallenberg virus in bull semen. *Veterinary research* 45(1), 37.

430. Van Der Poel, W., Parlevliet, J., Verstraten, E., Kooi, E., Hakze-Van Der Honing, R., & Stockhofe, N. (2014). Schmallenberg virus detection in bovine semen after experimental infection of bulls. *Epidemiology and Infection* 142(7), 1495-1500.

431. OIE. (2013). Fiche technique de l'OIE: le virus de Schmallenberg. 2016, from www.oie.int/fileadmin/Home/fr/Our_scientific_expertise/docs/pdf/F_Schmallenberg_virus.pdf

432. Pollock, J., & Neill, S. (2002). Mycobacterium bovis infection and tuberculosis in cattle. *The Veterinary Journal* 163(2), 115-127.

14

References

Alvarez, L.G., Webb, C.R. & Holmes, M.A. (2011). A novel field-based approach to validate the use of network models for disease spread between dairy herds. *Epidemiology and Infection* 139(12), 1863-1874.

Anderson, M.L., Andrianarivo, A.G. & Conrad, P.A. (2000). Neosporosis in cattle, *Animal Reproduction Science 60*, 417-431.

Barrington, G.M., Gay, J.M. & Evermann, J.F., (2002). Biosecurity for neonatal gastrointestinal diseases. *Veterinary Clinics of North America: Food Animal Practice 18*(1), 7-34.

Boelaert, F., Speybroeck, N., de Kruif, A., Aerts, M., Burzykowski, T., Molenberghs, G., et al. (2005). Risk factors for bovine herpesvirus-1 seropositivity. *Preventive Veterinary Medicine* 69(3-4), 285-295.

Brennan, M.L., Kemp, R. & Christley, R.M. (2008). Direct and indirect contacts between cattle farms in north-west England. *Preventive Veterinary Medicine 84*(3-4), 242-260.

Callan, R.J. and Garry, F.B. (2002). Biosecurity and bovine respiratory disease. *Veterinary Clinics of North America: Food Animal Practice 18*(1), 57-77.

Crookshank, H.R., Elissalde, M.H., White, R.G., Clanton, D.C. & Smalley, H.E. (1979). Effect of transportation and handling of calves on blood serum composition. *Journal of Animal Science 48*(3), 430-35.

Cuttance, W. and Cuttance, E. (2014). Analysis of individual farm investigations into bovine viral diarrhoea in beef herds in the North Island of New Zealand. *New Zealand Veterinary Journal* 62(6), 338-342.

Daugschies, A. and Najdrowski, M. (2005). Eimeriosis in cattle: current understanding. *Journal of Veterinary Medicine, Series B 52*(10), 417-427.

Edwards, T. (2010). Control methods for bovine respiratory disease for feedlot cattle. *Veterinary Clinics of North America: Food Animal Practice 26*(2), 273-284.

Foote, R. H. (2002). The history of artificial insemination: Selected notes and notables. *Journal of Animal Science 80*(E-Supplement 2), 1-10.

Fossler, C.P., Wells, S.J., Kaneene, J.B., Ruegg, P.L., Warnick, L.D., Bender, J.B., et al. (2005). Herd-level factors associated with isolation of Salmonella in a multi-state study of conventional and organic dairy farms: I. Salmonella shedding in cows. *Preventive Veterinary Medicine 70*(3-4), 257-277.

Gorden, P.J. and Plummer, P. (2010). Control, management, and prevention of bovine respiratory disease in dairy calves and cows. *Veterinary Clinics of North America: Food Animal Practice* 26(2), 243-259.

Griffin, D., Chengappa, M.M., Kuszak, J. & McVey, D.S. (2010). Bacterial pathogens of the bovine respiratory disease complex. *Veterinary Clinics of North America: Food Animal Practice 26*(2), 381-394.

Gulliksen, S.M., Jor, E., Lie, K.I., Løken, T., Akerstedt, J. & Østerås O., (2009). Respiratory infections in Norwegian dairy calves. *Journal of Dairy Science 92*(10), 5139-5146.

Hage, J., Schukken, Y. H., Schols, H., Maris-Veldhuis, M. A., Rijsewijk, F. A. M. & Klaassen C. H. L. (2003). Transmission of bovine herpesvirus 1 within and between herds on an island with a BHV1 control programme. *Epidemiology and Infection 130*(3), 541-552.

Harp, J. and Goff, J.P. (1998). Strategies for the control of Cryptosporidium parvum infection in calves. *Journal of Dairy Science 81*(1), 289-294.

Klein-Jöbstl, D., Iwersen, M. & Drillich, M. (2014). Farm characteristics and calf management practices on dairy farms with and without diarrhea: a case-control study to investigate risk factors for calf diarrhea. *Journal of Dairy Science 97*(8), 5110-5119.

Lassen, B. (2009). Diagnosis, Epidemiology and Control of Bovine Coccidiosis in Estonia. Dissertation. Estonian University of Life Sciences.

Lundborg, G., Svensson, E. & Oltenacu, P. (2005). Herd-level risk factors for infectious diseases in Swedish dairy calves aged 0-90 days. *Preventive Veterinary Medicine 68*(2-4), 123-143.

Maciorowski, K., Herrera, P., Jones, F., Pillai, S. & Ricke, S. (2007). Effects on poultry and livestock of feed contamination with bacteria and fungi. *Animal Feed Science and Technology, 133*(1), 109-136.

Maunsell, F., Woolums, A.R., Francoz, D., Rosenbusch, R.F., Step, D.L., Wilson, D.J., et al. (2011). Mycoplasma bovis infections in cattle. *Journal of Veterinary Internal Medicine 25*(4), 772-783.

Maunsell, F.P. and Donovan, G.A. (2008). Biosecurity and risk management for dairy replacement. *Veterinary Clinics of North America: Food Animal Practice 24*(1), 155-190.

Maunsell, F.P. and Donovan, G.A. (2009). Mycoplasma bovis infections in young calves. *Veterinary Clinics of North America: Food Animal Practice 25*(1), 139-177.

Mee, J.F. (2008). Prevalence and risk factors for dystocia in dairy cattle: A review. *The Veterinary Journal 176*(1), 93-101.

Mee, J.F., Garaghty, T., O'Neill, R. & More, S.J. (2012). Bioexclusion of diseases from dairy and beef farms: Risks of introducing infectious agents and risk reduction strategies. *The Veterinary Journal 194*(2), 1443-150.

Meganck, V., Hoflack, G., Piepers, S. & Opsomer, G. (2015). Evaluation of a protocol to reduce the incidence of neonatal calf diarrhoea in dairy herds. *Preventive Veterinary Medicine 118*(1), 64-70.

Mohammed, H., Wade, S. & Schaaf, S. (1999). Risk factors associated with Cryptosporidium parvum infection in dairy cattle in southeastern New York State. *Veterinary Parasitology 83*(1), 1-13.

Nafstad, O. and Grønstøl, H. (2001). Eradication of lice in cattle. *Acta Veterinaria Scandinavica 42*(1), 81-89.

Nielsen, L.R., Warnick, L. & Greiner, M. (2007). Risk factors for changing test classification in the Danish surveillance program for Salmonella in dairy herds. *Journal of Dairy Science 90*(6), 2815-2825.

Nöremark, M., Frossling, J. & Lewerin, S.S. (2013). A survey of visitors on Swedish livestock farms with reference to the spread of animal diseases. *BMC Veterinary Research 9*, 184.

Pardon, B., Catry, B., Boone, R., Theys, H., De Bleecker, K., Dewulf, J., et al. (2014). Characteristics and challenges of the modern Belgian veal industry. *Vlaams Diergeneeskundig Tijdschrift, 83*(4), 155-163.

Pardon, B., De Bleecker, K., Hostens, M., Callens. J., Dewulf, J. & Deprez, P. (2012). Longitudinal study on morbidity and mortality in white veal calves in Belgium. *BMC Veterinary Research 8*, 26.

Raaperi, K., Orro, T. & Viltrop, A. (2014). Epidemiology and control of bovine herpesvirus 1 infection in Europe. *The Veterinary Journal 201*(3), 249-256.

14

Renault, V., Damiaans, B., Sarrazin, S., Humblet, M., Lomba, M., Ribbens, S., et al. (2017). Classification of adult cattle diseases: a first step towards prioritization of biosecurity measures. Submitted

Ribbens, S., Dewulf, J., Koenen, F., Mintiens, K., De Kruif, A. & Maes, D. (2009). Type and frequency of contacts between Belgian pig herds. *Preventive Veterinary Medicine* 88(1), 57-66.

Robertson, A. and Rendel, J. (1950). The use of progeny testing with artificial insemination in dairy cattle. *Journal of Genetics* 50(1), 21-31.

Salisbury, G.W. and Vandemark, N.L. (1961). *Physiology of reproduction and artificial insemination of cattle*. Libraries Australia.

Saegerman, C., Dal Pozzo, F. & Humblet, M.-F. (2012). Reducing hazards for humans from animals: emerging and re-emerging zoonoses. *Italian Journal of Public Health* 9(2), 13-24.

Sanderson, M.W., Dargatz, D.A. & Wagner, B.A. (2008). Risk factors for initial respiratory disease in United States' feedlots based on producer-collected daily morbidity counts. *Canadian Veterinary Journal* 49(4), 373-378.

Sarrazin, S., Cay, A.B., Laureyns, J. & Dewulf, J. (2014). A survey on biosecurity and management practices in selected Belgian cattle herds. *Preventive Veterinary Medicine* 117(1), 129-139.

Smart, J.L., Jones, T.O., Clegg, F.G. & McMurtry, M.J. (1987). Poultry waste associated type C botulism in cattle. *Epidemiology and Infection* 98(1), 73-79.

Svensson, C., Lundborg, K., Emanuelson, U. & Olsson, S.O. (2003). Morbidity in Swedish dairy calves from birth to 90 days of age and individual calf-level risk factors for infectious diseases. *Preventive Veterinary Medicine* 58(3-4), 179-197.

Sweiger, S.H. and Nichols, M.D. (2010). Control methods for bovine respiratory disease in stocker cattle. *Veterinary Clinics of North America: Food Animal Practice* 26(2), 261-271.

Synge, B.A., Chase-Topping, M.E., Hopkins, G.F., McKendrick, I.J., Thomson-Carter, F., Gray, D., et al. (2003). Factors influencing the shedding of verocytotoxin-producing Escherichia coli O157 by beef suckler cows. *Epidemiology and Infection* 130(2), 301-312.

Valle, P., Martin, S.W., Tremblay, R. & Bateman, K. (1999). Factors associated with being a bovine-virus diarrhoea (BVD) seropositive dairy herd in the Møre and Romsdal County of Norway. *Preventive Veterinary Medicine* 40(3-4), 165-177.

Villarroel, A., Dargatz, D.A., Lane, V.M., McCluskey, B.J. & Salman, M.D. (2007). Suggested outline of potential critical control points for biosecurity and biocontainment on large dairy farms. *Journal of the American Veterinary Medical Association* 230(6), 808-819.

Virtala, A.M., Gröhn, Y.T., Mechor, G.D. & Erb, H.N. (1999). The effect of maternally derived immunoglobulin G on the risk of respiratory disease in heifers during the first 3 months of life. *Preventive Veterinary Medicine* 39(1), 25-37.

Wells, S.J., Dee, S. & Godden, S. (2002). Biosecurity for gastrointestinal diseases of adult dairy cattle. *Veterinary Clinics of North America: Food Animal Practice* 18(1), 35-55.

Wouda, W. (2000). Diagnosis and epidemiology of bovine neosporosis: a review. *Veterinary Quarterly* 22(2), 71-74.

Wright, C. L. (2007). Management of water quality for beef cattle. *Veterinary Clinics of North America: Food Animal Practice*, 23(1), 91-103.

Photo credits

All pictures by Faculty of Veterinary medicine, University of Ghent

CHAPTER 15

BIOSECURITY FOR HORSE FACILITIES

J. Scott Weese

Department of Pathobiology, Ontario Veterinary College, University of Guelph, Guelph, ON, Canada

1 Introduction

It is undeniable that infectious diseases pose substantial risks to the equine industry. Whether it is a sporadic infectious disease in an individual, cluster of infections on a farm or a regional or national outbreak, the impact on horses and their owners can be substantial. The burden of infectious diseases in poorly quantified and is to a large degree unquantifiable given the high occurrence of sporadic disease and the disparate nature of the equine industry. While there have been some notable outbreaks in veterinary hospitals and equine events, with rare but profound large national outbreaks (e.g. equine herpesvirus type I (EHV-1) in the US, equine influenza in Australia), (Burgess et al., 2012; Cummings et al., 2014; Dallap Schaer et al., 2010; Firestone et al., 2011; Traub-Dargatz et al., 2013) it is likely that the impact of sporadic endemic disease markedly outweighs that of higher profile outbreaks. This does not suggest that prevention of outbreaks is not important; it highlights the importance of approaching equine infectious disease control from individual horse, farm, event and (inter-)national perspectives in order to ensure the broadest impact.

2 Biosecurity challenges in the equine industry

Description of biosecurity challenges and goals for the equine industry is difficult, if not impossible, because of the highly varied nature of equine management. While there is variability in management in all animal sectors, the degree of variability in horses is likely unsurpassed. In some situations, horses are managed in closed facilities with strict biosecurity practices. At the other extreme we have facilities with widespread mixing of horses (and species), lots of contact with horses and people from other facilities, infrastructure and practices that are not amenable to biocontainment and that have little regard for pathogen transmission. It is likely that many more horses are kept under the latter conditions than under intense biosecurity, and that most horses are managed under conditions with enhanced risk.

The nature of the use of horses also poses unique risks compared to most other animal sectors. Unlike livestock and companion animals, where contact between groups is less common or more avoidable, inter-horse and inter-farm contacts are an inherent aspect involving a tremendous number of horses that travel to participate in races, shows and other events for example. These situations create considerable risk but are largely unavoidable. However, that does not mean that risk mitigation measures are not needed or practical (a perception that is too prevalent), on the contrary attention should be drawn to the importance of a practical yet effective, proactive infection control or biosecurity plan to reduce risks.

3 Principles of biosecurity applied to horses

The approach to preventing and controlling infection can be crudely divided into three main areas; reducing exposure, reducing susceptibility and increasing resistance.

3.1 Reducing exposure

Reducing exposure to pathogens is the ultimate goal as it is the most protective measure. Simply put, if a horse is not exposed to a pathogen, it will not develop disease, regardless of any other factors. The ability to reduce exposure is highly variable between pathogens and horses. Pathogens that can be shed by healthy horses (e.g. equine herpesvirus type-1 (EHV-1), *Salmonella, Streptococcus equi equi,* methicillin-resistant *Staphylococcus aureus,* various intestinal parasites), shed prior to the onset of disease (e.g. equine influenza), shed transiently after resolution of clinical disease (e.g. *Streptococcus equi, Salmonella*) or that are present as a latent infection (e.g. EHV-1) are more difficult to control because high-risk individuals cannot be detected through observation alone. This is compounded in situations where subclinical shedding is prolonged or intermittent (e.g. *S. equi*), as it limits the impact of measures such as quarantine.

Preventing exposure is the ultimate goal, but reducing the likelihood or level of exposure (i.e. inoculum size) is sometimes a more practical goal. Both should be strived for, and most infection control and biosecurity practices focus on reducing the risk of exposure.

3.2 Reducing susceptibility

Absolute prevention of exposure to infectious agents is rarely feasible. Fortunately, disease occurs following only a minority of horse-pathogen encounters thanks to various protective mechanisms (e.g. local and systemic immunity, skin barrier) that horses possess. These protective mechanisms may vary between individuals and be influenced by a wide range of factors. In some situations, a horse's susceptibility to infection may be elevated. Situations that could plausibly increase risk of disease include extremes of age, pregnancy, antimicrobial exposure, immunosuppressive treatment, underlying disease, endocrinopathy, presence of invasive devices (e.g. intravenous catheters), pain, transportation, poor nutrition, diet changes and various stressors. Some factors (e.g. age) cannot be modified, while others (e.g. pregnancy) are an inherent requirement of some horses and are unavoidable therefore. However, others such as concurrent disease (e.g. endocrinopathy), antimicrobial use, pain or diet changes can sometimes be reduced or eliminated. Good general management and healthcare play an important and often overlooked role in biosecurity therefore.

3.3 Increasing resistance

In some situations, the host's resistance to pathogens can be enhanced, which will reduce the risk of disease should a pathogen be encountered. Efforts to increase host resistance mainly involve vaccinations that target selected pathogens, and a wide range of commercially available vaccines can play an important role in preventing disease.

The role of vaccination in biosecurity on farms or among populations is more difficult to establish. There is no information about the degree of vaccine coverage needed to confer effective herd immunity (i.e. the percentage of horses that must be vaccinated to provide protection against those that cannot be or are not vaccinated) against equine diseases. Furthermore, while vaccines may reduce the risk or severity of disease in individual horses, they often do not provide sterilising immunity and some exposed horses can still shed the pathogen after exposure. These issues highlight the concept that vaccination should be positioned as an important component of biosecurity, but as a third line of defence in order to provide protection when measures to reduce exposure and reduce susceptibility have failed.

Other measures to increase host resistance could include immunomodulators and probiotics, but clinical efficacy of commercial products is currently disappointing.

4 Biosecurity considerations for equine facilities and personnel

A wide range of areas must be considered when designing and implementing effective equine biosecurity programmes. The disparate nature of the equine industry means that it is impossible to design one 'standard' plan. This means that a specific plan has to be drawn up for each facility and horse owner. A comprehensive overview of this subject is beyond the scope of this chapter, but examples of important areas are discussed below. Additional information can be obtained from a variety of resources (Table 15.1, see p. 396).

15

Table 15.1: Examples of equine biosecurity resources

Source	Location
National Farm and Facility Level Biosecurity Standard for the Equine Sector (Canada)	http://www.inspection.gc.ca/DAM/DAM-animals-animaux/WORKAREA/DAM-animals-animaux/text-texte/terr_biosec_standards_equine_1461274012655_eng.pdf
American Association for Equine Practitioners Biosecurity Guidelines (US)	http://www.aaep.org/custdocs/biosecurityguidelinesfinal030113.pdf
Biosecurity Toolkit for Equine Events (US)	https://www.cdfa.ca.gov/AHFSS/Animal_Health/pdfs/Biosecurity_Toolkit_Full_Version.pdf

4.1 Risk assessment

The first component in developing a biosecurity programme is determining the risks that are present. This is the premise behind a risk assessment, a practice that often sounds more daunting than it actually is. Ideally, a risk assessment is a joint effort by facilities owners or managers and their veterinarians, with input from other individuals (e.g. trainers or boarders at a public facility). Identification of risks and consideration of the likelihood and impact of those risks can help tailor an effective yet practical biosecurity programme that meets the needs of the individual facilities.

4.2 Quarantine

Quarantine is the practice of separating and monitoring healthy individuals. This may be used for a new arrival or an individual that has potentially been exposed to a pathogen but which is clinically normal. Quarantine allows time to observe the horse for development of signs of disease, time for elimination of pathogens that are shed transiently (e.g. equine influenza virus), time for provision of preventive medicine (e.g. vaccination, deworming) and time for any diagnostic testing results (e.g. *Streptococcus equi* screening) to become available, all before the individual is exposed to the rest of the population. Quarantine can be relatively basic, with physical and procedural separation of new arrivals for a short period of time, or intensive, with close monitoring, testing for various pathogens, vaccination and deworming. The approach taken varies according to the risk of pathogen shedding (e.g. return of horses from events with high levels of biosecurity vs purchase of a horse from a sale), implications of entry of a pathogen onto the farm (e.g. closed herd vs one with significant horse movement, farm with actively competing horses vs broodmares vs companion horses), the availability of a location for quarantine (e.g. separate barn or paddock, separate area in a main barn that can be adequately contained), risk tolerance and cost.

Each facility should have a quarantine plan, no matter how rudimentary. Routine quarantine of horses that have left the property is ideal but is often impractical for performance or show horses, where there is a routine movement of large numbers of horses. Facilities where there is considerable horse movement should also have a quarantine plan that addresses higher risk scenarios (e.g. entry of a new horse of unknown or potentially low health status). Duration and specific practices of quarantine are ill-defined and to a large degree indefinable, since duration and practices vary depending on different pathogens. Quarantine duration, location and practices need to be facility-specific and take into consideration the risks, risk tolerance, costs and practicality.

Quarantine can be an effective tool, but cannot guarantee total prevention of entry of pathogens because of factors such as the potential for long-term subclinical or latent carriage of pathogens such as *S. equi* or EHV-1.(Allen et al., 2008; Sweeney et al., 1989) Notwithstanding, short-term (e.g. 7-28 d) quarantine with the use of physical (e.g. housing in a quarantine area) and procedural (e.g. higher level of hygiene, personal protective equipment, dedicated items such as water buckets, contact with quarantined horses after other horses) separation methods can serve as a practical and effective tool.

15

4.3 Cohorting

Cohorting involves identification and separation of groups with a different risk status. This includes considering the likelihood of shedding infectious agents and the susceptibility or implications of infections. For example, this may include separation of resident horses from horses that routinely leave the property (because of different risks of pathogen exposure) or separation of broodmares from other populations (because of the greater risk to broodmares should they be exposed to a pathogen such as equine herpesvirus type I). On some farms, all horses might fit into one single cohort, while on others there may be many different risk groups. The ability to implement cohorting depends on the ability to identify separate risk groups and to implement physical and procedural separation practices.

4.4 Zoning

While cohorting involves identification and separation of different groups of *horses*, zoning applies a similar concept to the facility through the identification of high-, medium- and low-risk *areas*. Zoning requires assessing the risks of pathogen incursion or presence thereof in different areas of the farm, controlled access points that delineate different zones and control of access by horses, people, vehicles, equipment and animals.

There are two general levels of zoning. One is at facility level, where measures can be taken to prevent any unnecessary movement onto the property and to ensure that any entrance onto the property (people, equipment, animals) is carried out in a controlled manner. Thus, the zoning is essentially 'the farm' compared to 'anywhere else'. The other level is zoning within the farm, identifying different biosecure zones and implementing movement and access restrictions (Figures 15.1 and 15.2). On some farms, it may not be possible to delineate different zones, and all that can be done is zoning of the farm versus anywhere else. However, there is often the ability to identify and control two to three (and in some cases, more) zones on a facility. For example, a high-risk zone could be

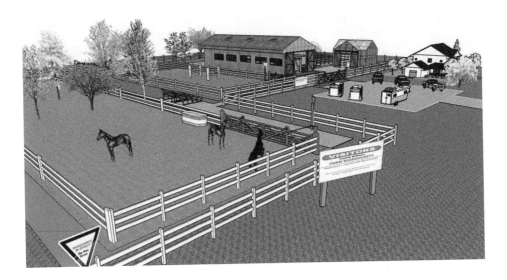

▲

Fig. 15.1: Basic zoning of an equine facility. The yellow fenced area indicates the boundary between horse care and management areas, and the rest of the facility. All aspects of routine horse care take place within the boundary. The visitors' parking and trailer storage area is outside the secure zone, which is controlled by an access point (purple gate).

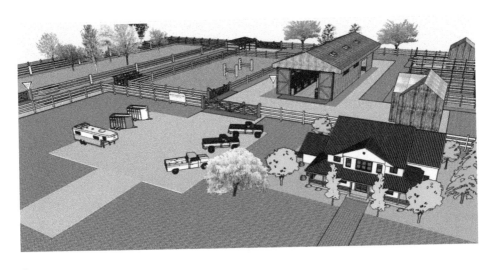

▲

Fig. 15.2: Alternate view of a basic zoning approach to an equine facility. In addition to the controls described in Fig. 15.1, this image depicts a small barn and paddock to the right of the main stable. This lies within the overall control zone and is a restricted area within that zone for quarantine or isolation. A feed storage barn is present within the secure zone. A covered manure storage facility is present in the back on the left, with its own access point to allow for removal of manure with limited entry into the property.

the area where various people (veterinarians, farriers, feed suppliers) enter and leave their vehicles. It could also include quarantine and isolation areas. At the opposite end of the spectrum would be barns and outdoor areas housing horses that do not leave the property and are therefore the most biosecure. Physical barriers between zones may include fencing, gates, structures that prevent movement of vehicles and general farm layout that provides distance between areas. Procedural barriers include signs and procedures to restrict or control access to different zones, particularly more biosecure zones. The concept of zoning can also be applied nationally or internationally, such as declaring endemic and free countries or regions. Zoning was also part of the response to the 2007 Australian equine influenza outbreak, which involved dividing the state of Queensland into different infection status zones with different movement restrictions (Kung et al., 2011).

4.5 Access management

An important aspect of successful cohorting, isolation and zoning is access management. This involves control of the entry of people, horses, other animals and items such as vehicles both onto and within a facility. It may consist of physical barriers (e.g. fences, gates) and procedures, and should be clearly outlined. The default for any access management strategy should be 'no access', with access granted as indicated. This is preferable to an approach based on access restriction, as the initial response to any undefined scenario is 'no access' versus a restriction-based approach where lack of a specific prohibition can be interpreted as indicating that access is permitted.

4.6 Isolation

Where quarantine is applied to apparently healthy horses, isolation is used to contain horses that are known or suspected to be shedding an infectious agent. Confirmation of an infectious disease should not be required for initiation of isolation. Identification of syndromes (see below) that suggest the presence of an infectious disease should be enough to trigger a response. Concurrent diagnostic testing may be useful, but waiting for confirmation of a diagnosis before initiating isolation practices is unacceptable.

The ability to provide strict isolation varies greatly between facilities and a comprehensive description of isolation practices is beyond the scope of this chapter. As with quarantine, the goal is to provide as much physical and procedural separation as possible. Physical separation is important because relying mainly on procedural separation (e.g. keeping an isolated horse in a common barn while using enhanced barrier practices) is highly dependent on compliance, and human factors tend to be the weak link of any control programme. Physical separation alone is not effective and needs to be supplemented with procedural separation; however, the less reliance on procedural separation and human activities, the better.

4.7 Syndromic surveillance

Prompt recognition of problems is critical, particularly for highly infectious pathogens that can spread rapidly. For some pathogens, signs of disease may be evident prior to the onset of infectivity (e.g. a horse exposed to *Streptococcus equi equi* will develop a fever 2-3 days prior to the time it sheds the bacterium and is able to infect other horses)(Sweeney et al., 2005). Prompt identification of abnormalities therefore can allow for early intervention and containment. Even when horses are infectious at or before the time of the onset of a clinical disease (e.g. equine influenza), rapid identification can reduce the amount of time that other horses might be exposed.

Syndromic surveillance is the act of identifying certain syndromes that suggest the presence of an infectious disease (Box 1).(Burgess and Morley, 2014; Ruple-Czerniak et al., 2013) While causes may be non-infectious, identification of these signs allows for rapid assessment and intervention, and is a cost-effective and practical measure that can be used at any facility. Since these signs are readily identified by lay personnel, everyone on the farm can be involved in this form of surveillance, provided they know to look for these syndromes and understand the required response (e.g. notify barn manager, isolate horse, call a veterinarian). Clear written guidance outlining the syndromes and the response should be available to reduce the risk of failing to identify relevant syndromes or to initiate the proper response.

Examples of syndromes that are easily identified and indicate the potential for an infectious disease

- New cough
- Depression/lethargy
- Nasal discharge
- Anorexia
- Abortion
- Neurological disease
- Limb oedema

4.8 Active surveillance

While syndromic surveillance takes advantage of broad but readily identifiable signs, active surveillance uses specific approaches to obtain information.(Burgess and Morley, 2014) This mainly involves diagnostic testing to screen for the presence of selected pathogens in clinically normal individuals. Potentially the most widely used (but still uncommon) approach is screening new arrivals for *S. equi* shedding. While syndromic surveillance would identify signs consistent with *S. equi* disease (strangles), it cannot detect subclinical carriers. Active surveillance therefore aims to identify infectious but clinically normal horses, ideally prior to their introduction to the general population. Other pathogens that have been targets for active surveillance on farms or in equine hospitals include *Salmonella* and methicillin-resistant *Staphylococcus aureus* (MRSA).(Tillotson et al., 1997; Weese et al., 2006) Because testing is never 100% sensitive, active surveillance cannot guarantee that horses are not shedding the agent of concern; however, negative results from properly collected and tested samples can provide a greater level of assurance.

Despite the potential benefits, active surveillance is rarely used at equine facilities. Perhaps the main barrier is cost, since diagnostic testing can be expensive. Logistical challenges may also be present in facilities with ample horse movement and/or limited quarantine facilities, as testing without concurrent quarantine is less effective. Yet, in some situations, particularly involving closed, high-health status herds with infrequent entry of new horses, active surveillance can be cost-effective and practical.

4.9 Event attendance procedures

Any situation where a horse leaves its premises and may encounter another horse poses some degree of risk. However, avoiding events (e.g. races, shows, trail rides, sales) is impossible in most sectors of the equine industry. By their nature, horses from different facilities will converge at events. While this creates some degree of inevitable risk, this risk can be reduced through measures performed by the event organiser and the horse owner. Comprehensive guidance is available for event organisers.(California Department of Food and Agriculture, 2012) Individual horse owners play an important role by encouraging events to use such guidelines and by complying with event guidelines. Aspects such as keeping sick horses (and horses exposed to potentially infectious horses) away from events, restricting contact between their horses and other horses and people at the event and avoiding sharing equipment (e.g. water buckets) with horses from other facilities are practical and should be implemented. Consideration must also be given to quarantining horses upon return (something that is often impractical, as discussed above), or to cohorting risk groups.

15

4.10 Personal hygiene

Anyone who comes into contact with horses or their environment has the potential to act as a source of infection. This includes transmission of pathogens carried by people (e.g. MRSA), transmission of pathogens between horses via the person's body (especially hands) or clothing or cross-contamination of pathogens from the environment. The risk of transmission from horses or the environment is present both within and between farms. Examples of basic hygiene measures to reduce the risk of transmission are listed in Box 2.

Examples of personal hygiene measures to reduce the risk of pathogen transmission to and from horses:

- Change clothing and footwear between facilities
- Perform hand hygiene (hand washing or application of an alcohol-based hand sanitiser), particularly after contact with horses at increased risk of shedding pathogens, before contact with horses with an increased risk of disease (e.g. neonatal foals), between cohorts and after having contact with respiratory secretions or faeces
- Change clothing and footwear (or donning and doffing additional protective outerwear) after handling isolated or quarantined horses, or potentially when moving between cohorts
- Use additional barriers for high-risk procedures, such as wearing disposable gloves when handling wounds
- Work with lower-risk cohorts first and highest-risk individuals or groups last

---

4.11 Cleaning and disinfection

Cleaning and disinfection are two separate but closely related activities that are widely used and often misused (Box 3).(Dwyer, 2004) The entire process is designed to reduce (not necessarily eliminate) pathogen burdens in the environment and on equipment. Cleaning is the most important and often overlooked step. Effective disinfection is not possible without effective cleaning, as disinfectants are typically inactivated or ineffective in the presence of abundant organic debris. Cleaning the environment is a routine (e.g. daily) part of facility and equipment management. Disinfection may be performed on a routine, periodic (e.g. weekly) or as needed (e.g. after suspected contamination) basis, depending on the site and other factors.

Common errors with cleaning and disinfection

- Failure to clean adequately before disinfection
- Attempting to disinfect surfaces that are impossible to disinfect (e.g. dirt)
- Use of a poor quality disinfectant
- Use of a cleaner instead of a disinfectant
- Improper disinfectant concentration
- Inadequate disinfectant contact time
- Inactivation of bleach by light or organic contamination
- Failure to have a written protocol to ensure consistency and accuracy

Cleaning is the first step and removes 90% or more of the microbial burden and other substances (e.g. organic material), creating a site that is more amenable to disinfection. Thorough cleaning is also critical for removal of microorganisms that are resistant to most disinfectants, such as clostridial spores and protozoa. Simply rinsing or wiping surfaces is rarely adequate. Combinations of physical removal of debris (e.g. removing bedding or manure), scrubbing and washing may be required. Detergents can help remove debris. High-pressure water can also help remove debris, but should be avoided because of the potential for aerosolisation of pathogens and the potential for damage to surfaces (which might compromise disinfection efficacy). (Dwyer, 2004)

Disinfection is designed to further reduce the bioburden by eliminating a large percentage of the microbes that remain after clean-

15

ing. This step involves application of a disinfectant, in the correct concentration and for the appropriate contact time. Not all disinfectants are alike and they must be chosen for their properties such spectrum, activity in residual organic debris, safety and cost. Optimal disinfectants are those with a broad spectrum of activity that work in the presence of moderate organic debris (e.g. accelerated hydrogen peroxide).

The approach to disinfection of equipment is similar to that of the general environment. However, additional factors sometimes need to be considered. The potential for contact irritation exists with some disinfectants, so rinsing items such as tack and water buckets may be required after the appropriate disinfectant contact time. Additionally, surface tolerance is often an issue with tack, since disinfectants could damage or alter materials such as leather, particularly with repeated use. There is very little information available about material tolerance.. Testing disinfectants on hidden parts of tack to look for visible change and rinsing after disinfection are the main recommended measures for these types of surfaces.

4.12 Surface materials

Cleaning and disinfection should be considered when choosing materials for flooring, walls and other areas. Optimal surfaces for cleaning and disinfection are non-porous, sealed surfaces such as metal and some plastics. Dirt and gravel are essentially impossible to clean and disinfect. Unsealed concrete is similarly challenging because of its porosity. Wood that is unsealed or where the treated surface has been damaged is similarly difficult to address. Rubber floor mats may be amenable to upper surface disinfection but unless they are permanent and completely sealed, water and pathogens can accumulate under them.

While smooth, sturdy and non-porous surfaces are ideal from a disinfection standpoint, many other aspects such as grip (for flooring) and cost must be considered, and there are very few optimal surfaces that balance cost, safety, comfort and biosecurity. There will always be significant challenges for cleaning and disinfection in equine facilities because of the need to balance all these factors. The goal is to achieve an optimal environment with easy-to-clean and disinfect surfaces, with the understanding that not all surfaces will be ideal. Measures to increase disinfection efficacy include sealing wood and concrete surfaces (e.g. coating wood with marine epoxy), regularly inspecting surfaces to identify damage, and avoiding damaging activities such as power washing. Where cost prohibits the use of certain surfaces throughout a facility, limited use in high-risk (e.g. quarantine, isolation, foaling) areas might be practical.

Outdoor areas are difficult or impossible to disinfect because of size, (e.g. fencing), surface (e.g. dirt, rough wood) or access zones. This is one reason for trying to keep infectious or otherwise high-risk horses away from outside areas as much as possible. However, ultraviolet light is a highly effective disinfectant and many pathogens will die quickly upon exposure to sunlight.(Weese et al., 2009) While it is difficult to provide any objective guidance about the time required for different pathogens to die outdoors because of variations in temperature, degree of exposure to sunlight, protection of organic debris and inherent pathogen susceptibility, most vegetative bacteria and non-enveloped viruses that are exposed to direct sunlight will probably die within days.

Sheltered indoor environments such as riding arenas can be particularly challenging because of a lack of sunlight and impossible-to-disinfect surfaces such as dirt. This means that farm practices to prevent potentially infectious horses accessing those areas are a key control measure.

4.13 Manure management

Manure is obviously a potential source of pathogens. While manure from horses with known enteric infectious disease (e.g. salmonellosis) is of major concern, all horses can shed one or more potentially pathogenic bacteria, viruses or parasites at any time.

15

All manure should be considered as posing an element of risk therefore to humans, horses and other animals. Storage and handling of manure should be performed in such a way as to reduce the risk of exposure to other individuals. Some basic aspects of manure management are listed in Box 4.

Considerations for manure management:

- Do not use items used for manure removal on feedstuffs
- Dedicate manure removal equipment (e.g. pitchforks, wheelbarrow) to specific cohorts (i.e. do not share manure removal items between groups)
- Store manure where runoff will not contaminate pastures, paddocks or water sources
- Compost manure if it is to be used on horse pastures, and only spread manure that has been properly composted
- Prevent horses gaining direct access to manure piles
- Try to restrict wildlife access to manure piles
- Wash hands and clean footwear after manure removal
- Consider having a separate handling area or process (e.g. contracted removal) for manure from high-risk areas such as treatment areas, isolation and quarantine

4.14 Pasture management

Pastures are a possible source of various pathogens, particularly intestinal parasites. While a facility-specific deworming regimen (ideally with targeted treatment and faecal egg count reduction testing) is a key component of parasite prevention, pasture management is an essential consideration. Good pasture management practices include preventing overstocking, ensuring that all horses turned out to pasture are included in a deworming programme, preventing overgrazing, only spreading composted manure on pastures and, ideally, manure removal.

4.15 Transportation

Moving horses between facilities is associated with the risk of pathogen exposure. This risk is also present when horses are being transported, something that may be overlooked. Transporting horses by trailer or airplane can create opportunities for direct and indirect contact between individuals and exposure to pathogens in the environment or on handlers. When this involves individuals from different farms or different health statuses, there is an increased risk. Various measures can be taken to reduce the risk of pathogen exposure during transportation (Table 15.2).

Table 15.2: Examples of practical measures to reduce the risk of pathogen exposure during transportation

Pathogen source	Mitigation
Transported horses	Try to limit transport to horses from the same farm and same cohort
	Prevent direct contact between horses during transit
	Prevent mingling with other horses if rest stops are provided in areas where other horses may be present
Trailer	Clean and disinfect trailer between all shipments
	Maintain trailer surfaces in a good state of repair to facilitate cleaning and disinfection
	Avoid surfaces in horse contact areas that are difficult to clean and disinfect
Handlers	Ensure handlers do not wear clothing that was used when handling other shipments of horses
	Encourage hand hygiene
Equipment	Provide farm- (and cohort-) specific equipment such as hay nets and water buckets
	If equipment such as water buckets is used between shipments, clean and disinfect each time

15

4.16 Personnel

In equine veterinary facilities, as in human healthcare, there is increasing use of 'infection control practitioners', individuals with specific roles pertaining to infection control in the facility. The training of these individuals varies, but their common characteristic is that they are the central resource for infection control. They coordinate infection control activities, conduct surveillance, educate, communicate and perform a variety of routine tasks. A similar model can be applied to equine facilities. This is rarely a full time position occupied by someone with specialised training, although that would certainly be desirable. More usually and practically this is someone interested in infection control, who can oversee day-to-day infection control practices as a minor component of their other duties. They can help identify issues, communicate and educate. They act as the central resource on the facility for any questions, problems or concerns that arise. In most instances, this requires limited time and financial commitment, as day-to-day requirements in most circumstances are not excessive. However, by centralising communications and knowledge, it is possible to ensure a more efficient and effective infection control programme. For example, this person would be promptly notified following identification of a potentially worrying syndrome (e.g. fever). With centralised reporting, a cluster of infections might be more rapidly identified, as would happen if different owners with different veterinarians identified horses with a fever on the same day. With multiple cases reported to the infection control practitioner in real time, a rapid response can be initiated to identify the problem, identify other potentially infected (and/or infectious) horses and to coordinate the response.

4.17 Auditing

Periodic auditing of procedures and practices is a useful tool. This may involve use of a generic checklist of procedures and practices, a checklist developed specifically for the facility, observation of practices, a review of written materials, or combinations thereof.

Auditing can be performed by facility personnel, a facility veterinarian or an independent third party. The goal of auditing is not to lay blame, but to identify gaps in protocols and practices, so that improvements can be made.

4.18 Communication

Since human factors, particularly poor compliance, are at the root of many breakdowns in biosecurity, it is important to implement measures to improve communications. Poor compliance may be intentional, but more often than not it is associated with a lack of understanding of appropriate biosecurity measures. Intentional non-compliance may also have its roots in poor communications as people will be less motivated to comply if they do not understand why they are being asked to do something. Optimising communications is critical therefore for effective biosecurity. Various groups may be involved, such as farm managers, horse owners, farm personnel, farriers, feed suppliers, transporters and anyone else who has contact with horses or the farm. Communications must be clear, consistent and understandable, and interpersonal factors, language barriers, education, and numerous other factors can impact the effectiveness of communications. Biosecurity practices should be communicated through different approaches and on a regular basis. A written biosecurity manual is critical for consistency and depth, but cannot be relied on as the sole method of providing information. It can be supplemented with conversations, demonstrations, inspections (with feedback), concise written information (e.g. fact sheets) and meetings, depending on the facility and the issue.

15

References

Canadian Food Inspection Agency. National Farm and Facility Level Biosecurity Standard for the Equine Sector. 2016. Available at http://www.inspection.gc.ca/animals/terrestrial-animals/biosecurity/standards-and-principles/equine-sector/eng/1460662612042/1460662650577. Last accessed Sept 27, 2017.

Allen, G.P., Bolin, D.C., Bryant, U., Carter, C.N., Giles, R.C., Harrison, L.R., Hong, C.B., Jackson, C.B., Poonacha, K., Wharton, R., Williams, N.M., 2008. Prevalence of latent, neuropathogenic equine herpesvirus-1 in the thoroughbred broodmare population of central Kentucky. Equine Vet J 40, 105-110.

Burgess, B.A., Morley, P.S., 2014. Veterinary hospital surveillance systems. Vet Clin North Am Small Anim Pract doi: 10.1111/evj.12234.

Burgess, B.A., Tokateloff, N., Manning, S., Lohmann, K., Lunn, D.P., Hussey, S.B., Morley, P.S., 2012. Nasal shedding of equine herpesvirus-1 from horses in an outbreak of equine herpes myeloencephalopathy in Western Canada. J Vet Int Med 26, 384-392.

California Department of Food and Agriculture, 2012. Biosecurity toolkit for equine events. https://www.cdfa.ca.gov/AHFSS/Animal_Health/pdfs/Biosecurity_Toolkit_Full_Version.pdf (accessed Mar 8 2017).

Cummings, K.J., Rodriguez-Rivera, L.D., Mitchell, K.J., Hoelzer, K., Wiedmann, M., McDonough, P.L., Altier, C., Warnick, L.D., Perkins, G.A., 2014. Salmonella enterica serovar Oranienburg outbreak in a veterinary medical teaching hospital with evidence of nosocomial and on-farm transmission. Vector-borne and zoonotic diseases (Larchmont, NY) 14, 496-502.

Dallap Schaer, B.L., Aceto, H., Rankin, S.C., 2010. Outbreak of salmonellosis caused by Salmonella enterica serovar Newport MDR-AmpC in a large animal veterinary teaching hospital. J Vet Intern Med 24, 1138-1146.

Dwyer, R.M., 2004. Environmental disinfection to control equine infectious diseases. Vet Clin North Am Equine Pract 20, 531-542.

Firestone, S.M., Schemann, K.A., Toribio, J.-A.L.M.L., Ward, M.P., Dhand, N.K., 2011. A case-control study of risk factors for equine influenza spread onto horse premises during the 2007 epidemic in Australia. Preventive veterinary medicine.

Kung, N., Mackenzie, S., Pitt, D., Robinson, B., Perkins, N.R., 2011. Significant features of the epidemiology of equine influenza in Queensland, Australia, 2007. Australian Veterinary Journal 89 Suppl 1, 78-85.

Ruple-Czerniak, A.A., Aceto, H.W., Bender, J.B., Paradis, M.R., Shaw, S.P., Van Metre, D.C., Weese, J.S., Wilson, D.A., Wilson, J., Morley, P.S., 2013. Syndromic surveillance for evaluating the occurrence of healthcare-associated infections in equine hospitals. Equine Veterinary Journal 46, 435-440.

Sweeney, C.R., Benson, C.E., Whitlock, R.H., Meirs, D.A., Barningham, S.O., Whitehead, S.C., Cohen, D., 1989. Description of an epizootic and persistence of Streptococcus equi infections in horses. Journal of the American Veterinary Medical Association 194, 1281-1286.

Sweeney, C.R., Timoney, J.F., Newton, J.R., Hines, M.T., 2005. Streptococcus equi infections in horses: guidelines for treatment, control, and prevention of strangles. J Vet Intern Med 19, 123-134.

Tillotson, K., Savage, C.J., Salman, M.D., Gentry-Weeks, C., Rice, D., Fedorko-Cray, P.J., Hendrickson, D.A., Jones, R.L., Nelson, A.W., Traub-Dargatz, J.L., 1997. Outbreak of *Salmonella infantis* infection in a large animal veterinary teaching hospital. J Am Vet Med Assoc 211, 1554-1557.

Traub-Dargatz, J.L., Pelzel-McCluskey, A.M., Creekmore, L.H., Geiser-Novotny, S., Kasari, T.R., Wiedenheft, A.M., Bush, E.J., Bjork, K.E., 2013. Case-control study of a multistate equine herpesvirus myeloencephalopathy outbreak. J Vet Int Med 27, 339-346.

Weese, J.S., Jarlot, C., Morley, P.S., 2009. Survival of Streptococcus equi on surfaces in an outdoor environment. Can Vet J 50, 968-970.

Weese, J.S., Rousseau, J., Willey, B.M., Archambault, M., McGeer, A., Low, D.E., 2006. Methicillin-resistant *Staphylococcus aureus* in horses at a veterinary teaching hospital: frequency, characterization, and association with clinical disease. J Vet Intern Med 20, 182-186.

Photo credits

National Farm and Facility Level Biosecurity Standard for the Equine Sector, Canadian Food Inspection Agency: figures 15.1, 15.2

15

CHAPTER 16

BIOSECURITY MEASURES FOR DOG MERCHANTS AND CANINE BREEDING KENNELS

Pierre-Alexandre Dendoncker [1]

Hilde de Rooster [2]

Eline Abma [2]

Eline Wydooghe [3]

Jeroen Dewulf [1]

[1] Faculty of Veterinary Medicine, Department of Reproduction, Obstetrics and Herd Health, Veterinary Epidemiology Unit, University of Ghent, 9820 Merelbeke, Belgium
[2] Faculty of Veterinary Medicine, Small Animal Department, University of Ghent, 9820 Merelbeke, Belgium
[3] Faculty of Veterinary Medicine, Department of Reproduction, Obstetrics and Herd Health, Unit for companion animal reproduction, University of Ghent, 9820 Merelbeke, Belgium

1 Introduction

More than 20% of households in Western countries own one or more dogs. The main origins of these dogs, apart from private individuals, are breeding facilities (i.e. breeding kennels, commercial breeders, merchants) and shelters. Every year approximatively 1% of all pet dogs end up in a shelter and up to 5% of dogs live in semi-permanent facilities such as day-care or boarding kennels. This chapter is written for professionals exploiting, managing or assisting the above-mentioned facilities where dogs are housed in groups. Our aim is to enumerate and classify the scarce literature on biosecurity and disease prevention and to describe recommendations while assessing evidence of their impact and feasibility.

Although veterinarians have cooperated with shelters and kennels for decades, until recently there was little scientific interest in the discipline of preventive companion animals' veterinary medicine for shelters and kennels. Currently, however, we have seen an increase in interest in this field as the need for expertise in risk assessment and disease management has now been acknowledged. Numerous canine pathogens that impact on health, welfare or economics have been described and emerging diseases are still being reported. Furthermore, some canine pathogens represent an important hazard for public health. To avert animal and human health risks, poor animal welfare and economic losses, biosecurity measures need to be implemented to prevent the introduction, persistence and transmission of infectious agents.

In-depth knowledge and understanding of the different transmission pathways provide guidance for the development of biosecurity measures that should be implemented in kennels and other canine facilities.

2 General Biosecurity Guidelines

In describing the biosecurity measures a distinction will be made between external biosecurity measures aimed at preventing the introduction of pathogens into the facility, and internal biosecurity which aims at preventing the spread of pathogens between different animals, groups or compartments within the facility. For more details on the general principles of biosecurity please consult chapter 2.

2.1 External biosecurity

2.1.1 Purchase of animals/semen

The biggest risk associated with the acquisition of new animals is the introduction of pathogens. Anecdotal evidence shows the purchase of puppies and adult dogs by dog breeders is common practice and purchasing puppies is an essential element in the business of dog merchants. The number of origins should be limited as much as possible. Nevertheless, different origins are intrinsic when running a shelter, introducing new bloodlines or running a pet store. In such circumstances, the incoming dogs should be divided into smaller risk groups according to origin among other things.

New animals should always be fully assessed by a veterinarian prior to or on admission. Inconsistent vaccination status, presence of parasites and symptoms of illness are risk factors and should be managed accordingly. Prophylactic treatments to support the new animals and/or to protect the other animals in the facility should be provided and should be performed according to protocols adapted to the group at risk, as well as geographical and seasonal parameters. Merchants trading puppies from different origins may find themselves with puppies that have a different immune status. They should at least insist that the same vaccination protocols are followed by all suppliers for both puppies and breeding adults. Detailed recommendations for vaccination and deworming can be found further in box 16.1 and box 16.2.

Although the risk of pathogen introduction in a breeding facility through semen is much smaller than via the introduction of new animals, transmission of diseases through semen is a possibility (Silva et al., 2009). The prevalence of venereal transmission of canine diseases is well known (i.e. Brucellosis, Canine Herpesvirosis, venereal tumours, Leishmaniosis, Toxoplasmosis); canine breeding professionals should always be aware of the risk of transmission not only via mating but also during artificial insemination (AI). Since AI is common in dog breeding, especially in brachycephalic breeds, it is recommended that sires from endemic areas on particular diseases be tested (e.g. Brucella canis in Canada, Europe and subtropics or anecdotally canine visceral leishmaniasis in Southern Europe, North Africa and Latin America).

Vaccination recommendations:

Multiple organisations and workgroups have developed vaccination guidelines (Davis-Wurzler, 2014; Day et al., 2016; Moore and Glickman, 2004; Welborn et al., 2011). The contracting veterinarian plays a key role in choosing the most appropriate vaccination programme for each particular animal, depending on its needs, and taking into account the essentials for puppy immunization.

Core vaccines should be administrated prior to or directly on admission, as early as at four weeks of age. Adults should be revaccinated after two weeks, while puppies should be vaccinated until the age of twenty weeks with intervals of two weeks.

Deworming recommendations:

Recommendations for most endoparasites have been published. In addition to American recommendations (CAPCVET), European recommendations are also readily available (ESCCAP, 2010; W.V.P.N., 2008). Regarding the prevention of worm infestations (e.g. Toxacara canis, *Toxascaris leonina, Uncinaria stenocephala, Trichuris vulpis*), it is recommended to deworm puppies with a broad spectrum anthelminthic product from the age of 2 weeks onwards and repeat every 2 weeks until weaning. Thereafter, puppies should be dewormed monthly until the age of 6 months. Adult dogs should be treated monthly (ESCCAP, 2010b; ESCCAP_Deutschland, 2014).

Prevention is crucial in the combat against protozoa (e.g. *Giardia duodenalis, Cryptosporidium isospora*), especially in shelters and large kennels. Meticulous cleaning and drying of the environment, constant removal of faeces and the use of disinfection-proof objects are necessary. Although curative treatments are available, chronic cases are typically caused by reinfection (Dupont et al., 2013; ESCCAP, 2010).

2.1.2 **Quarantine**

The principle of quarantine consists of segregation of suspicious animals in a fully separated location (Gensini et al., 2004).

Quarantine is essential and should always be implemented even for dogs that appear healthy at the time of purchase since they may be incubating infectious diseases. During this period, the quarantined dog is monitored carefully by the veterinarian and staff for any signs of illness.

Besides the evident risks associated with direct contact between newly acquired and other dogs, one should be aware of indirect disease transmission through people, vehicles, material, food and water as a result of contact with the different animals. Access must be easy, closed off from other accesses and restricted to dedicated staff with specific regulations. When animal caretakers visit the quarantine house, they should wear special clothing and footwear and wash and disinfect their hands at entry and when leaving the facility. Separate cleaning equipment, grooming accessories, and feeding bowls must also be used. Quarantined dogs should only be given access to specific separate outdoor spaces. Additional exposure to social stimuli is necessary since quarantined dogs are kept confined. The duration of the quarantine period should be no shorter than the longest incubation period of the diseases being screened for. For particular diseases like rabies, antibody screening has been proven to be a valid alternative to long quarantine periods (>6 months) (Cliquet et al., 2003), so animals only need to be isolated until the results of the test are negative. Evidence from outbreaks recommends adhering to a quarantine period of at least four weeks (Bohm et al., 1989; Hollett, 2006). On the ground however, the legal minimum quarantine between countries does not exceed 10 to 14 days (Simmons and Hoffman, 2016), but this is subject to prior prophylaxis (for external and internal parasites)

16

and vaccination or serological testing (i.e. rabies, leptospirosis, brucellosis) being carried out before admission (Australian Government – Department of Agriculture, 2013; European Commission – Food Safety, 2017).

2.1.3 Animal flow patterns

Animal flow (e.g. acquisition, reintroduction, visits, exhibition, mating) is undoubtedly a major cause of the spread of disease. Vehicles are often omitted when establishing a biosecurity plan for facilities; yet vehicles must be considered as potential vectors for disease transmission.

Transport can cause an increase in stress, resulting in higher shedding of pathogens and a lower immunity (Beerda et al., 1997).

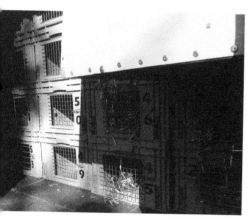

▲
Fig. 16.1: Vehicle transporting dogs

In most pet shops and larger kennels, dogs are delivered in groups. Transport is also often organised by third parties (i.e. specialised carriers) in vehicles with limited to moderate compartmentalisation, as shown in Fig. 16.1. Transporting dogs from different origins in the same vehicle should be avoided.

To limit transmission between facilities, each animal transport should be limited to one destination. In reality, unfortunately, delivery vehicles with smaller deliveries commonly travel to multiple facilities. Measures such as ensuring separate and easy access, cleaning and/or disinfecting the vehicle between each kennel, requiring couriers to wear disposable clothing and footwear, limiting access of staff to the transport vehicle, and confining access of the carrier to the quarantine site should be taken. Facilities for cleaning and disinfecting vehicles should be provided at every stopover. Kennels and pet stores with a high intensity of shipments should definitely implement a dirty road principle. This will ensure that dogs transported to the quarantine site are physically separated from the normal working lines and healthy dogs.

What is the dirty road principle?

The dirty road principle is the concept designed to ensure movement categorised as a risk is directed towards one specific route.
This passage should only be used for movement of other elements
at similar risk and must not cross normal working paths at any point in
time. Dirty road is the extension therefore of the compartmentalisation and workflow from arrival to departure from the kennel.

There may be different reasons for reintroduction of a dog to the
facility. Anecdotal evidence shows pedigree breeders regularly
attend exhibitions or shows or exchange animals for mating. Dogs
are also sometimes relinquished to the facility. Reintroduction of
animals should always be managed in the same way as acquisition
of a new animal, including assessment, testing for immunisation
and quarantine.

2.1.4 Supply of food, water and equipment

Food and accessories (e.g. bedding material, apparel, tools) for
several facilities are often transported in the same truck. Deliveries
and storage should be processed in a place therefore that is easily
accessible and where there is no contact with the animals. All food
should be processed during production and dispensed in such a
way as to guarantee a low risk of contamination of pathogens.
From a sanitary point of view, raw food is not recommended as a
large number of surveys have shown evidence of risks (e.g. pseudorabies, salmonellosis, toxoplasmosis) (Finley et al., 2008; Jones
et al., 2009; LeJeune and Hancock, 2001). Drinking water should
be of suitable for consumption and should be assessed on a regular
basis. Rain water is not recommended. (Lye, 2002). Food bowls
and drinking devices should be washed daily. Access to standing
water should be avoided at all times as water can be contaminated by rats (i.e. *Leptospira* spp.) (Ghneim et al., 2007). All tools
and equipment used in daily care should be cleaned on a regular
basis. Grooming equipment (i.e. brushes, scissors, shavers) must
be cleaned and disinfected every time they are used.

16

Canine facilities are frequently visited by visitors from outside. In addition to professional visitors (contracting veterinarians, inspectors), private visitors frequently ask to see the facility, not only to see the dog they might want to buy, but also to see breeding adults. Some visitors even request to bring their own dog when visiting. Since a considerable number of visitors are frequently in contact with dogs, they all present a potential risk of disease transmission. Generally, access should only be possible after notification, preferably accompanied by a member of the personnel. Fences, doors, windows, room dividers with clear signs that delimit the restricted area are certainly an easy way to limit free access. Pet shops, which tend to have unregulated access to at least the dogs they are selling, can limit physical access to puppies through the layout of the showroom and if no contained division is available, visitors should be supervised at all times. Compartmentalisation and workflow (see further in this chapter) should be respected at all times.

If people want contact with an animal, sanitary measures can be imposed such as hand and footwear hygiene in order to limit the introduction of pathogens, contain diseases in the occurrence of an outbreak, and limit the zoonotic risks (Glickman and Shofer, 1987). Visitors should be informed about general health measures and about the consequences of not following them. Since hands are the most important part of the body to come in contact with dogs, hands should be washed with soap and water and then disinfected or a sanitizing gel should be applied between each compartmentalisation group and this should be mandatory for every visitor. Footwear hygiene can be achieved by using disposable boot covers or footbaths.

Additional measures such as wearing protective clothing are also advised for visitors who have intensive contact with other kennels, i.e. professional visitors. The use of a transition zone (i.e. hygiene lock) is an effective way to remind visitors that they enter another unit. As a general rule, biosecurity measures directed at visitors should always be easily accessible, feasible and unambiguously applicable.

The Hygiene Lock?

A hygiene lock is a separate room or part of a room where staff and visitors apply biosecurity measures such as changing clothes or putting on protective clothing, washing and disinfecting hands, ... before entering the premises or when moving between different units. A hygiene lock must be located at the entrance or in between the different units, and it should be as effortless as possible to use.

2.1.6 Vermin/birds and other animals

You will always find rodents or small birds where animals are kept and food is stored. Apart from anecdotal data there is no evidence of canine disease transmission through birds. Rodents, on the other hand, are a known reservoir and vector for canine diseases. A rodent control programme is strongly recommended therefore (see chapter 11).

In an ideal situation, no household dogs should be allowed. It is evident that pet dogs following staff everywhere will negate all other biosecurity measures. Kennel keepers with pet dogs (e.g. retired breeding bitches) should be aware of the risks of transmission and always avoid (in)direct contact between pet dogs and the kennel dogs.

Depending on geographical and seasonal differences, some insects and arachnids (e.g. sand-flies, ticks) can be vectors of diseases. A good insect control programme should also be installed therefore (see chapter 10). Contact with external dogs, feral animals or wildlife should be avoided at all times.

2.2 Internal biosecurity

The goal of internal biosecurity is to control the spread of disease within the facility. One of the key factors influencing internal biosecurity is the time spent by a particular dog in a facility (Stavisky et al., 2012). The design of the facility can contribute consider-

16

ably to reducing transmission if it allows segregation (separation of animals into different groups based on their susceptibility to infectious diseases). General measures for the group of adults or breeding dogs should be discussed. When considering breeding facilities, pregnant dogs represent another separate group as pregnancy, whelping and lactating incur specific needs. Puppies under five months of age need more protection from exposure to infectious diseases because they are generally more susceptible than older dogs; both age groups should therefore be segregated. And last but not least, diseased dogs should be confined during treatment or recovery.

2.2.1 General measures

2.2.1.1 Direct transmission

Direct spread of pathogens between multiple dogs in one facility is the result of animal flow and the potential for contact between dogs. The former can be limited via management planning of the facility. The latter is a consequence of housing. Well-designed housing will make it possible to limit and control transmission. Dogs can be housed in rooms, pens, stables, cages, and indoors or outdoors. Individual buildings are a preferred guarantee of segregation. When housing multiple groups in the same building, physical contact (e.g. nose to nose, urinary and defaecation) has to be limited. Housing must meet the physical and psychological needs of dogs. Inadequate management and housing of dogs will increase the incidence of acute and chronic stress (Beerda et al., 1999). Chronic stress has been linked to negative effects on a dog's health and immunity, by altering tissue physiology and damping immune responses to invasive pathogens, hence influencing the appearance and transmission of diseases (Radek, 2010).

2.2.1.2 Indirect transmission

The spread of disease is not just a result of direct contact; fomites can also play an important role in disease transmission. All objects and materials have to be resistant to cleaning, disinfection but also resistant to urine and wear (i.e. dogs biting and scratching). Enrichment material, food bowls and water dispensers must be cleaned and disinfected if used among the different dog groups or, preferably, must be used separately for each particular group. Disease can also be transmitted via vectors such as insects (i.e. flies, mosquitoes) and arachnids (Beugnet and Marié, 2009), rodents (i.e. rats and mice) (Jansen et al., 2005), birds (Song et al., 2008), other domestic animals (dogs or other) (Crawford et al., 2005), and feral animals (Kapel et al., 2006). Finally, disease may also be transmitted indirectly through mechanical vectors such as vehicles, staff, and visitors. Transmission paths are inherent to a pathogens' ability to survive in the environment and vice-versa. Non-enveloped viruses (e.g. Canine Parvovirus), mycobacteria, bacterial spores and coccidia in particular can survive for months and are largely resistant to disinfectants (McDonnell and Russell, 1999).

2.2.2. Work flow

Healthy animals should always be taken care of at the beginning of the daily routine, and staff should gradually move down the working line, finishing with diseased animals. Young animals should be taken care of before adults so that exposure to pathogens is kept to a minimum. All upstream paths (e.g. from diseased animals to clinically healthy young animals) should be avoided at all costs. However, maintaining a strict downstream path is not always feasible (e.g. having to administer medical treatments at the beginning of the working day). In these instances, different staff members should take care of diseased and healthy animals and hygienic measures should be respected even more strictly.
Ideally a sanitary transition zone (disposables, hand hygiene) should be provided for each group and be used correctly. It is important to extend the principles of the working lines for each movement or action (e.g. professional visitors).

2.2.3 Cleaning and disinfection

When discussing cleaning and disinfection, the first thing that comes to mind are the different pens and units. This is particularly

16

true since faeces are an important risk factor for enteric disease if the oro-faecal cycle is sustained. Since dirty animals have been reported as risk factors (Nagy et al., 2011), regular bathing or brushing coats if bathing is not possible, are good measures for removing dirt and soiling. Most uncapsulated viruses (e.g. Canine Parvovirus, CPV) and sporulated cysts can survive for months and are largely resistant to disinfectants. But capsulated viruses, spores and cysts can also demonstrate strong resistance when surrounded by organic material. Rapid or at least daily removal of all debris, faeces or other organic material before cleaning with water and detergents and disinfecting is of utmost importance therefore. Product guidelines should be followed thoroughly (molecule, dilution, formulation, contact time). Surface-dried viruses are generally more resistant to disinfection; a single stage disinfection might not be sufficient. Soaking surface-dried viruses prior to disinfection is recommended. Obviously, care should be taken with handling, during and after rehydration, as this waste contains infectious viruses (Terpstra et al., 2007). Since dogs are – at least partly – housed outdoors and most dogs have daily outdoor access, the outdoor areas should follow the same principles as indoor areas. It is advised to use separate materials toys and equipment for each group within the kennel (e.g. puppies, breeding adults). Distinction between specific materials can easily be achieved by labelling or using different colours. More detailed info on cleaning and disinfection procedures can be found in chapter 6.

2.2.4 Management of sick animals and removal of dead animals

Animals with clinical signs of illness represent potential risks for others dogs. In addition, diseased animals are more susceptible to other diseases, resulting in complicated diseases with increased morbidity, mortality and/or health expenses (e.g. coronavirus and parvovirus). Since cleaning outdoor areas is more limited, diseased animals should not be kept outside.

2.2.4.1 Direct transmission

Animals with suspected (presenting one or several risk factors) or proven (by laboratory data) presence of infectious diseases should be physically isolated to allow for further investigation and treatment before coming into contact with other animals. The isolation unit should be secluded from other animal groups and individual isolation within the unit or isolation per type of disease should be implemented and the same precautionary measures should apply as in the quarantine unit.

When an animal dies it is advisable to remove the animal from the kennel as quickly as possible. If infectious disease is the cause of death, the carcass might as act as a source of infection for the remaining animals. Carcasses should be stored in a cooled unit (the mortuary) until disposal can be carried out. Removal by a rendering company is recommended. As an alternative, the treating veterinarian can dispose of the carcass. Burying, local incineration or removal with everyday rubbish are not recommended and are legally prohibited in most countries.

2.2.4.2 Indirect transmission

Healthy dogs should always be looked after before animals with clinical signs. Biosecurity measures that apply to the isolation unit are similar to those described for the quarantine unit: the use of disposables, specific clothing, hand and footwear hygiene and dedicated material are strongly recommended.

When manipulating dead animals, it is advisable to use disposable gloves and/or clean and disinfect the hands afterwards. Routine cleaning and disinfection of the mortuary is essential. Care should be taken to prevent access to the mortuary by vermin, rodents or other animals.

2.2.5 Maternity

The maternity unit is the part of the kennel where pregnant bitches are housed during the short period around whelping. Immunity of whelping bitches drops significantly around the time of parturition and new-born puppies have a low immunity (Day, 2007; Evermann and Wills, 2011). It is of utmost importance therefore to maintain a clean, controlled environment.

2.2.5.1 Direct transmission

Transmission of disease towards the maternity unit can be limited by avoiding contact with other dogs. Compared to males, bitches are not only more susceptible to acute stress, but also to chronic housing stress (Beerda et al., 1999). Several degrees of isolation can be achieved although pregnant bitches will show reduced stress if they are able to interact with other dogs until partum when social withdrawal is observed. Transmission of pathogens to puppies can occur vertically, meaning through placenta or, to a lesser extent, milk. The maternity unit also serves as a housing for the puppies until they reach a minimum age of four weeks. If feasible, and necessary, social exposure is can be achieved; puppies can be housed in the maternity unit until weaning, at the age of seven or more week.

2.2.5.2 Indirect transmission

The abovementioned principles of hand and footwear hygiene also applies to the maternity unit.

Since the shedding of pathogens 2 (in particular enteric parasites) dramatically increases during the late pregnancy (Lloyd et al., 1983), a whelping box can serve as transmitter of diseases. Whelping boxes should not only be practical and sturdy therefore, but also easy to clean and disinfect (Fig. 16.2). Painted plywood or polyethene are more resistant to detergents, wear, water and are better alternatives to solid wood, Oriented Strand boards (OSB) and Medium Density Fibre (MDF) boards.

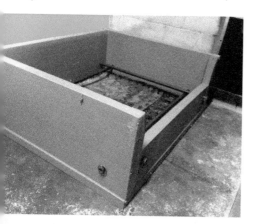

Fig. 16.2: Whelping box in polyethene
▼

What are Whelping Boxes?

Whelping boxes are commonly used by breeders as a safe place for pregnant bitches during late pregnancy and parturition and they are also used as housing for the puppies until they are weaned. This confined space creates a safe place for dams, while the presence of (removable) rails at approximatively 10cm (4inches) of the side walls and floor helps to avoid them lying on top of new-born puppies.

2.2.6 Puppy management

Housing conditions must be adapted to the physiology and needs of puppies, with particular focus on ambient temperature. Automatic thermo-regulation should only be used at the end of the fourth week (Lawler, 2008). Puppies build up a major part of their immunity by drinking colostrum during the first hours of life; placental transfer of antibodies is negligible.

These maternal antibodies will start to decline after three to four weeks. Meanwhile, immunity will be taken over by the pup's own immune system and prime vaccination of core vaccines (Root Kustritz, 2011).

Infectious diseases, particularly bacterial diseases, are the second cause of neonatal death in dogs. Necropsy of the pups mostly resulted in isolation of bacteria that originate in the environment or the dam (Münnich and Lübke-Becker, 2004; Nielen et al., 1998; Schäfer-Somi et al., 2003). The combination of maternal immunity, primary vaccination and a fast-developing immunity progressively decreases the risk of infection.

2.2.6.1 Direct transmission

Puppies are housed in groups together with the dam and other litter-mates in order to ensure maternal care and social exposure needed for behavioural development (Wilsson, 1984). Depending on the degree of immunisation, contact with other litters, adult dogs, and other animals can be progressively increased from four weeks to twelve weeks of age as part of the socialisation process.

16

If we look at pet shops however, we see that puppies are housed with dogs of other origins for a short time after they have often been shipped across a number of different countries. In these conditions, puppies can be more susceptible to disease; stress will inhibit their immune system while at the same time promoting pathogen shedding. In these instances high density should be avoided and puppies should be segregated by supplier, origin and age (Buonavoglia and Martella, 2007).

2.2.6.2 Indirect transmission

Daily cleaning and regularly disinfecting of the pen, food bowls and equipment is effective in countering oro-faecal transmission and environmental accumulation of pathogens. No pen or object should be reused for a new litter until it has been completely disinfected. Airborne spread of diseases can be controlled even further by extending compartmentalisation to individual ventilation, waste water and heating/cooling of every pen. Housing puppies from different litters (and even different countries) together in one pen or remixing puppies left over from one litter is not recommended. When a litter has been sold, housing should be completely cleaned and disinfected before introducing new puppies.

3 Conclusion

Biosecurity is a cornerstone of infectious disease control in facilities where large numbers of dogs are housed together. As recent sources show, scientific interest in disease prevention and management of pet dogs is finally increasing. Measures for disease management in (semi-) permanent canine groups have long been underrated; however, preventive medicine is an essential step in companion animal veterinary medicine. The environment is often the determining factor in the development and harbouring of infectious diseases (e.g. giardiasis, worm infestation, parvovirosis). However, it appears to be difficult to implement the environmental factor into health management of canine facilities. The leading cause seems to be that the majority of contracting veterinarians of canine facilities have trained as small animal veterinarians and are not familiar with risk assessment in herd management and have not been trained in designing comprehensive infection-control plans (Miller and Zawistowski, 2013).

Because there are large variations in the size and purpose of different types of canine facilities, it is impossible to develop a one-size-fits-all protocol. Never has it been more essential to use a tailored approach to assess and implement feasible and practical biosecurity measures in (semi-)permanent canine facilities.

Biosecurity measures will only have an impact if they are applied correctly and consistently. Further improvement can be achieved by training and accompanying staff. Each facility should have a trained person who develops and controls the biosecurity measures as well as a consulting veterinarian who is familiar with the management and purpose of the facility. This veterinarian should be willing to adapt general guidelines to practical protocols.

Meanwhile, specific training should be offered to companion animal veterinarians who are eager to work as consulting vets in canine facilities. This training should encompass the principles of disease management in larger populations and familiarisation with risk assessment. This could result in an increased surveillance of infectious diseases enabling professionals to evaluate, adapt and optimise the implemented protocols and to react proactively to possible outbreaks, thus improving the welfare and quality of care.

16

References

Australian Government – Department of Agriculture, 2013. Importation of dogs and cats and their semen from approved countries.

Beerda, B., Schilder, M.B.., Bernadina, W., Van Hooff, J.A.R.A.., De Vries, H.W., Mol, J.A., 1999. Chronic Stress in Dogs Subjected to Social and Spatial Restriction. II. Hormonal and Immunological Responses. Physiol. Behav. 66, 243-254. doi:10.1016/S0031-9384(98)00290-X

Beerda, B., Schilder, M.B.H., van Hooff, J.A.R.A.M., de Vries, H.W., 1997. Manifestations of chronic and acute stress in dogs. Appl. Anim. Behav. Sci. 52, 307-319. doi:10.1016/S0168-1591(96)01131-8

Beugnet, F., Marié, J.-L., 2009. Emerging arthropod-borne diseases of companion animals in Europe. Vet. Parasitol. 163, 298-305. doi:10.1016/j.vetpar.2009.03.028

Bohm, J., Blixenkrone-Møller, M., Lund, E., 1989. A serious outbreak of canine distemper among sled-dogs in northern Greenland. Arctic Med. Res. 48, 195-203.

Buonavoglia, C., Martella, V., 2007. Canine respiratory viruses. Vet Res 38, 355-373. doi:10.1051/vetres:2006058

Cliquet, F., Verdier, Y., Sagné, L., Aubert, M., 2003. titration in 25,000 sera of dogs and cats vaccinated against rabies in France, in the framework of the new regulations that offer an alternative to quarantine. Rev. Sci.

Crawford, P., Dubovi, E., Castleman, W., 2005. Transmission of equine influenza virus to dogs.

Davis-Wurzler, G.M., 2014. 2013 update on current vaccination strategies in puppies and kittens. Vet Clin North Am Small Anim Pr. 44, 235-263. doi:10.1016/j.cvsm.2013.11.006

Day, M.J., 2007. Immune System Development in the Dog and Cat. J. Comp. Pathol. 137, S10-S15. doi:10.1016/j.jcpa.2007.04.005

Day, M.J., Horzinek, M.C., Schultz, R.D., Squires, R.A., 2016. WSAVA Guidelines for the vaccination of dogs and cats. J. Small Anim. Pract. 57, E1-E45. doi:10.1111/jsap.2_12431

Dupont, S., Butaye, P., Claerebout, E., Theuns, S., Duchateau, L., Van de Maele, I., Daminet, S., 2013. Enteropathogens in pups from pet shops and breeding facilities. J. Small Anim. Pract. 54, 475-480. doi:10.1111/jsap.12119

ESCCAP, 2010. Worm Control in Dogs and Cats – ESCCAP Guidelines 2nd edition.

European Commission – Food Safety, 2017. Imports from non-EU countries [WWW Document]. URL https://ec.europa.eu/food/animals/pet-movement/eu-legislation/non-eu-imports_en (accessed 8.14.17).

Evermann, J.F., Wills, T.B., 2011. Immunologic development and immunization. Peterson ME, Kutzler MA 104-112.

Finley, R., Reid-Smith, R., Ribble, C., Popa, M., Vandermeer, M., Aramini, J., 2008. The Occurrence and Antimicrobial Susceptibility of Salmonellae Isolated from Commercially Available Canine Raw Food Diets in Three Canadian Cities. Zoonoses Public Health 55, 462-469. doi:10.1111/j.1863-2378.2008.01147.x

Gensini, G., Yacoub, M., Conti, A., 2004. The concept of quarantine in history: from plague to SARS. J. Infect.

Ghneim, G.S., Viers, J.H., Chomel, B.B., Kass, P.H., Descollonges, D.A., Johnson, M.L., 2007. Use of a case-control study and geographic information systems to determine environmental and demographic risk factors for canine leptospirosis. Vet. Res. 38, 37-50. doi:10.1051/vetres:2006043

Glickman, L.T., Shofer, F.S., 1987. Zoonotic Visceral and Ocular Larva Migrans. Vet. Clin. North Am. Small Anim. Pract. 17, 39-53. doi:10.1016/S0195-5616(87)50604-0

Hollett, R.B., 2006. Canine brucellosis: Outbreaks and compliance. Theriogenology 66, 575-587. doi:10.1016/j.theriogenology.2006.04.011

Jansen, A., Schöneberg, I., Frank, C., Alpers, K., Schneider, T., Stark, K., 2005. Leptospirosis in Germany, 1962-2003. Emerg. Infect. Dis. 11, 1048-54. doi:10.3201/eid1107.041172

Jones, J.L., Dargelas, V., Roberts, J., Press, C., Remington, J.S., Montoya, J.G., 2009. Risk Factors for *Toxoplasma gondii* Infection in the United States. Clin. Infect. Dis. 49, 878-884. doi:10.1086/605433

Kapel, C.M.O., Torgerson, P.R., Thompson, R.C.A., Deplazes, P., 2006. Reproductive potential of Echinococcus multilocularis in experimentally infected foxes, dogs, raccoon dogs and cats. Int. J. Parasitol. 36, 79-86. doi:10.1016/j.ijpara.2005.08.012

Lawler, D.F., 2008. Neonatal and pediatric care of the puppy and kitten. Theriogenology 70, 384-392. doi:10.1016/j.theriogenology.2008.04.019

LeJeune, J.T., Hancock, D.D., 2001. Public health concerns associated with feeding raw meat diets to dogs. J. Am. Vet. Med. Assoc. 219, 1222-1225. doi:10.2460/javma.2001.219.1222

Lloyd, S., Amerasinghe, P.H., Soulsby, E.J.L., 1983. Periparturient immunosuppression in the bitch and its influence on infection with Toxocara canis. J. Small Anim. Pract. 24, 237-247. doi:10.1111/j.1748-5827.1983.tb00437.x

Lye, D.J., 2002. Health risks associated with consumption of untreated water from household roof catchment systems. J. Am. Water Resour. Assoc. 38, 1301-1306. doi:10.1111/j.1752-1688.2002.tb04349.x

McDonnell, G., Russell, A.D., 1999. Antiseptics and disinfectants: activity, action, and resistance. Clin. Microbiol. Rev. 12, 147-79.

Miller, L., Zawistowski, S., 2013. Shelter medicine for veterinarians and staff. Wiley-Blackwell.

Moore, G.E., Glickman, L.T., 2004. A perspective on vaccine guidelines and titer tests for dogs. J. Am. Vet. Med. Assoc. 224, 200-203.

Münnich, A., Lübke-Becker, A., 2004. Escherichia coli infections in newborn puppies—clinical and epidemiological investigations. Theriogenology.

Nagy, A., Ziadinov, I., Schweiger, A., Schnyder, M., Deplazes, P., 2011. [Hair coat contamination with zoonotic helminth eggs of farm and pet dogs and foxes]. Berl. Munch. Tierarztl. Wochenschr. 124, 503-11.

Nielen, A., Gaag, I. Van der, Knol, B., 1998. Investigation of mortality and pathological changes in a 14-month birth cohort of boxer puppies. Vet.

Radek, K.A., 2010. Antimicrobial anxiety: the impact of stress on antimicrobial immunity. J. Leukoc. Biol. 88, 263-77. doi:10.1189/jlb.1109740

Root Kustritz, M. V, 2011. Chapter 4 – History and Physical Examination of the Weanling and Adolescent, in: Kutzler, M.E.P.A. (Ed.), Small Animal Pediatrics. W.B. Saunders, Saint Louis, pp. 28-33. doi:http://dx.doi.org/10.1016/B978-1-4160-4889-3.00004-8

16

Schäfer-Somi, S., Spergser, J., Breitenfellner, J., Aurich, J.E., 2003. Bacteriological status of canine milk and septicaemia in neonatal puppies--a retrospective study. J. Vet. Med. B. Infect. Dis. Vet. Public Health 50, 343-6.

Silva, F., Oliveira, R., Silva, T., Xavier, M., 2009. Venereal transmission of canine visceral leishmaniasis. Veterinary.

Simmons, K., Hoffman, C., 2016. Dogs on the Move: Factors Impacting Animal Shelter and Rescue Organizations' Decisions to Accept Dogs from Distant Locations. Animals 6, 11. doi:10.3390/ani6020011

Song, D., Kang, B., Lee, C., Jung, K., Ha, G., Kang, D., Park, S., Park, B., Oh, J., 2008. Transmission of avian influenza virus (H3N2) to dogs. Emerg. Infect. Dis. 14, 741-6. doi:10.3201/eid1405.071471

Stavisky, J., Pinchbeck, G., Gaskell, R.M., Dawson, S., German, A.J., Radford, A.D., 2012. Cross sectional and longitudinal surveys of canine enteric coronavirus infection in kennelled dogs: A molecular marker for biosecurity. Infect. Genet. Evol. 12, 1419-1426. doi:10.1016/j.meegid.2012.04.010

Terpstra, F.G., van den Blink, A.E., Bos, L.M., Boots, A.G.C., Brinkhuis, F.H.M., Gijsen, E., van Remmerden, Y., Schuitemaker, H., van 't Wout, A.B., 2007. Resistance of surface-dried virus to common disinfection procedures. J. Hosp. Infect. 66, 332-338. doi:10.1016/j.jhin.2007.05.005

Welborn, L. V, DeVries, J.G., Ford, R., Franklin, R.T., Hurley, K.F., McClure, K.D., Paul, M.A., Schultz, R.D., 2011. 2011 AAHA canine vaccination guidelines. J Am Anim Hosp Assoc 47, 1-42.

Wilsson, E., 1984. The social interaction between mother and offspring during weaning in German shepherd dogs: individual differences between mothers and their effects on offspring. Appl. Anim. Behav. Sci.

CHAPTER 17

BIOSECURITY IN VETERINARY PRACTICES AND CLINICS

Claude Saegerman[1]

Marie-France Humblet[2]

[1] Faculty of Veterinary Medicine, Fundamental and Applied Research in Animals Health (FARAH) Centre, Research Unit in Epidemiology and Risk Analysis applied to Veterinary Science (UREAR-ULg), University of Liège, 4000 Liège, Belgium
[2] Department for Occupational Safety and Health, Biosafety and Biosecurity Unit, University of Liège, 4000 Liège, Belgium

1 Introduction

After a short presentation of the general principles of biosecurity that apply to veterinary clinics/practices, we will present two case studies to illustrate the implementation thereof. The first one focuses on the hospitalisation of a dog with methicillin-resistant *Staphylococcus aureus* (MRSA) in a small animal clinic while the second focuses on consultation involving a horse with salmonellosis.

As biosecurity measures are applicable at any time, two additional sections have been included covering biosecurity audits and internal audits as well as biosecurity-related veterinary education.

2 General principles of biosecurity applicable to veterinary clinics/practices

Biosecurity consists of implementing measures that reduce the risk of the introduction (bio-exclusion) and spread of disease agents (bio-containment); it involves adopting a set of attitudes and behaviour to reduce the risk in all activities involving domestic, captive exotic species and wild birds and their by-products (World Organisation for Animal Health, 2008). Biosecurity is based on the prevention of and protection against infectious agents. The measures to be established should not be seen as constraints but rather as part of a process aimed at improving the health of animals, humans and the environment.

Fig. 17.1: Biosecurity principles in an animal facility (Saegerman et al., 2012)

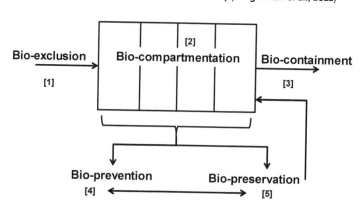

Biosecurity as applied to veterinary medicine is based on 5 main principles (Saegerman et al., 2012), as shown in Fig. 17.1.

Legend: All stages specified in the figure above are part of a biosecurity approach and contribute to reducing the risk of introduction and spread of infectious agents: 1) to limit the risk of introduction (bio-exclusion); 2) to limit the spread of the pathogen within the same facility, e.g. by isolating excreting animals (bio-compartmentation); 3) to limit the spread of the disease agent outside the facility (inter-herd transmission) (bio-containment); 4) to prevent the risk of human contamination (bio-prevention); 5) to prevent any environmental bio-contamination and persistence of the pathogen (bio-preservation). Humans can contaminate animals as well (e.g., *Mycobacterium bovis*) (Fritsche et al., 2004). Animals can become re-infected by a contaminated environment, which is especially true for pathogens presenting a high environmental persistence such as *Bacillus anthracis* or *Mycobacterium bovis,* when ecological conditions are optimal (Courtenay & Wellington, 2008; OIE-WHO-FAO, 2008).

Implementing biosecurity amounts to the prevention and control of infections. The main goals of a biosecurity programme in a hospital setting are to optimise hygiene, break transmission cycles and protect hospitalised individuals (in case of zoonotic pathogens).

Fig. 17.2: Yellow line may be crossed with certain restrictions ▼

At the Faculty of Veterinary Medicine (FVM), University of Liege (ULg), Belgium, biosecurity has been implemented in different ways, motivated by the European Association of Establishments for Veterinary Education (EAEVE) agreement; these concepts are also completely appropriate for private practices/clinics:

- **Floor markings:** green lines may be crossed without restrictions, yellow lines (Fig. 17.2) may be crossed but with certain restrictions (with particular account being taken of strict biosecurity measures, such as wearing the appropriate personal protective equipment) and red lines may not be crossed other than with the explicit permission of supervisors (e.g. operating theatre). For example, at the Faculty of Veteri-

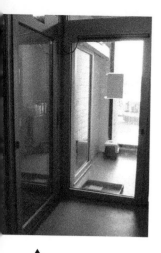

▲

Fig. 17.3: Red line may not be crossed without the explicit permission of supervisors (e.g. entrance of the isolation unit)

nary Medicine, University of Liege, a red line is painted just in front of the entrance of the isolation unit for small animals (Fig. 17.3). Access is thus limited and only allowed with staff authorisation and subject to wearing appropriate additional personal protective equipment.

- The principle of 'onward march' must be respected. This type of concept is generally used in the food industry; it is based on a movement from the least contaminated to the most contaminated sectors. For example, in a practice, infectious animals are treated last to avoid contaminating non-infected patients. Daily visits should be scheduled according to the same principle. Another example is provided in the Clinic of Ruminants (FVM, ULg): animal caretakers (staff and students) have to respect the order of visits: first, they look after the non-infectious calves (hospitalised for surgery, etc.), which are usually more susceptible to infections, then the adults hospitalised for non-infectious diseases, and finish with infectious animals, i.e. class 3 (infectious disease with a moderate risk of transmission; see below) (Fig. 17.4).

Fig. 17.4: The principle of onward march in a clinic of ruminants

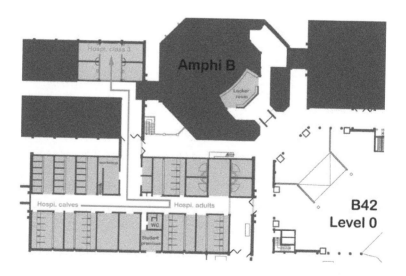

BIOSECURITY IN ANIMAL PRODUCTION AND VETERINARY MEDICINE

- **Classes of risk** have been defined in function of the pathogens involved (Table 17.1):
  - CLASS 1: non-infectious condition
  - CLASS 2: infectious disease with a low or non-existent risk of transmission
  - CLASS 3: infectious disease with a moderate risk of transmission; these patients are suspected of having an infectious disease and being contagious for other patients and/or for humans
  - CLASS 4: infectious diseases with a significant risk of transmission; any patient suspected of suffering from a notifiable disease falls in this category.

Classes of risk determine the way patients are housed. Class 1 and Class 2 patients are held in normal housing. Class 3 patients are housed in a dedicated aisle of the practice/clinic and handled with **barrier nursing** precautions. Barrier nursing is a concept intending to protect other patients and/or the medical staff from contamination. It relies on the implementation of a 'barrier' between the patient and medical staff in order to prevent cross-contamination of the body, clothing and footwear, which, in turn, decreases the risk of nosocomial transmission to other patients (Sheridan, 2009, Manuel SOP). Barrier nursing precautions include, among others:

- Visible information on the animal status (display on the stall/cage door)
- Wearing specially designated personal attire (e.g. specific/additional personal protective equipment such as disposable overalls, over-boots, etc.)
- Using material and equipment totally dedicated to the animal (e.g. for cattle: halter and rope, examination equipment such as thermometer, stethoscope, etc.)
- Minimising the movements of patients (and ensuring the 'onward march') and avoiding unnecessary contact with them
- Hosting in a separate unit (but not in the isolation unit), if possible, with implementation of foot bath/mat. In a small animal hospitalisation unit, if it is not possible to dedicate a unit to moderately infectious patients, leave at least one cage unoccupied on either side of the patient's cage.

17

o   Management of waste as being biologically contaminated
Appropriate decontamination protocols when the patient leaves
the unit. Sometimes the use of a different biocide might be necessary, depending on the pathogen. For example, a horse might be
hospitalised in the class 3 unit of the equine clinic for a contagious
dermatologic infection such as mange (see Table 17.1), in this
instance a specific insecticide must be used (e.g. phoxim[1]). Class 4
patients should be housed in the specific isolation unit and barrier-
nursing precautions must also be taken of course.

Table 17.1: Classification of infectious risks, as implemented in the Veterinary
Teaching Hospital, University of Liege (some practical examples)

SMALL ANIMAL HOSPITAL	EQUINE HOSPITAL
CLASS 1 – normal housing	
Non-infectious diseases or infectious diseases caused by agents with no likelihood of transmission to other animals and no potential for human infection	
Pre- and post-operative patients	No fever, no respiratory problem, no history of fever or respiratory problems during the last 6 months Trauma, wounds Pre- and post-operative patients, excluding colic patients (without contagious complications) Ophthalmologic patients Non-contagious neonates And other similar conditions
CLASS 2 – normal housing	
Infectious diseases caused by agents with a low level of transmission and with the likely inclusion of non-resistant bacterial infections	
Feline leukaemia virus Feline immunodeficiency virus (FIV) Feline infectious peritonitis (FIP) Any wound infected with non-resistant bacteria Chronic coryza Aspergillosis Leukopenia Severe immunosuppression Sepsis	Wounds infected with non-resistant bacterial infections Bacterial pneumonia, pleuro-pneumonia with no suspicion of contagious bacteria Bacterial corneal ulcers with non-resistant bacterial infections And other similar animal conditions

[1] https://www.vetcompendium.be/fr/node/3732

CLASS 3 – barrier nursing	
Subclass A: (multi)resistant bacteria	
Subclass B: infectious diseases caused by agents with a moderate level of transmission and/or potential human pathogens	
Leptospirosis Patients carrying multi-resistant bacteria	Fever and/or leukopenia of unknown origin Viral respiratory disease: cough, nasal discharge (< 2 weeks), possibly with fever *Rhodococcus equi* (foals < 10 months with respiratory problems and fever) Diarrhoea without fever and/or leukopenia Non-surgical digestive problem with haemorrhagic reflux OR non-haemorrhagic reflux with fever and/or leukopenia MRSA or other multi-resistant bacterial infections Contagious skin infections (dermatophytosis, dermatophilosis, chorioptic mange, phtiriasis and other parasitic conditions)
CLASS 4 – isolation	
Infectious diseases caused by agents that are considered to have a high level of transmission and/or are extremely serious human pathogens; housing in the isolation unit	
Feline panleukopenia Canine parvovirus Rabies Canine distemper virus Acute coryza Acute diarrhoea in dogs and cats (*Salmonella* spp., *Campylobacter* spp., *Cryptosporidium* spp., *Giardia* spp.)	Strangles Salmonellosis Acute diarrhoea with leukopenia and/or fever Acute, rapidly deteriorating neurological disease or acute neurological disease accompanied by fever (e.g. suspicion of EHV1-myelocencephalopathy) Abortion (150-300 days of gestation) Perinatal death (>300 days of gestation) without dystocia, premature placental separation, congenital abnormality or twins explaining the perinatal death Zoonotic diseases: rabies, glanders, brucellosis, anthrax, tuberculosis, etc.

17

- **Personal protective equipment (PPE):** in order to avoid the risk of transferring pathogens through contact with contaminated clothing and specific attire is often required; it can vary depending on the zone or activity at risk. Wherever possible, equipment for handling contagious patients (barrier nursing) should be furnished on site. For example, horses housed in the isolation unit should only be handled after donning white coveralls, gloves and special rubber boots (as well as a respiratory mask and safety goggles if necessary). It is crucial to remember that wearing gloves does not exempt from hand washing. Some people might be concerned by the cost and waste generated by disposable PPE, and might opt for re-using potentially contaminated PPE. It is strongly advised not to do so. The risk represented by handling contaminated PPE is high and requires particular skills and strong discipline to avoid it.
- **Personal hygiene:** basic hygiene principles reduce risk. For example, everyone involved should have short nails and not wear jewellery; hair should be tied back. Waterproof shoes are highly recommended in order to limit potential damage due do foot baths/mats solutions.
- **Hygiene of patients:** keeping animals as clean as possible helps reduce infection pressure. It is also essential to keep the environment of the cage/stall tidy and clean.
- **Use of disposable material** (syringes, needles, PPE)
- **Behaviour:** specific behaviour should be adopted, while other types of behaviour should be avoided (e.g. using a mobile phone or smoking). Hand hygiene is a cornerstone of biosecurity as it reduces the risk of transmitting pathogens between patients and it protects oneself against zoonotic pathogens (World Health Organisation, 2009). Food and beverages should not be consumed or stored in the hospital, except in designated areas (cafeteria, offices).
- **Minimise unnecessary contact with patients:** anyone involved in the care of animals should minimise contact with patients in order to reduce the risk of nosocomial exposure to them. This is particularly important when dealing with class 3 and class 4 patients. Video surveillance could be seen as an option.

- **Management of visitors:** animal owners are discouraged from visiting their animal when hospitalised, especially if housed in the isolation unit. If necessary (e.g. in event that an animal has to be euthanized), visitors should only be allowed if they wear the appropriate attire and they should always be accompanied by a staff member.
- **Waste management:** waste can be broken down into specific categories. Contaminated waste is managed via specific routes: an accredited company is charged with collecting waste for further incineration. Specific containers are either yellow or red, depending on the company and the country.

  Sharp objects such as needles and scalpel blades are disposed of in small puncture-resistant containers provided by the official collector, for further incineration as well. Precautions should be taken to prevent injury by sharp objects, so needle recapping should be avoided.
- **Cleansing and disinfection protocols:** specific protocols are implemented in practices/clinics. These are sometimes adapted in the case of specific pathogens that are more resistant in the environment (e.g. canine parvovirus or *Leptospira* spp. [Gordon &Angrick, 1986; Levett, 2001]). The decontamination process consists in: (1) removing all waste as organic material (faeces, in particular), which inactivates most disinfectants; (2) washing with water and detergent, then rinsing to remove all residual detergent as some biocides may be inactivated by detergents; (3) leave the area to dry; (4) apply the appropriate biocide (e.g. http://www.cfsph.iastate.edu/Disinfection/Assets/AntimicrobialSpectrumDisinfectants.pdf) and respect the contact time; (5) remove all residual biocide and leave the surface to dry. Due to the toxic and irritant potential for people and animals, several biocides such as bleach (sodium hypohlorite), phenols, oxidizing agents and quaternary ammonium compounds should only be applied on equipment or facility surfaces. If contact with skin or other tissues is unavoidable, it is advised, depending on the spectrum of activity, to use biocides such as alcohols, povidone-iodine and chlorhexidine (Biosecurity SOP, 2010).

17

- **Communicating about risks:** efficient communication about the potential infective status of patients is crucial. This can be done through labelling the doors of premises in which they are hosted; patients' hospitalisation cards; any biological samples as well as any requests for complementary examinations. In addition, displaying pictograms also encourages individuals to follow biosecurity guidelines.

- **Exclusion criteria for patient admission:** wherever possible, animals with a suspected officially reportable disease should be refused. Admission can also be refused if the potential contagion to other patients and/or humans is too important.

3 How to implement biosecurity in a veterinary practice/clinic – case-study #1: dog with methicillin-resistant *Staphylococcus aureus*

A dog came for a routine surgery but developed a surgical site infection during post-operative hospitalisation. A sample taken from the wound revealed the presence of methicillin-resistant *Staphylococcus aureus* (MRSA). The pathogen is considered to be an emerging zoonotic pathogen (Weese, 2005). Furthermore, nasal and intestinal carriage of MRSA by clinically healthy animals as well as nasal colonisation of veterinarians are frequent, (Loeffler et al., 2005; Hanselman et al., 2006). This means that it is a reverse zoonosis that can be transmitted from human to animals and from animals to humans (Van Duijkeren et al., 2004; Weese et al., 2005; 2006; 2007). Upon receiving lab results, the patient fell into the class 3 category; barrier nursing precautions were implemented to minimise the risk of transmission to other patients and humans.

3.1 Patient care

The first step consisted in moving the patient to another unit on a specific medical cart to avoid contaminating the floor. Low-traffic route was preferred for transit. The cart was completely cleaned then disinfected after use.

The dog was given a yellow collar, to remind others of the class 3 status (Fig. 17.5). A dedicated leash was allocated to the patient. Movements of the patients were restricted to a minimum, and only allowed on a gurney. If the patient had to undergo a special clinical examination which could only be performed in the main hospital, e.g. in the Medical Imaging Unit, procedures were scheduled for the end of the day, after all the other patients. Barrier nursing precautions were also taken in the Medical Imaging Unit. A specific antimicrobial susceptibility test was carried out along with a sample analysis in order to select the appropriate antibiotic. The patient was cared for after all the other patients hospitalised in the class 1-class 2 hospitalisation area, in order to prevent cross-contamination. Unconsumed feed was discarded as contaminated waste. Any biological samples were handled with the same barrier nursing precautions as the patient itself, and stored in a sealed plastic bag. The risk of infection was clearly identified on the plastic bag and on the analysis request.

Prior to discharge, the dog's owners were informed about the potential zoonotic risk of MRSA and recommendations were provided to minimise the risk at home. Any surplus medication was sent home with the patient, and not returned to the pharmacy.

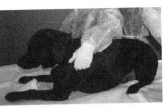

▲
Fig. 17.5: The dog was given a yellow collar to identify its class 3 status. Additional PPE (disposable yellow apron and examination gloves) were used).

Fig. 17.6: The dog was moved to another unit and the adjacent cage was kept unoccupied
▼

3.2 Personal protection when handling the patient

All personal hygiene recommendations, as already mentioned, were strictly followed. Special attire was worn by anyone coming into contact with the patient. The personal protective equipment (PPE) consisted of a disposable yellow apron and single-use gloves (Fig. 17.6). A surgical mask and protective eyewear, two classical items of PPE, were worn only when procedures that generated droplets and splashes of blood or any other fluids were performed. Appropriate clothing was worn for cage/unit decontamination as well.

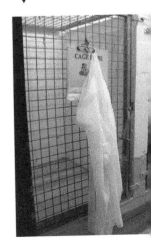

Contact with the patient was kept to a minimum, in order to limit the risk of nosocomial exposure to the patient. The owners' visits were restricted to the minimum, but barrier nursing rules were observed at each visit.

Special emphasis was laid on hand hygiene, as MRSA is a risk for other patients and humans; people can act also as vectors and contaminate other patients. Thorough hand washing and disinfection (hydro-alcoholic solution) was mandatory after removing gloves, following any contact with the patient, its direct environment, its dedicated material, any equipment for complementary examinations and any contaminated waste.

3.3 Management of premises

The cage was located at the end of an aisle, away from all traffic routes (Fig. 17.6). Cages on both sides of the cage housing the patient were left empty. The risk and diagnosis were clearly identified on the cage. Yellow tape was stuck on the ground to delimit a buffer area. A foot mat was placed at the entrance of the unit and refilled as soon as dry. Any contaminated surface outside the cage (secretions/excretions such as faeces, urine, blood, etc.) was immediately decontaminated. When the patient left the area, the bed pad was disposed of in a yellow container (contaminated waste). All organic materials were removed before proceeding to decontamination, as they could inactivate many disinfectants. A thorough cleaning of the cage and surrounding areas was performed before disinfection. After decontamination, the unit was labelled as 'disinfected' so that people knew that the process had been completed.

3.4 Equipment and materials

A ready-to-use and specific class 3 box was brought to the unit: it contained all classical and reusable equipment such as a thermometer and a stethoscope required for caring of a class 3 patient. As such equipment is dedicated to the patient; it was left next to the cage during its hospitalisation, and went through a decontamination process before further use. If surplus disposable material was brought in the unit (e.g. bandages), it was put into the class 3 box and reused for this animal only. When the animal left the unit, all single-use materials remaining in the premises were processed as contaminated waste (yellow bin).

Yellow bowls for food and water were specifically labelled with the patient's name to be sure that they were not used for another patient.

After the patient's discharge, all instruments, equipment and other objects (bowls, leash, etc.) were collected in the cage, then decontaminated by using 0.5% chlorhexidine (if they had come into contact with animal), then sterilised as soon as possible.

3.5 Waste management

All contaminated waste was disposed of in yellow containers. These containers were then brought to the temporary storage facility through low traffic areas that could be easily cleaned and disinfected.

4 How to implement biosecurity in a veterinary practice/clinic – case-study #2: horse with salmonellosis

Salmonellosis is a very contagious bacterial disease affecting several animal species and humans. The disease is reportable at national level if diagnosed by a laboratory in an animal sample (Anonymous, 2014). Our case-study focused on a horse that had come to the equine hospital for routine surgery. During the post-operative period, while hospitalised in the class 1-class 2 area of the equine hospital, it developed clinical signs suspicious of salmonellosis, mainly characterised by diarrhoea, along with fever and leukopenia. The combination of these clinical signs led the horse to be categorised as a class 4 patient, requiring hospitalisation in the isolation unit. *Salmonella* spp. are carried asymptomatically in intes-

17

tines of many animals.[2] Any stress or immunosuppressive state (e.g. surgery) can lead to reactivation of the bacteria and the development of clinical signs (Weese, 2002).

4.1 Patient care

As soon as the suspected clinical signs appeared, the horse was moved to the isolation unit. Two people were required to carry out the transfer, both of them wearing appropriate PPE: one person led the horse while the other followed it, holding a bag under the tail to collect any faeces discharged during the transfer. The horse was led to the isolation unit through a low-traffic route, and avoiding any contact with other patients or humans.

In the main hospital (class 1-class 2), the premises in which it was housed was identified as unavailable before complete cleaning and disinfection had been carried out. Once in the isolation unit, the horse did not leave it under any circumstances during the whole stay. Any complementary examination would have been performed in the unit itself (e.g. x-ray or ultrasound).

4.2 Personal protection

Anyone coming into contact with the patient had to wear appropriate PPE. Before entering the isolation unit, people had to go through an air lock (or cloakroom) where all necessary protective equipment was available: basic PPE equipment to be worn in the isolation unit are water-resistant coveralls, rubber boots (dedicated to the isolation unit) and disposable gloves. Face masks and protective eyewear (goggles) are also available for procedures where there is a risk of generating droplets and splashes of body fluids. If infrastructures are unable to provide a specific dedicated room as an air lock, a special area dedicated to dressing must be made available to ensure the 'onward march' (form the clean to the dirty area).

---

[2] http://www.cfsph.iastate.edu/Factsheets/pdfs/nontyphoidal_salmonellosis.pdf

Air locks should generally be designed to ensure the 'onward march principle', with clean and dirty areas separated by a bench (Fig. 17.8 and 17.9): (1) people remove clothes/coveralls worn outside the isolation unit and leave them in a locker, along with their personal belongings, (2) they put on waterproof disposable coveralls, (3) they step over the bench to enter the dirty area and put on a pair of rubber boots (stored in the air lock and dedicated to the isolation unit), (3) they wash and disinfect their hands at the sink then put on disposable gloves, (4) they walk through the foot bath then leave the air lock and enter the animal air lock, then access the isolation ward.

After handling the animal, and before leaving the isolation unit, they will follow the same path, but in the reverse direction. Boots should be washed (boot-washing station) before leaving the animal air lock and before walking through the footbath.

It was crucial to limit the number of people looking after the patient in the isolation unit, to minimise the zoonotic risk and the potential dissemination outside the isolation unit. People at risk, such as young, old, pregnant and immunosuppressed people (YOPI's), were forbidden to enter the unit. The patient's owners were not allowed in either; usually, they are authorised to enter the isolation unit only should their animal need to be euthanized, in which instances they are required to observe all the procedures to be adopted in terms of PPE, hygiene, etc. Whenever and wherever possible, only a few people (always the same) should be allowed in the risk area; after caring for the isolated patients, they should not go back to the main hospital. If such an approach is not possible (i.e. if one or two people cannot be dedicated to the isolation unit), the isolated patient should be taken care of after all the other animals, based on the 'onward march' principle.

Hand hygiene is especially important when dealing with *Salmonella* spp., due to the zoonotic risk and the main route of transmis-

Fig. 17.8: In the large animal isolation unit, the special air lock for people is split up into two separate parts, the clean area (grey floor) and dirty area (red floor), both being separated by a bench.

▼

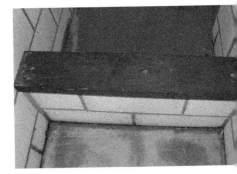

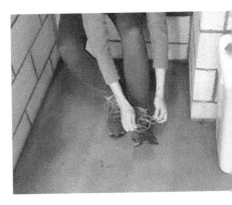

▲

Fig. 17.9: People just sit down on the bench to remove their shoes then turn around to put on the boots

17

sion, i.e. faecal-oral.[3] As wearing gloves is not sufficient, a special emphasis was made on hand washing and disinfection (with a hydro-alcoholic solution).

4.3 Premises – isolation unit

The isolation unit was prepared before the patient arrived (bedding in the stall, all equipment ready, etc.). Doors remained closed at all times. Once the patient had left the unit, it was completely emptied, cleaned and disinfected, using the appropriate biocide. *Salmonella* spp. is susceptible to a wide variety of biocides, e.g. 2% bleach, 70% ethanol, 2% glutaraldehyde, iodine-based disinfectants, phenolics and peroxygen disinfectants (Wheeler and Dallap, 2008). Formaldehyde is efficient as well, but due to its carcinogenic potential, its use is now discouraged (U.S. Department of Health and Human Services, 2016). A stall that housed a patient with a *Salmonella* positive-culture should be sampled after cleaning and decontamination to assess the effectiveness of the process, and before being made available to another patient.

4.4 Equipment and material

Any equipment used in the isolation unit was disinfected before leaving the area. This is especially important for x-ray and ultrasound equipment that needs to be thoroughly cleaned then disinfected before leaving the unit. Specific grooming material was left in the unit and dedicated to the patient during its stay. The unit has its own cleaning equipment (wheelbarrow, brooms, etc.), that is not used in the main hospital.

---

[3] http://www.cfsph.iastate.edu/Factsheets/pdfs/nontyphoidal_salmonellosis.pdf

4.5 Waste management

A special emphasis was put on the management of manure as it is highly contagious for other horses and humans. Furthermore, *Salmonella* spp. is quite resistant in the environment: it was determined that *Salmonella* Typhimurium could survive in cattle slurry during 19 to 60 days, and in cattle manure for 48 days (vs. 231 days in the soil and maximum 152 days in water).[4] Manure was put directly into resistant plastic bags dedicated to contaminated waste, and these were disposed of in specific containers. The containers are collected by a specific and accredited company for further incineration. All PPE and single-use equipment was disposed of in a similar way. It is important to minimise the amount of equipment and material introduced into the unit for economic reasons. Any remaining feed and medicine were eliminated via the same procedure.

5 Biosecurity audits – internal audit

The standard operating procedures (SOP) in each clinic/practice should be promoted and needs regular audits to monitor its practical application and to identify any shortcomings that could compromise the level of biosecurity. When a shortcoming is identified, corrective action should be taken.
Moreover, an independent annual audit of each clinic/practice is recommended in order to validate/approve the process. In addition, all results of internal and external audits should be centralised in a biosecurity unit. The role of this type of unit is to anticipate problems and resolve them before they appear.

6 Biosecurity and veterinary education

Prevention is better than cure and hints at changes taking place in veterinary education, especially with the introduction of biosecurity concepts and methods as new skills (Saegerman et al., 2009).

---

4 http://www.phac-aspc.gc.ca/lab-bio/res/psds-ftss/salmonella-ent-eng.php

17

In order for veterinary students to acquire the above information the introduction of a course in biosecurity and veterinary good practices in the curriculum is recommended. As an example, one such course was introduced in the FVM-ULg in 2010. The course includes a theoretical introduction (2 hours) and 30 hours of e-learning. This eLearning is hosted on the University website, largely illustrated by video capsules. Furthermore, an associated open website illustrating the biosecurity SOP was developed for students and all potential visitors to the various clinics and 'high-risk' areas (from a biosecurity point of view) in the Faculty (http://www.fmv-biosecurite.ulg.ac.be/?langue=en).

Each chapter includes written notes (FVM Biosecurity manual and Good Veterinary or Farming Practices codes) and multimedia data (a video or Power Point presentation illustrating the main points to be memorised). After studying each chapter, the student has to pass an on-line questionnaire in order to test his or her knowledge (max. 5 questions) before moving on to the next chapter. Chapters are organised as follows: necropsy room, dissection room, equids, ruminants, swine, small animals, birds, rabbits and rodents, food industry [slaughterhouse, cutting plants and industries], microbiology labs and imaging unit.

It is also essential to maintain an awareness about veterinary biosecurity through continuing education. A good example is the Biosecurity Day that the FVM-ULg has held every year since 2013. Continuing education is essential, as infection control procedures need regular revision. Furthermore, the continuous (re)emergence of potentially zoonotic infectious diseases also highlights the importance of staying up-to-date with developments through conference/meeting attendance, and even briefings organised within the veterinary structure itself. The One Health approach is totally justified in such context. In order to ensure continuing education in a veterinary private structure or teaching hospital, a veterinarian responsible for infection control should be designated (Australian Veterinary Association, 2011).

7 Conclusion

Biosecurity is an important key component of disease prevention. It should be part of the educational programme of each veterinary student as it applies everywhere, at every stage of the food chain (from primary production, processing, distribution, consumption and management of waste and by-products). In the context of a veterinary teaching hospital, it relates to clinical activities, visits to farms, dissection rooms and visits to abattoirs and food industry companies. The main concepts are completely applicable in any private practice or clinic.

17

References

Anonymous (2014). Royal Decree Feb 3 2014 [Arrêté royal désignant les maladies des animaux soumises à l'application du chapitre III de la loi du 24 mars 1987 relative à la santé des animaux et portant règlement de la déclaration obligatoire] [in French]

Australian Veterinary Association (2011). Guidelines for Veterinary Personal Biosecurity. 59 pp. Available from: https://www.ava.com.au/sites/default/files/AVA_website/pdfs/Biosecurity_Guidelines_ad.pdf [Accessed on Jul 18, 2017].

Biosecurity SOP (2010). Biosecurity SOP applied to the Faculty of Veterinary Medicine of the University of Liege, pp. 146. Available from: http://www2.fmv.ulg.ac.be/actualites/Biosecurity_Manual_Final_6Jan10.pdf [Accessed on Apr 19, 2016].

Courtenay, O. and Wellington, E.M.H. (2008). *Mycobacterium bovis* in the environment: towards our understanding of its biology. *Cattle Practice* 16, 122-126.

Federation of Veterinarians of Europe (FVE) (2002). Code of good veterinary practices. Federation of Veterinarians of Europe, Brussels, pp. 23.

Fritsche, A., Engel, R., Buhl, D., Zellweger, J.P. (2004). *Mycobacterium bovis* tuberculosis: from animal to man and back. International Journal of Tuberculosis and Lung Disease. 8, 903-904.

Gordon, J.C. and Angrick, E.J. (1986). Canine parvovirus: environmental effects on infectivity. *American Journal of Veterinary Research* 47, 1464-7.

Hanselman, B.A., Kruth, S.A., Rousseau, J., Low, D.E., Willey, B.M., McGeer, A., Weese, J.S. (2006). Methicillin-resistant *Staphylococcus aureus* colonization in veterinary personnel. *Emerging and Infectious Diseases* 12, 1933-1938.

Levett, P.N. (2001). Leptospirosis. *Clinical Microbiology Reviews* 14, 296-326.

Loeffler, A., Boag, A.K., Sung, J., Lindsay, J.A., Guardabassi, L., Dalsgaard, A., Smith, H., Stevens, K.B., Lloyd, D.H. (2005). Prevalence of methicillin-resistant *Staphylococcus aureus* among staff and pets in a small animal referral hospital in the UK. *Journal of Antimicrobial Chemotherapy* 56, 692-697.

Saegerman, C., Lancelot, R., Humblet, M.F., Thiry, E., Seegers, H. (2009). Renewed veterinary education is needed to improve the surveillance and control of OIE-listed diseases, diseases of wildlife and rare events. *In*: Proceedings of the First OIE Global Conference on Evolving Veterinary Education for a Safer World, Oct 12-14, 2009, Paris, France, 63-77.C.

Saegerman, C., Dal Pozzo, F., Humblet, M.-F. (2012). Reducing hazards for humans from animals: emerging and re-emerging zoonoses. *Italian Journal of Public Health* 9, 13-24.

Sheridan, L. (2009). Considerations for Isolation and Barrier Nursing. *Veterinary Nursing Journal* 24, 12-14.

U.S. Department of Health and Human Services (2016). Formaldehyde. In: 14th report on carcinogens [https://ntp.niehs.nih.gov/ntp/roc/content/profiles/formaldehyde.pdf]

van Duijkeren, E., Wolfhagen, M.J., Box, A.T., Heck, M.E., Wannet, W.J., Fluit, A.C. (2004). Human-to-dog transmission of methicillin-resistant *Staphylococcus aureus*. *Emerging and Infectious Diseases* 10, 2235-2237.

Weese, J.S. (2002). A review of equine zoonotic diseases: risks in veterinary medicine. In: Proceedings of the Annual convention of the American Association of Equine Practitioners (AAEP), Dec. 4-8, 2002, Orlando, USA. pp. 362-369.

Weese, J.S. (2005). Methicillin-resistant *Staphylococcus aureus*: an emerging pathogen in small animals. *Journal of the American Animal Hospital Association* 41, 150-7.

Weese, J.S., Rousseau, J., Traub-Dargatz, J.L., Willey, B.M., McGeer, A.J., Low, D.E. (2005). Community-associated methicillin-resistant *Staphylococcus aureus* in horses and humans who work with horses. Journal of the American Veterinary Medical Association 226, 580-583.

Weese, J.S., Dick, H., Willey, B.M., McGeer, A., Kreiswirth, B.N., Innis, B., Low, D.E., (2006). Suspected transmission of methicillin-resistant *Staphylococcus aureus* between domestic pets and humans in veterinary clinics and in the household. *Veterinary Microbiology* 115, 148-155.

Weese, J.S., Faires, M., Rousseau, J., Bersenas, A.M., Mathews, K.A. (2007). Cluster of methicillin-resistant *Staphylococcus aureus* colonization in a small animal intensive care unit. Journal of the American Veterinary Medical Association 231, 1361-1364

Wheeler Aceto, H. and Dallap Schaer, B. (2008). Chapter 3.3 Biosecurity for equine hospitals: protecting the patient and the hospital. In: The Equine Hospital Manual, 1st edition. Corley K. and Stephen J., Eds. Blackwell Publishing, Oxford, UK, 2008, p.180-199.

World Health Organisation (WHO) (2009). Hand Hygiene: why, how and when? Available at: http://www.who.int/gpsc/5may/Hand_Hygiene_Why_How_and_When_Brochure.pdf?ua=1 [Accessed on Feb 14, 2017].

World Organisation for Animal Health (OIE) – Food and Agriculture Organisation of the United Nations (FAO) (2010) Guide to good farming practices for animal production food safety, FAO, Roma, Italy, pp. 55

World Organisation for Animal Health (OIE) – World Health Organisation (WHO) – Food and Agriculture Organisation of the United Nations (FAO) (2008) Anthrax in humans and animals, 4th edition. WHO Press, Geneva, Switzerland, pp 219.

17

CHAPTER 18

BIOSECURITY IN LABORATORY ANIMAL RESEARCH FACILITIES

Patty H. Chen[1]

Robin Trundy[2]

[1] Department of Pathology, Microbiology, and Immunology, Division of Comparative Medicine, Vanderbilt University Medical Center

[2] Vanderbilt Environmental Health & Safety

The development of therapeutic agents and advances in biomedical research would not be possible without the use of animal models. Responsible conduct of animal research starts with an effective animal care and use programme as described in the Guide for the Care and Use of Laboratory Animals (the Guide) (National Research Council (US), 2011). Although this is an American guidance document, it is a cornerstone resource used by the Association for Assessment and Accreditation of Laboratory Animal Care International (AAALAC International), which accredits lab animal programmes that maintain a high level of quality animal care. Animal biosecurity programme criteria are described in the Guide as a preventive medicine function. The Guide also outlines expectations for an occupational health and safety programme which includes the safe and contained research use of biological agents as well as other research-related hazards.

While a broad spectrum of species may be used to support biomedical research, this chapter focuses primarily on 'traditional' lab animal models (i.e., rodents) commonly used in academic or pharmaceutical research settings. The first part focuses on animal biosecurity from the veterinary care perspective. Best practices for assuring that incoming animals are pathogen-free as well as monitoring and hygiene practices used to prevent spread of infections within animal colonies will be discussed. The second part discusses animal biosecurity as it relates to the introduction of biological agents in animal models, and the principles behind determining and applying biosafety or biocontainment measures to ensure that pathogens are not spread beyond their intended study population.

1 Biosecurity & the lab animal holding facility

Disease transmission in laboratory animal facilities can arise from multiple sources. Contamination could occur from direct animal contact, cell lines, tissue transplants, or fomites. Preventing disease transmission requires addressing all potential sources of infection. Preventive measures include the use of clean, sanitised supplies, purchasing animals free from specific pathogens, introducing pathogen-free products into live animals, and practising strict hygiene processes.

Establishing and maintaining the appropriate health status of an animal colony involves a comprehensive preventive approach. Sources of pathogen introduction need to be identified and preventive practices need to be developed and implemented to address each source. The ideal practice to ensure the exclusion of specific pathogens within the animal colony is to only permit animals of acceptable disease status from reputable sources into the colony. In addition to sourcing quality animals, a culture of heightened biosecurity practices is necessary. These factors will support a comprehensive health monitoring programme that provides an effective mechanism to verify the disease status of the colony.

The style of rodent housing will also affect disease transmission and containment. Each system has advantages and limitations that need to be considered as outlined below.

Fig. 18.1: Caging Systems: Biosecurity Advantages & Limitations

CAGING SYSTEM	ADVANTAGES	LIMITATIONS
Conventional (open top, wire bar lid)	• Low cost of equipment • Effective pathogen transmission between cages	• High biosecurity risk • Unable to contain pathogens within a cage
Microisolator –style (filter lid)	• Cost effective design • Effective in containing pathogens within a cage	• Increased labor cost from increased cage change • Accumulation of waste gases within the cage
Individually ventilated caging (forced Ventilation)	• Good allergen control • Effective in containing pathogens within a cage • Decrease labor cost from decreased cage change frequency	• High equipment cost • Poor pathogen detection at low prevalence levels

Reference: (Smith & Szczepan, 2013)
Source: Smith J, B. Szczepan. Rodent Housing Methodologies. 2013.ALN Magazine. Advantage Media. https://www.alnmag.com/article/2013/07/rodent-housing-methodologies)

2 Animal acquisition considerations

Given the need of specific animal models and the variety of research focuses, institutional animal colonies generally originate from commercial vendors, internal breeding and animals bred in other research facilities. A reputable commercial vendor adheres to strict practices in order to minimise the introduction of pathogens; provides timely notification to clients when excluded pathogens are identified; and adheres to transportation practices that further protect the disease status of the animals during delivery. The descriptions and results of their health monitoring programme should be readily available for review. Commercial vendor health monitoring programmes are not standardised resulting in variability between companies with regards their excluded agent list and testing frequency. Institutions should carefully review commercial vendor health monitoring programmes therefore as well as disease status reports and delivery practices to establish an approved vendor list of commercial suppliers that meet the institution's expectations.

When commercial vendors do not have specific animal models readily available, research requirements will drive the need to acquire animals from non-approved research or commercial sources. To protect the integrity of the health of the colony, institutions should only consider accepting animals that either meet or exceed their colony's disease status. Evaluating the originating animal colony disease status involves reviewing the description of their health monitoring programme and the health monitoring reports from the previous year or a longer historical perspective. Biosecurity of these animals also needs to be considered for the transportation procedure in order to minimise disease. A quarantine programme to verify that the disease status meets the receiving institution's requirement is highly recommended for these animals prior to introducing them into the colony.

If the health report from the originating institution identifies the presence of an excluded agent, the receiving institution will need to assess the potential risk of receiving infected animals. The risk assessment should be based on the originating institution's husbandry practices, biosecurity practices, eradication response, and colony health status testing in response to the detected presence of the excluded agent. If the receiving institution agrees to accept these animals, the quarantine programme will provide an opportunity to directly assess the health status of the animals.

3 Maintaining biosecurity in the facility

Maintaining the appropriate health status of an animal colony involves taking a comprehensive approach to pathogen prevention within the institution, as well as by the manufacturers and distributors of animal supplies. The manufacturers and distributors need to establish processes that eliminate pathogens and protect their products from contamination. Many control points within the institution can be implemented to protect the colony health status including:

- a pest management programme to control the introduction of feral animal pathogens;
- an animal supply in-processing sanitation programme to control the introduction of pathogenic agents on packaging surfaces;
- a thorough animal housing sanitising programme to eliminate contaminants in the animal environment;
- microisolation practices in animal handling to prevent cross-contamination (Fig. 18.2);
- implementing a room entry order from the cleanest to the least clean animal area;
- discouraging the practice of returning animals back into the colony after leaving the animal facility to reduce the introduction of contaminants;
- sanitising research equipment and support areas, and using biological products in animal that are certified or tested free of specific pathogens to reduce the risk of pathogen introduction into the animal colony.

Fig. 18.2: Best Practice: Microisolation Technique

GOAL: protect animals from contamination during handling procedures

Process: prevent cross contamination of surfaces in direct contact with the animal

Technique:
When available, only open cages and work with animals in cage change stations or biosafety cabinets
Liberally apply animal-safe sanitizer on surrounding surfaces that come in contact with cage
Only allow the outside surfaces of the cage to contact table surfaces
Liberally apply animal-safe sanitizer to gloved hands when handling animals
Sanitize equipment that has direct contact with animals
Change gloves when soiled, damaged and/or between study groups

4 Health monitoring programme considerations

In conjunction with the preventive practices currently in place, a health monitoring programme is also needed to actually detect the presence of any pathogenic agents within the animal colony. There are multiple strategies that involve the use of live animals, testing fomites, or a combination of both. The dirty bedding sentinel programme is commonly implemented, and the advancements in molecular biology with polymerase chain reaction technology have enabled the exploration of fomite testing to represent the colony disease status, which could potentially replace the use of sentinel animals. Institutions could strategically use both systems to optimise disease detection.

Dirty bedding sentinel programmes are practical. This type of programme depends on faecal oral pathogen transmission and is reliable for the detection of many viral, bacterial, and parasitic agents of concern. However, it is not be reliable for detecting certain pathogens such as Sendai virus (Smith & Szczepan, 2013) or murine fur mites (de Bruin et al., 2016). Sentinel animals allow direct testing for parasites and bacterial presence, and serology analysis as an indirect method for evidence of viral pathogen exposure. PCR is highly sensitive because it identifies DNA sequences of pathogenic vectors and is fully dependent on the specificity of primers to control cross-reactions to similar agents (Leblanc et al.,

2014). PCR can also be used exclusively for fomite testing but this strategy is dependent on the ventilated rack technology where the rack exhaust design allows full representation of the colony (Exhaust Air Dust (EADTM), 2016; Höfler et al., 2014; Jensen et al., 2013; Leblanc et al., 2014). For example, exhaust plenum particulate samples from rack designs where exhaust air is not pre-filtered prior to entering the plenum are ideal for this technology. The current cost of PCR analysis and its specificity for detecting DNA limits its choice as a surveillance strategy.

The design of health monitoring programmes is driven by multiple considerations that include pathogens of concern, testing modality, frequency of testing, cost, and practicality. In the end, decisions are primarily based on balancing cost and practicality. The goal of the health monitoring programme is to provide a surveillance method for disease detection. For general disease surveillance, quarterly testing of immunocompetent sentinel animals is commonly practised. Direct parasitology and bacterial analysis with serology testing to detect exposure to viral vectors is cost-effective and addresses the most common pathogens of concern. Once a pathogen is identified, a more targeted approach can be developed to address the specific characteristics of the pathogen. For example, a targeted approach could involve using immunocompromised animals to identify viral presence via PCR that offers a direct testing method for identifying a specific pathogen such as Murine Parvovirus where intermittent shedding in immunocompotent mice confounds accurate detection (de Bruin et al., 2016).

Fig. 18.3: Health Monitoring Program

COMPONENT	STRENGTH	LIMITATION
Serology	Cost	Indirect testing; detects exposure to pathogen; does not detect presence
PCR	Highly sensitive; direct testing	Expensive; relies on primer specificity; detects DNA – not viability
Immunocompetent Sentinel Animal	Healthy status; reasonable cost to purchase; direct parasitology	Viral detection – serology detects exposure to pathogen
Immunocompomised Sentinel Animal	Does not clear infections; detect presence of pathogen	Become unhealthy over time; expensive to purchase
Plenum Testing	PCR detects presence of pathogen; replace the use of live animals	PCR testing cost; requires cage level prefilter exhaust rack design

A quarantine programme designed to assess the diseases status of animals from non-approved sources will protect the integrity of the colony's health. A quarantine programme can be managed in-house or through a commercial resource. An all-in, all-out process that houses quarantine animals geographically separate from the general population minimises the potential for cross-contamination between shipments and the general colony animals. Alternative systems can be managed successfully by using appropriate practices and equipment. Breeding can be included or excluded. The quarantine-excluded pathogen list determines the testing strategy options primarily between serology or molecular biology in addition to direct testing. The choice of testing strategy determines if a sentinel programme is needed in quarantine. Sentinel animals allow direct testing without risk to the quarantine colony animals, but time is needed in order to detect infective pathogens among sentinel animals. PCR permits low-risk direct testing of quarantine animals thus potentially reducing the total quarantine time, but at a much higher financial cost. A combination of serology and PCR can also be developed in order to collect samples directly from quarantine and/or sentinel animals.

Best practices and strict adherence to biosecurity measures will minimise inadvertent pathogen introduction into a colony. The goal of the health monitoring programme is to identify the presence of excluded pathogens in order to permit timely response, containment, and eradication from the colony.

5 Biosecurity & animal research activities

In addition to the aforementioned biosecurity measures to obtain and maintain animals free of pathogens, biomedical lab animal research facilities must also plan for the biosecurity challenges introduced as a consequence of research being conducted. Many research models employ immunocompromised animals, genetically-modified animals, animals administered with human-derived cells or tissues, or with wild-type or genetically modified infectious agents. These models increase the potential for infectious agents to be introduced in the facility and possibly to the external environment in a manner that transcends natural occurrence. These agents may be infectious to naïve animals, humans, or both. Therefore, additional measures to prevent cross-contamination, personnel exposure, and environmental release are required when working with these models. Employing such measures is commonly referred to as biosafety or biocontainment depending on the regulatory standards applicable to specific countries. The remainder of this chapter is devoted to understanding and applying biosafety/biocontainment measures to use in research of biological agents in animal models.

6 Biological material risk considerations

In order to determine effective practices for working with animal models without spreading contamination beyond the study animals, one must first classify the risk of infectious disease caused by the microbiological agent used (or possibly present) in the study. The World Health Organization breaks down agents into 4 groups based on the probability of the agent causing disease in humans or animals, the transmissibility and severity of the infection, and the availability of treatment measures (World Health Organization (Geneva), 2004). The risk groups are further described in the table below, and this classification system is recognised worldwide. Some countries have generated lists of specific agents and their risk group assignment (Department of Health and Human Services, 2016; European Commission, 2000) as part of their biosafety/biocontainment standards, and these lists are a valuable frontline reference for those involved in determining biosafety/biocontainment measures.

Fig. 18.4: WHO Risk Group Classification of Infectious Agents

RISK GROUP	PUBLIC HEALTH RISK	PATHOGEN & DISEASE FEATURES
1	no or low individual and community risk	A microorganism that is unlikely to cause human or animal disease.
2	moderate individual risk, low community risk	A pathogen that can cause human or animal disease but is unlikely to be a serious hazard to laboratory workers, the community, livestock or the environment. Laboratory exposures may cause serious infection, but effective treatment and preventive measures are available and the risk of spread of infection is limited.
3	high individual risk, low community risk	A pathogen that usually causes serious human or animal disease but does not ordinarily spread from one infected individual to another. Effective treatment and preventive measures are available.
4	high individual and community risk	A pathogen that usually causes serious human or animal disease and that can be readily transmitted from one individual to another, directly or indirectly. Effective treatment and preventive measures are not usually available.

As a general rule, the higher the risk group designation, the greater the hazard controls and biosafety/biocontainment measures needed for working with the agent in a manner that is safe for personnel, other animals in the facility and the outside environment. While it may seem that risk group designation is applied mostly in the administration of infectious agents in animal studies, it is also applied to viable biological materials that may be administered in the study. For instance, human cells are frequently administered in cancer-related studies. Human cells are generally assumed to be potentially infectious for blood-borne pathogens. Most blood-borne pathogens are considered to be Risk Group 2 agents. Therefore, as a minimum standard, all human-derived cells in animal studies (both when administered and harvested) should be regarded as Risk Group 2 materials. In the case of viral vectors, consideration should be given to the risk group designation of the virus of origin. The potential for a recombination event resulting in a functional replicating virus may warrant a risk group assignment equal to the parent strain. Finally, one must not overlook the zoonotic infectious disease risk associated with animal species sometimes used in biomedical research. Common examples of agents that may be shed include: Herpes B virus from macaques, *Toxoplasma gondii* from cats, and *Coxiella burnetii* from sheep. An extensive table of global zoonoses can be found in the Merck Veterinary Manual (Spickler, 2016). When zoonotic agents are likely to be present in research animal groups, the risk group associated with the pathogen should be considered when determining biosafety or biocontainment measures for working with potentially or endemically infected species.

7 Procedure-related hazards & hazard control

In addition to the risk group designation for different agents, other factors that may impact the risk of a study include: the dose of the agent to be administered, the agent's host range, genetic modification features of the agent being studied (or the animals receiving the agent) that will impact disease severity, and the potential for shedding the agent. If previous research outcomes for use of an agent in the proposed animal model are not well-established or are unknown, biocontainment practices should err on the side of caution and assume that agents may be shed or present in the animal holding environment.

Hazard identification, assessment and adoption of hazard controls during the planning phase of the study can reduce the likelihood of an accidental break in biocontainment that could result in cross-contamination or lab-acquired infection. In addition to the aforementioned biohazard aspects, the physical hazards of animal research must be considered.

The use of live animals in research presents risk of exposure for personnel that are different from (and in some cases greater than) those encountered during in vitro life science research activities. Regardless of the size of animal, they are living beings that will behave in accordance with their instincts. Biting, scratching and urinating are examples of ways in which traditional terrestrial lab animals will respond to handling stress. Other less traditional species may hiss, spit, throw items, or flap their wings or tails. All of these actions can generate aerosols and disperse potentially infectious body fluids or residues when present. It is essential for the welfare of the animals and also for the safety of personnel to ensure that individuals handling research animals are well-trained, and deemed proficient by experienced staff in husbandry, handling and restraint techniques before they are permitted to work independently with the animals.

Procedures required in order to support biological agent-related research often include the use of sharps such as needles, scalpels, and punches. Needles are commonly used to administer test agents, therapeutics or analgesics. Sharp devices may be used in surgery and are also necessary for blood and tissue collection. By the nature of their intended use, sharps present a significant risk of exposure for personnel using them in animal studies. Compromising the skin barrier creates an opportunity for infectious material to be introduced. Therefore, sharp devices must be properly selected and appropriately used in order to reduce this risk.

A common occupational safety tool for minimising risks when planning activities is the hierarchy of hazard controls (Centers for Disease control and Prevention, 2015). This system involves considering each of the hazards identified and determining first if there is a means of removing the hazard completely or replacing it with a lesser hazard. The remaining hazards then need to be considered in the context of equipment and procedures designed to protect workers. Because these all require staff to be trained and because they need to constantly meet established biosafety/biocontainment policies and procedures, they are more prone to failure.

Fig. 18.5: Hierarchy of Hazard Controls

MOST EFFECTIVE

CONTROL	DESCRIPTION	EXAMPLES
Elimination	Physically remove the hazard	Needle-less systems
Substitution	Replace the hazard with a lesser one	Nonpathogenic or vaccine strain instead of wildtype agent; species selection
Engineering Controls	Isolate the hazard from personnel	Biosafety cabinets, restraint cages/shutes, self-shielding sharps
Work Practice Controls	Change the way personnel work	Training & proficiency programs; signage; restricted access
Personal Protective Equipment	On-body barrier to protect from injury/exposure	Safety glasses, face shields, respirators, fluid-resistant disposable gloves, fluid-resistant body coverings

LEAST EFFECTIVE

8 Biosafety/Biocontainment levels & principles

The basic goal of biosafety is to employ hazard control measures in order to work with potentially infectious biological materials without contaminating the people working with the agent, other people (or susceptible animals) in the surrounding area, or without allowing contaminants to escape outside of the facility. In other words, all necessary actions are taken to 'contain' the contaminant. These actions include a combination of facility design features, safety equipment, work practices, personnel training and qualifications, and personal protective equipment (PPE).

Like the 4 risk group classification system for pathogens, many countries have adopted a 4-level system to define biosafety/biocontainment combinations (Public Health Agency of Canada, 2016; Public Health Service, Centers for Disease Control and Prevention, 2009; World Health Organization (Geneva), 2004). Additionally, standards exist that specifically address biocontainment levels and considerations for genetically modified microorganisms (Department of Health and Human Services, 2016; European Commission, 2009). In many instances, the risk group assignment and the biosafety/biocontainment level will correlate (i.e., RG 1 agents are typically handled using biosafety level 1 (BSL-1)/containment level 1 (CL-1) conditions). Under the BSL/CL system, as the level increases, so do the facility requirements, need for safety equipment and PPE, work practices and level of training and qualification of personnel. As a basic reference, BSL-2/CL-2 is usually be assigned for work with mammalian cells or common pathogens transmitted primarily through contact (such as *Staphylococcus aureus*). This is work that is carried out routinely in academic research lab settings. BSL-3/CL-3 is usually assigned for work with Mycobacterium tuberculosis and many pathogens deemed to present a security risk. This work may be carried out at academic research institutions but requires facilities that are segregated from the public and with enhancements to contain the risk of aerosols and airborne transmission.

Animal biosafety levels/containment levels apply to the in vivo portion of studies. The size of the animals and caging conFiguration are drivers for determining containment practices.

Containment measures required for handling infected animals housed in microisolation caging (such as mice and rats) are similar to the measures one would use in a lab setting. Cages should be opened only in a biological safety cabinet, personnel must follow good standard microbiological practices and use PPE prescribed for the biosafety/containment level. The animal room serves as a secondary containment barrier. Under these circumstances, the potential for cross-contamination or escape of contaminants depends largely on the person handling the infected animals. Rodent work can be highly repetitive and may not be perceived as 'risky'. If the person does not consistently follow through with all required biosafety/biocontainment procedures, a breach of containment may result. By way of an example, this scenario occurred in 2015 when *Burkholderia pseudomallei* was discovered in a breeding colony of non-human primates (NHPs) at a U.S. institution (Centers for Disease control and Prevention, 2015). The strain identified in the NHPs was the same as that used in a mouse study at the time. Investigation findings by the Centers for Disease Control (CDC) indicated that lapses and lack of use of PPE could have resulted in the transfer of the contaminant via personal clothing from the rodents to the NHPs.

In the case of species that are housed in open cage systems (i.e., stalls, dog runs, rabbit cages, etc.), the animal room serves as the primary containment barrier. Personnel working in these settings must be mindful to use a containment approach when performing husbandry procedures. Husbandry and cleaning techniques that may be acceptable for rooms housing naïve animals of the same species may undermine contamination containment. Examples include dry sweeping and liberal use of water for washing rooms down.

Because there is no true separation between the room surfaces and the animal and its waste products, every surface in the room has a strong potential for contamination. Physical handling of the animals (which is not likely to be carried out in a biosafety cabinet or BSC) will result in more widespread contamination of PPE. Regardless of BSL/CL in an open cage environment, it is essential that personnel regard the exit of the biocontainment room or area as a true barrier for potential contamination. Accessible surfaces of all items and equipment should be disinfected before removal from the room. PPE should be removed in a designated doffing area within the containment zone.

Fig. 18.6: Protecting Animals & Personnel at all Levels

LEVEL	DESCRIPTION	CONTAINMENT ESSENTIALS
Cage	Preventing transmission through cage-to-cage handling interactions	Microisolation technique, BSC use, rack hygiene, cage identification
Room	Minimizing potential for spread of contamination via equipment and common work surfaces	BSC use, secondary containment of agents/samples, room & equipment cleaning methods, segregation of groups/agents, restricted access
Facility	Minimizing potential for contaminant escape/release outside the animal containment area	Directional airflow, room entry order, secondary containment, decontamination of outgoing items
Outside Facility	Preventing escape of viable research agents to the surrounding community	Waste treatment/disposal practices, personnel exposure prevention/management, adoption practices

Note: To be effective, containment essentials beginning at the room level must be supported by facility design and construction standards. Two key references for those who are planning to build or refurbish animal containment facilities are the NIH Design Requirements Manual (Division of Technical Resources (Office NSW Government), 2010) and the USDA ARS Facilities Design Standards (United States Department of Agriculture Research, Education, Economics, & ARS, 2002). Both standards are available online at no cost.

Waste management from animal biocontainment areas warrants specific consideration because it is a means of contamination release to environments beyond the animal facility. Waste categories and applicable practices to support containment include:

- **microisolation cage contents-** should be autoclaved prior to bedding removal
- **open cage pan liners-** should be carefully rolled and placed in a hard-walled, cleanable container lined with a biohazard bag; autoclave treatment (or equivalent approved sterilisation technique) prior to disposal
- **urine/faeces/body fluids in room environment-** minimise water and pressure used during waste removal process; effluent decontamination may apply to higher containment levels
- **procedural wastes (non-sharps) generated in BSC-** these should be collected in a biohazard bag in the BSC; autoclave treatment (or equivalent approved sterilisation technique) prior to disposal

- **PPE and procedural waste generated in open-cage procedures-** collect in a hard-walled, cleanable container lined with a biohazard bag; autoclave treatment (or equivalent approved sterilisation technique) prior to disposal
- **carcass and tissue waste-** collect in a biohazard bag that is securely closed; store in a hard-walled cleanable container in cold storage; dispose of via incineration.

To eliminate both public relation issues and potential containment breaches, animals (living or dead) that have been in the containment environment should not be permitted to leave the facility as anything other than pathological/biohazardous waste for treatment and disposal.

As biomedical research priorities evolve and infectious diseases emerge, some research entities will be likely to employ less traditional animals for these studies. Biocontainment levels and practice standards/guidelines have been developed for fish (Kent et al., 2009) and insects (Liebert, 2003). These standards/guidelines echo the principles of biocontainment found in the biosafety/biocontainment standards/guidelines previously discussed. The potential for environmental release of fish and insects presents unique challenges that are comprehensively addressed in these species-specific resource documents.

9 Human factors impacting biocontainment

There are two ways in which human behaviour can directly undermine biocontainment in such a way that e agents are able to escape from animal facilities. The first of these is intentional removal for criminal purposes; the actions to prevent this are often referred to as biosecurity. The United States and Canada are examples of countries that have implemented regulations identifying specific pathogens and toxins of biological origin which require governmental approval and specific security measures to possess such agents (Legal Information Institute US (Cornell Law School), 2017; Minister of Justice of Canada, 2014). Listed agents are those that have been identified as having the potential to be weaponised, and should be maintained under secure conditions therefore. Common biosecurity measures include: background checks, security plans, incident response plans, cybersecurity measures, inventory procedures, validated inactivation procedures, locked storage, and restricted lab access. When used in animals, access to the infected animals will likely require the same additional security measures as access to the agent itself.

The second way that human behaviour can result in a release of biological agents outside of the laboratory animal research setting is through lab-acquired infections LAIs). It is entirely possible for someone to acquire an infection through contaminant splashes or inadvertent contact with the eyes, nose or mouth. While inhalation is also a potential route of exposure, airborne agents are typically not handled without respiratory protection, and usually under BSL-3/CL-3 conditions. Regardless of the containment level, the use of animals almost always involves the use of sharp devices. Puncturing or breaking the skin with a contaminated object is an efficient way of administering the contaminant into the body and starting an infection. Unfortunately, in animal research applications, literature suggests that the risk of exposure via sharp objects is underestimated.

Fig. 18.7: Best Practices: Sharps Handling

GOAL: reduce lab-acquired infections and animal injury

Process: prevent accidental exposures/injuries through safe sharps handling practices

Technique:
Eliminate use of devices sharp enough to puncture skin when possible
Select devices that are self-shielding if feasible to minimize recapping as practice
Use luer-lock or fixed needle syringes; avoid the use of slip-tip needles
Do not apply excessive force to a sharp device; if force is required, suspend activity and consult with senior personnel regarding technique
Do not attempt to use a sharp unless the animal is effectively restrained; avoid manual restraint that places the hand near or in front of the sharp edge
Place sharps disposal container within arm's reach of the point of use; deposit the sharp immediately after using without recapping/resheathing
Assure that sharps disposal containers are configured for the size and number of sharps to be used; do not fill sharps containers more than 3/4 full
If a sharps-related injury occurs, suspend operations and flush/cleanse the injured body part immediately; report the injury to occupational health department

Between 2005 and 2013, seven cases of lab-acquired vaccinia infections were reported in the U.S. Morbidity and Mortality Weekly Report (Davies et al., 2009; Hsu et al., 2015; Melchreit et al., 2008). All seven involved animal procedures, and six had recognised incidents involving exposure to sharps -. One of the exposures occurred through a needle scratch. Three exposures were sustained during/after injecting the mouse. One exposure was the result of recapping. The last of the six cases of exposure involved a clean needle stick, but the individual did not change their gloves or wash their hands until after the work was finished. Of the seven LAIs, only two were reported before medical intervention was needed to treat infection. Of the seven LAIs, four had not been previously vaccinated. Based on these details, we can conclude that the laboratory animal research community should take action to emphasise the importance of safe handling procedures for sharps, exposure response and reporting procedures, and vaccination programmes.

10 Animal biosecurity: preventive medicine and research biocontainment partnership

In this chapter, the elements and best practices of animal biosecurity from both the veterinary and biosafety perspectives were discussed. In many cases, the practices used to maintain pathogen-free facilities and those employed for biocontainment purposes are complementary. If procedures do conflict, it is important for veterinary care, biosafety and research personnel to communicate openly and determine together how procedures can be carried out so that it achieves the goal of protecting both personnel and the susceptible animal colonies.

References

Centers for Disease control and Prevention. (2015). Hierarchy of controls.

Centers for Disease control and Prevention. (2015). Conclusion of select agent inquiry into Burkholderia pseudomallei release at Tulane national primate research center. News Release.

de Bruin, W. C. C., van de Ven, E. M. E., & Hooijmans, C. R. (2016). Efficacy of Soiled Bedding Transfer for Transmission of Mouse and Rat Infections to Sentinels: A Systematic Review. PLoS ONE, 11(8), e0158410. https://doi.org/10.1371/journal.pone.0158410

Department of Health and Human Services (National Institutes of Health). (2016). NIH Guidelines for Research Involving Recombinant or Synthetic Nucleic Acid Molecules. NIH Guidelines, (April).

Division of Technical Resources (Office NSW Government). (2010). Design requirements manual., 2016(5.2), 2-81.

E Davies, L Peake, D Woolard, C Novak, K., & Hall, RT Leonard, R Allen, M Reynolds, W Davidson, C Hughes, V Olson, S Smith, H Zhao, Y Li, K Karem, I Damon, A. R. (2009). Laboratory-acquired vaccinia virus infection – Virginia, 2008. MMWR. Morbidity and Mortality Weekly Report, 58(29), 797-800.

European Commission. (2000). Directive 2000/54/EC of the European Parliament and of The Council of 18 September 2000 on the protection of workers from risks related to exposure to biological agents at work (seventh individual directive within the meaning of Article 16(1) of Directive. Official Journal of the European Communities, L262, 21-45.

European Commission. (2009). Directive 2009/41/EC of the European Parliament and of the Council of 6 May 2009 on the contained use of genetically modified micro-organisms (Recast). Official Journal of the European Union, 125, 75-97.

Exhaust Air Dust (EADTM). (2016). FAQs: Plenum Swabbing and Allentown Sentinel TM EADTM – Charles River Technical Sheet.

Höfler, D., Nicklas, W., Mauter, P., Pawlita, M., & Schmitt, M. (2014). A Bead-Based Multiplex Assay for the Detection of DNA Viruses Infecting Laboratory Rodents. (S. Bereswill, Ed.), PLoS ONE. San Francisco, USA. https://doi.org/10.1371/journal.pone.0097525

Hsu, C. H., Farland, J., Winters, T., Gunn, J., Caron, D., Evans, J., … Barry, M. A. (2015). Laboratory-acquired vaccinia virus infection in a recently immunized person--Massachusetts, 2013. MMWR. Morbidity and Mortality Weekly Report, 64(16), 435-438.

Jensen, E. S., Allen, K. P., Henderson, K. S., Szabo, A., & Thulin, J. D. (2013, January). PCR Testing of a Ventilated Caging System to Detect Murine Fur Mites. Journal of the American Association for Laboratory Animal Science: JAALAS.

Kent, M. L., Feist, S. W., Harper, C., Hoogstraten-Miller, S., Law, J. Mac, Sanchez-Morgado, J. M., … Whipps, C. M. (2009). Recommendations for control of pathogens and infectious diseases in fish research facilities. Comparative Biochemistry and Physiology. Toxicology & Pharmacology : CBP, 149(2), 240–248. https://doi.org/10.1016/j.cbpc.2008.08.001

Leblanc, M., Berry, K., Graciano, S., Becker, B., & Reuter, J. D. (2014). False-Positive Results after Environmental Pinworm PCR Testing due to Rhabditid Nematodes in Corncob Bedding. Journal of the American Association for Laboratory Animal Science: JAALAS, 53(6), 717-724.

Legal Information Institute US (Cornell Law School). (2017). US Law: select agents and toxins.

Liebert, M. A. (2003). Arthropod containment levels (Acls). Vector-Borne and Zoonotic Diseases, 3(2), 75-90. https://doi.org/10.1089/153036603322163439

Melchreit, R., Lewis, F., Quinlisk, P., Soyemi, K., DesJardin, L., Kirchhoff, L. V., ... Dufficy, D. (2008). Laboratory-acquired vaccinia exposures and infections--United States, 2005-2007. MMWR. Morbidity and Mortality Weekly Report, 57(15), 401-404.

Minister of Justice of Canada. (2014). Human pathogens and toxins act.

National Research Council (US) Committee for the Update of the Guide for the Care and Use of Laboratory Animals. (2011). Guide for the Care and Use of Laboratory Animals. Guide for the Care and Use of Laboratory Animals (8th editio, Vol. 46). Washington (DC): National Academies Press (US). https://doi.org/10.17226/12910

Public Health Agency of Canada. (2016). Canadian Biosafety Handbook (2nd editio).

Public Health Service, Centers for Disease Control and Prevention, N. I. of H. (2009). Biosafety in Microbiological and Biomedical Laboratories. US Department of Health and Human Services, 5th Edition (April), 1–250. https://doi.org/citeulike-article-id:3658941

Smith, J., & Szczepan, B. (2013). Rodent Housing Methodologies. ALN Magazine (Advantage Media).

Spickler, A. R. (2016). Zoonotic Diseases. MSD Manual – Public Health – Veterinary Manual.

United States Department of Agriculture Research, Education, Economics, & ARS. (2002). ARS Facilities Design Standards.

World Health Organization (Geneva). (2004). Laboratory biosafety manual. (3th editio). https://doi.org/10.1007/SpringerReference_61629

CHAPTER 19

BIOSECURITY IN AQUACULTURE: PRACTICAL VETERINARY APPROACHES FOR AQUATIC ANIMAL DISEASE PREVENTION, CONTROL, AND POTENTIAL ERADICATION

Dušan Palić [1,2]

A. David Scarfe [1,3,4]

[1] International Aquatic Veterinary Biosecurity Consortium
[2] Chair for Fish Diseases and Fisheries Biology, Faculty of Veterinary Medicine, Ludwig-Maximilians-Universität-München, Germany
[3] Department of Paraclinical Sciences, Faculty of Veterinary Medicine, University of Pretoria, South Africa.
[4] Aquatic Veterinary Associates International, LLC, Bartlett, Illinois, USA

1 Introduction

Developing effective, practical and economically viable approaches to prevent, control and potentially eradicate infectious and contagious diseases in aquaculture operations, have eluded those involved in farmed aquatic animals for some time. An approach for meeting these objectives using sound scientific veterinary principles outlined in the World Organisation for Animal Health (O.I.E. 2017a) and elsewhere, was developed by the International Aquatic Veterinary Biosecurity Consortium (IAVBC) (Palić et al. 2015), and offers a solution that should meet the needs of producers and government regulatory agencies. Developed over a number of years with input from a wide variety of collaborators from around the world, the IAVBC approach focuses on applying several important core OIE processes aimed at determining and maintaining freedom from disease in any epidemiological unit (EpiUnit) – from individual farms to whole countries.

These processes include: identifying and assessing risk and prioritising hazardous diseases important to a clearly defined EpiUnit; identifying and correcting critical points via which these diseases might enter or leave the EpiUnit; developing contingency plans should a disease be discovered in the EpiUnit through disease surveillance and monitoring; periodic auditing of EpiUnit biosecurity programmes and records; and, where necessary, certifying the absence of these diseases in the EpiUnit, with government agency oversight and endorsement (Palić et al. 2015, Scarfe and Palić 2017).

The primary objective of this chapter therefore is to introduce readers to key concepts that can help prevent, control and eradicate infectious and contagious diseases in aquaculture in any epidemiological unit – what we refer to as *biosecurity*.

1.1 Disease 'Management' vs. Disease Prevention, Control and Eradication

While a number of publications refer to 'managing' disease, or 'best management practices', we purposefully and intentionally try to avoid the use of these passive terms. Our intent is to clearly demonstrate that if the correct approaches are *actively* taken, all stakeholders will benefit from the prevention control and eradication of disease in *Epidemiological Units*. Indeed, if one were to carefully examine how smallpox and rinderpest were eradicated from all countries, we would not be surprised to discover that many of the procedures are the same as those mentioned here.

Many of the processes and procedures are included in the OIE Code and Manual (O.I.E. 2017i, O.I.E. 2017a) and, if implemented correctly, will significantly contribute to sustainable aquaculture development and economic growth, and meet government regulations aimed at protecting aquaculture industries from outbreaks of devastating diseases. Although implementing biosecurity procedures may seem daunting at first, the most important factor is to understand what is required of and what to include in a *written biosecurity plan*.

OIE defines a number of terms that are important in drawing up and implementing a biosecurity plan, including:

- *Biosecurity* in aquaculture is a set of management and physical measures designed to reduce the risk of introduction, establishment and spread of pathogenic agents to, from and within an aquatic animal population.
- A *Biosecurity Plan* is a plan that identifies significant potential pathways for the introduction and spread of disease in a zone or compartment, and describes the measures that are, or will be, applied in order to mitigate the risks of the introduction and spread of disease, based on the recommendations in the Aquatic Code. The plan should also describe how these measures are audited, with respect to both their implementation and their targeting, to

BIOSECURITY IN AQUACULTURE: PRACTICAL VETERINARY APPROACHES FOR AQUATIC ANIMAL DISEASE PREVENTION, CONTROL, AND POTENTIAL ERADICATION

499

19

ensure that the risks are regularly re-assessed and the measures adjusted accordingly.

- An *Epidemiological Unit* is a group of animals that share approximately the same risk of exposure to a pathogenic agent within a defined location. This may be because they share a common aquatic environment (e.g. fish in a pond, caged fish in a lake), or because management practices make it likely that a pathogenic agent in one group of animals would quickly spread to other animals (e.g. all the ponds on a farm, all the ponds in a village system).
- An *Aquaculture Establishment* is an establishment [e.g. farm] in which amphibians, fish, molluscs or crustaceans for breeding, stocking or sale are raised or kept.
- A *Compartment* is one or more aquaculture establishments [farms] under a common biosecurity management system containing an aquatic animal population with a distinct health status with respect to a specific disease or diseases for which required surveillance and control measures are applied and for which basic biosecurity conditions are met for the purpose of international trade. Such compartments must be clearly documented by the Competent Authority/authorities).
- A *Zone* is an area of one or more countries comprising of: an entire water catchment from the source of a waterway to the estuary or lake, or; more than one water catchment, or; part of a water catchment from the source of a waterway to a barrier that prevents the introduction of a specific disease or diseases, or part of coastal area with a precise geographical delimitation, or an estuary with a precise geographical delimitation, that consists of a contiguous hydrological system with a distinct health status with respect to a specific disease or diseases. The zones must be clearly documented (e.g. by a map or other precise locators such as GPS co-ordinates) by the Competent Authority/authorities).

Adapted from (O.I.E. 2017h)

1.2 The Epidemiological Unit – the Focus of All Biosecurity Activities

An epidemiological unit may be small (an individual farm or 'establishment', or parts of a farm), or large (several farms, a state or province, or a whole country). Any geographic area that somehow separates one group of animals from another may form an EpiUnit, *provided* that all animals in each unit are managed in the same way. The separation may be a physical barrier, or simply distance – but the animal population in each unit *must not co-mingle* with animals outside the unit.

1.3 Expanding the Process for Larger Units in a Country (Compartmentalisation and Zoning)

The OIE clearly extends the concepts of epidemiological units to include larger geographic units. Although this chapter focuses on individual farms (establishments) to illustrate how biosecurity programmes on a fish farm can prevent, control and eradicate a number of diseases, the same concepts (with some modifications) can be extended to larger geographical areas to eventually encompass a whole country or continent. These concepts can also be used to develop and implement biosecurity plans in order to prevent, control and eradicate *any* disease, on *any* type of operation or establishment.

2 The IAVBC Process Applied to Developing Biosecurity Plan on Individual Farms

The process we follow has been reduced to nine essential steps or key processes that are important for developing any biosecurity plan tailored to specific epidemiological units (from an individual tank or pond, to a whole country). These are illustrated in Figure 19.1.

BIOSECURITY IN AQUACULTURE: PRACTICAL VETERINARY APPROACHES FOR AQUATIC ANIMAL DISEASE PREVENTION, CONTROL, AND POTENTIAL ERADICATION

501

19

Fig. 19.1: IAVBC Aquaculture Biosecurity Concept Sheet

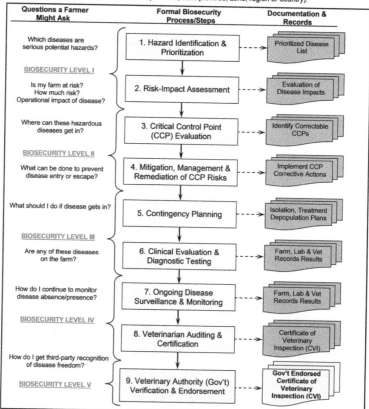

INTEGRATED COMPONENTS OF EFFECTIVE VETERINARY BIOSECURITY FOR AQUACULTURE

Steps for developing, implementing, auditing and certifying an effective biosecurity program intended to prevent, control and possibly eradicate disease in any epidemiological unit1 (a tank/pond, farm, compartment, state/province, zone, region or country).

Questions a Farmer Might Ask	Formal Biosecurity Process/Steps	Documentation & Records
Which diseases are serious potential hazards?	1. Hazard Identification & Prioritization	Prioritized Disease List
BIOSECURITY LEVEL I		
Is my farm at risk? How much risk? Operational impact of disease?	2. Risk-Impact Assessment	Evaluation of Disease Impacts
Where can these hazardous diseases get in?	3. Critical Control Point (CCP) Evaluation	Identify Correctable CCPs
BIOSECURITY LEVEL II		
What can be done to prevent disease entry or escape?	4. Mitigation, Management & Remediation of CCP Risks	Implement CCP Corrective Actions
What should I do if disease gets in?	5. Contingency Planning	Isolation, Treatment Depopulation Plans
BIOSECURITY LEVEL III		
Are any of these diseases on the farm?	6. Clinical Evaluation & Diagnostic Testing	Farm, Lab & Vet Records Results
How do I continue to monitor disease absence/presence?	7. Ongoing Disease Surveillance & Monitoring	Farm, Lab & Vet Records Results
BIOSECURITY LEVEL IV		
	8. Veterinarian Auditing & Certification	Certificate of Veterinary Inspection (CVI)
How do I get third-party recognition of disease freedom?		
BIOSECURITY LEVEL V	9. Veterinary Authority (Gov't) Verification & Endorsement	Gov't Endorsed Certificate of Veterinary Inspection (CVI)

1   Epidemiologic Unit—a defined population of animals, separated to some degree from other populations, in which infectious and contagious diseases can be transmitted

2.1 Teamwork in Developing and Implementing Biosecurity Programmes

Optimally, developing and implementing a biosecurity plan should involve a team of individuals that are well acquainted with the intimate workings of aquaculture operations, farms or EpiUnit/s. These should include farm owners, managers or employees specifically assigned to oversee all biosecurity activities, veterinarians or para-veterinary professionals with expertise in aquatic animal disease, diagnostics and epidemiology, and government officials. Inevitably, any disease prevention, control and eradication will involve government regulations. It is important therefore to include a government official who is familiar with local, national,

Fig. 19.2 (a): Example of Google Maps spatial layout of a 2017 IAVBC workshop case study aquaculture operation (35 Hectares).

▼

and international veterinary regulations, laws and OIE standards – particularly if any animals or their products are sold, traded or moved from the farm, or if there is a desire to have the farm certified free of any specific disease, pathogen or infectious agent. Following steps outlined in figure 19.1., the team should first gather as much information as possible about the EpiUnit and how the farm operates, as all subsequent activities revolve around this information. This can often be done by talking to the owner or actually visiting the farm. Maps or aerial views (e.g. Google maps) can be very useful in this as well as architectural plans, or

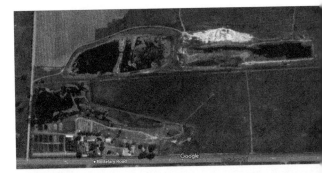

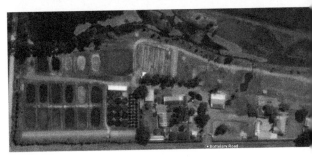

hand-drawn layouts of the farm and locations of buildings, tanks, ponds, feed, equipment and water sources (figure. 19.2 a-b). Particular attention should be given to how diseases can enter or leave the EpiUnit. Developing a set of standardised preliminary questions can help here (an example page from an IAVBC questionnaire© is provided in figure 19.2 c) and the owner or manager should complete it before the actual farm visit to get an idea of the operational set-up. This preliminary information will become part of the records that need to be kept and should be included in a biosecurity plan.

▲

Fig. 19.2 (b): Use of high-resolution satellite imagery (Google Maps) and owner-provided information to delineate aquaculture farm facilities layout: 18 clay ground dams for the rearing of fish; 44 'Porta Pools' for the breeding and rearing of fish; one 100 m greenhouse with 18 breeding and rearing ponds; one 30 m greenhouse with 40 concrete pools for breeding fish; a tropical hatchery housing 500 tanks for breeding, rearing and holding fish; covered display area with a wooden deck and 5 show ponds.

BIOSECURITY IN AQUACULTURE: PRACTICAL VETERINARY APPROACHES FOR AQUATIC ANIMAL DISEASE PREVENTION, CONTROL, AND POTENTIAL ERADICATION

503

19

Fig. 19.2 (c): Example questionnaire pages filled by the aquaculture establishment manager/owner and shared with veterinary biosecurity programme development team.

Preliminary Producer/Operation Biosecurity Questionnaire[†]

Some important risk considerations for introduction of catastrophic infectious and contagious diseases onto your farm include:

1. The movement of infected fish
2. Introduction of contaminated water or feed
3. Fomites including contaminated equipment, or vehicles
4. Vectors such as people, fish-eating birds or wildlife

Please Note:

- Each farm or operation is unique because of species cultured, the location of the operation, the diseases of concern, the types of production, management styles, available personnel and their understanding of these diseases, financial constraints and many other variable factors. Consequently, every biosecurity program developed is unique and must be tailored to the specific farm or operation.

- This questionnaire is designed to help you begin to identify and evaluate the areas of risk, and the impact of an introduction and/or spread of a disease on your farm.

- Not all questions are equal in identifying the risk of disease introduction and severity; however, answers to the following questions begin to identify critical points or procedures that can be controlled and should be considered in developing a written biosecurity plan for this farm or operation.

Your Disease Concerns

Please identify what diseases *you feel are most important to your farm*? List the top 5, in order of your priority:

1. KHV
2. External bacterial diseases
3. Malawi Bloat (internal bacterial infection)
4. Parasitic infections (internal & external
5. Fungal infections

Other diseases of concern: FUS

[†] This questionnaire is modeled after a checklist of critical elements, developed by the Center of Food Security and Public Health, Iowa State University, initially intended to address viral haemorrhagic septicemia biosecurity

Copyright © 2017, International Aquatic Veterinary Biosecurity Consortium – All Rights Reserved. *Copying or duplicating any information in this manual, without written permission of the IAVBC, is explicitly prohibited.*

Identifying the Critical Points where disease can enter or leave your farm

Check ☑ Yes or *No* for each question.

Fish Movement

Yes	No	
☐	☒	Have you restricted or stopped all fish movement on or off your farm to prevent entry or spread of any disease? No returns on stock, health certificate, quarntine
☒	☐	Have you implemented strict biosecurity measures for fish, water sources, equipment, vehicles, wildlife vectors and people on your farm? informal system
☒	☐	Are you closely and frequently monitoring your fish for signs of disease?
☒	☐	Do you limit contact between your fish stock and wild fish stocks?
☒	☐	Do you limit the frequency and number of new introductions of fish onto your farm?
☒	☐	Do you limit purchases to a few sources with known and trusted fish health programs?
☒	☐	Do you know the health status and the source of the fish brought onto your farm?
☒	☐	Do you only bring animals onto your farm, that have been inspected or tested to be free of the disease you listed above?
☒	☐	Do you request copies of treatment records (and vaccinations, if applicable) for all purchased fish? health certificate
☐	☐	Do you disinfect eggs upon arrival on the farm? NA
☒	☐	Do you require that newly acquired or returned fish for your farm are quarantined for at least 3 weeks upon arrival?
☒	☐	Are your quarantine facilities separate from all other fish areas?
☒	☐	Do you prevent the sharing of water, facilities or equipment between newly acquired or returned fish and your currently stocked fish?
☒	☐	If equipment must be used elsewhere on the farm, do you clean and disinfect the item before moving it from one location and another location?
12	1	Total Number of Yes and *No* answers

Farm Entrance

Yes	No	
☒	☐	Do you limit access to your farm?
☒	☐	Do you have only one gated entrance to fish production areas on your farm to better control and monitor visitors and vehicles?
☒	☐	Do you keep the gate locked when not in use?
☐	☒	Have you posted signs at the farm entrance to inform visitors to stay off your farm unless they have received permission?
☐	☒	Is traffic on or off your farm closely monitored and recorded? control not monitored
☐	☒	Do you maintain a log sheet to record any visitors or vehicles that come onto your farm? record through sales
☒	☐	Do you require delivery vehicles and visitors follow your farm biosecurity guidelines regarding parking and fish contact?
4	3	Total Number of Yes and *No* answers

Copyright © 2017, International Aquatic Veterinary Biosecurity Consortium – All Rights Reserved. *Copying or duplicating any information in this manual, without written permission of the IAVBC, is explicitly prohibited.*

BIOSECURITY IN ANIMAL PRODUCTION AND VETERINARY MEDICINE

2.2 Identifying, Prioritising and Determining the Impact of Hazardous Diseases for the Biosecurity Plan

Biosecurity programmes are best designed and tailored *for* specific EpiUnits and for diseases that are, or may be, encountered on those particular EpiUnits. Including diseases that will never be encountered in the animals used on the farm (e.g. mollusc disease on a finfish farm), or diseases that are documented but do not exist in the country where the farm is located are not a priority. In many cases, because developing and implementing biosecurity programmes will require resources (typically man hours, equipment, and money), developing biosecurity programmes for those diseases that have the greatest potential to negatively impact the farm is a prudent approach. If necessary, emerging disease(s) found elsewhere are better addressed in contingency plans. Furthermore, because a number of issues change over time, overall biosecurity programmes will need to be periodically revised and new diseases can be addressed at that time.

In many cases, the owners/managers of aquaculture operations are already familiar with the diseases that cause (or have caused) problems on the farms. It is therefore expedient for the producer to work with a veterinarian and government official to draw up a list of diseases that are of highest concern. This list can then be prioritised, based on the respective risk of introduction and the impact thereof on the farms.

Using a relatively simple semi-quantitative approach, the risks and impacts of each disease on a farm can be determined by estimating the probability of it occurring, and the consequences if it is discovered. Although complex quantitative risk analyses can be carried out, relatively simple semi-quantitative assessments usually provide sufficient information (Arthur et al. 2009, Moore et al. 2010, Oidtmann et al. 2013).

Simple, semi-quantitative risk-impact assessments can be based on scores (e.g. 1 to 10) on the relative 'weight' of the likelihood of

BIOSECURITY IN AQUACULTURE: PRACTICAL VETERINARY APPROACHES FOR AQUATIC ANIMAL DISEASE PREVENTION, CONTROL, AND POTENTIAL ERADICATION

505

19

a disease being introduced on a farm, and the impact based on the experience of the biosecurity team (the producer, veterinarian, and government official). Although it is often simpler to address in contingency plans many emerging diseases that are not currently found in the home country of the farm, if circumstances warrant it (such as importation of animals from countries known to be experiencing an epidemic), it might be wise to include these diseases in a risk-impact assessment. A hypothetical example of a risk-impact assessment is illustrated in figure 19.3 (Scarfe and Palić 2017).

Fig. 19.3: Example of risk-impact assessment sheet

Identifying & Prioritizing Disease Hazards Using a Simplified, Semi-quantitative Risk-Impact Analysis

Instructions: Based on the general knowledge of the group, quantify 3-4 viral, bacterial, parasitic, or other diseases that might impact this farm

Score: *1. Presence* (Not in Africa= 1, In country=5, On farm=10); *2. Affect farm* (0=no likelihood, 10=very likely); *3. Impact* (None=0, 10=very high)

1. Disease present?	2. Likelihood will affect farm?	3. Impact on farm?	Describe impacts on Farm (e.g. production, morbidity, mortality, zoonotic, regulatory depopulation, etc.)	Total Score (1x2x3)	Rank 1=highest
Viral Diseases					
Bacterial Diseases					
Parasitic Diseases					
Other Diseases					

Important elements used in a biosecurity risk-impact analysis.

1. Determine what diseases might present a hazard, and severely impact the EpiUnit;

2. Using a semi-quantitative (weighted) approach*, estimate the risks and impact of each disease, in order to prioritise the diseases for inclusion in the specific biosecurity plan; and,

3. Determine which important 'emerging' diseases might be considered for inclusion in a biosecurity programme for the EpiUnit.

4. Using cumulative scores (sum of risk and impact scores) select the highest ranking diseases to include in the biosecurity plan for this EpiUnit or farm.

* In more complex EpiUnits such as larger farms, compartments, zones or countries/regions, a more formal risk assessment process is probably needed in order to provide a better estimate of priorities and associated actions to be drawn up for disease control and prevention programmes (e.g. FAO Risk Assessment Arthur et al 2009).

The expected output from this step is a prioritised list of diseases with a historic, current or potential serious impact on the farm. i.e. ones that severely decrease production, zoonotic diseases, diseases that could cause unacceptable morbidity or mortality, could result in regulatory restrictions, negatively affect the reputation or economic viability of the farm, or that might have a serious impact on wild populations or other farms in the neighbourhood. The list should not only include those diseases that are reportable to a government agency, but should also include diseases the owner feels are important. Once this list of disease hazards has been prioritised, it will be possible to move on to the next step in drawing up the biosecurity plan.

3 Identifying, Prioritising and Mitigating Critical Points Where Disease can Enter or Leave an Epidemiological Unit

Identifying how diseases might enter (or leave) the farm, and which on-farm procedures might enable this, is an important step in preventing the introduction (or spread) of any unwanted diseases. Equally important are procedures or places that might provide a way for the disease to exit the farm. These are sometimes considered to be bio-exclusion and biocontainment priorities. Ensuring good procedures to accomplish either will reduce a farmer's liability for the potential spread of a disease. Inevitably all diseases or infectious pathogens that can enter and leave the EpiUnit are associated with vectors (animals or people), or inanimate fomites

BIOSECURITY IN AQUACULTURE: PRACTICAL VETERINARY APPROACHES FOR AQUATIC ANIMAL DISEASE PREVENTION, CONTROL, AND POTENTIAL ERADICATION

507

19

(non-living objects). Vectors and fomites should also be considered as critical points to be controlled (Karreman et al. 2015).

Overall, critical control points may be very diverse, and include (but not limited to): animals, people, pests, birds, water, feed, equipment, and a large number of other things. Drawing up processes or procedures to correct, mitigate, or eliminate these, contributes substantially to protecting farms. Prioritising these in terms of how easy or difficult it will be for diseases or pathogens to enter or leave the farm, helps to prioritise where to allocate resources. It is important to consider drawing up processes or procedures that can reduce (or even eliminate) the probability of diseases or pathogens entering or leaving a farm as an insurance policy to protect the farms and their owners (Huchzermeyer and Colly 2015).

After evaluating the information obtained from the farms' preliminary producer/operation biosecurity questionnaire as well as list of prioritised disease risks and hazards specific to the epidemiological unit the following objectives need to be met:

1. Identify procedures or locations, vectors and fomites (critical points) via which diseases can enter or leave the farm.
2. Determine and prioritise the level or risk for each critical control point, so that resources for correcting, mitigating, or eliminating risks, can be allocated.
3. Determine what needs to be done to correct, mitigate or eliminate these critical control points on the farm.

A completed output of this step should include a detailed list of all Critical Points (vectors, fomites, and on-farm procedures) that might allow a disease or pathogen to enter or leave this EpiUnit. An integral part of documenting this in the biosecurity plan, is a list of actions or measures that have or will be implemented in order to correct, mitigate or eliminate the problem for each vector, fomite and procedure. As these actions may use or require additional resources it is also advisable to: 1) decide how much effort (manpower, time or money) will be required; and, 2) prioritise (rank) the actions for each vector, fomite and on-farm procedure based on the level of risk and the resources needed to correct, mitigate or eliminate the problem.

4 Developing a Contingency Plan if Disease is Found

Irrespective of how diligent a farm is in ensuring that diseases or pathogens do not gain access, there is always the chance that this might happen. Preparing for this by drawing up contingency plans is not only prudent, but those farms that have developed contingency plans for possible disease outbreaks as a part of their written biosecurity plan, will have the advantage of rapid recovery. Furthermore, rapid recovery will inevitably save a considerable amount of money, enhance the reputation of the farm as a reliable source of disease-free animals, and minimise any regulatory impact (O.I.E. 2017d). *Think of contingency plans as an insurance policy to protect farms and their owners!*

Many countries have regulations that determine what is required if certain diseases are discovered. It is therefore prudent to include a government regulator in drawing up contingency plans, or to use information available from the respective national or international organisations (e.g. OIE). While requirements might vary between countries, they will inevitably require the owner, the attending veterinarian, and in some cases a diagnostic laboratory to report occurrences or suspicions of regulated diseases. Typically, regulations will also require isolating (quarantining) the affected animals, and all or parts of the farm or a larger EpiUnit, and placing some sort of barrier between the infected population and uninfected populations (E.U. 2006).

Depending on a wide variety of issues, options on which contingencies should be in place will always be specific to each disease. These may include depopulating all animals in EpiUnit and safely disposing of carcasses so the disease cannot spread. Also, if there are no food-safety or public-health concerns, the animals could be sent to a slaughter facility to be processed as seafood or animal feed. Further, fallowing or disinfecting the premises and disposing of all contaminated equipment and supplies, treating animals with appropriate therapeutic agents (drugs), vaccinating animals, or other options should be considered depending on the suspected disease and its potential impact (Gudding et al. 2015).

BIOSECURITY IN AQUACULTURE: PRACTICAL VETERINARY APPROACHES FOR AQUATIC ANIMAL
DISEASE PREVENTION, CONTROL, AND POTENTIAL ERADICATION

509

19

Using the available information collected or developed in earlier steps, a formal contingency plan should be drawn up in an attempt to meet the following objectives:

1. Which activities should be considered? Should a viral, bacterial, parasitic or other disease be discovered on this EpiUnit?
2. What is to be accomplished with these activities?
3. Who should oversee implementation of each activity?
4. The order in which the activities should be implemented.

The practical approach for ensuring an optimal response to a disease outbreak in an EpiUnit would be to draw up an operations manual as part of the written biosecurity plan including a detailed, comprehensive and practical description of all the actions, procedures, instructions and control measures to be implemented. Training staff to recognise clinical signs is imperative before any outbreak occurs. After an outbreak an epidemiological investigation to discover the source of the disease, and how and why it entered the EpiUnit, should be carried out. It is also important to ensure that if depopulation is necessary, the animals are killed or slaughtered in accordance with recommended sanitary and humane guidelines and that veterinary and environmental safety issues are properly coordinated (Lillehaug et al. 2015). If premises are depopulated, attention must be given to mass disposal of aquatic animal carcasses without endangering animal or human health, or increasing the possibility of spreading the disease.

Contingency plans should be designed therefore to detect and control the outbreak of a disease within an EpiUnit, and outline the 'who' and 'how' of immediate actions, particularly for: a) communications; b) containment; c) disposal procedures; and d) re-establishing freedom from disease. In order to ensure that contingency plans are an effective part of biosecurity programmes aimed at ensuring freedom from disease, all the steps in the contingency plans and respective actions during contingency must be documented and verified in the EpiUnit or farm, and personnel must be trained in their respective roles.

5 Determining if Priority Diseases (Hazards) are Present using Clinical Evaluation and Diagnostic Tests

The clinical evaluation and diagnostic testing procedures are imperative in determining the presence or absence of a particular disease within EpiUnits (Oidtmann et al. 2013). Decisions on which disease on which to perform laboratory diagnostic assays are based on the disease hazard and prioritisation list, and on which of these diseases might be suspected during the clinical evaluation. As stipulated in the biosecurity plan, the clinical evaluation of a disease situation in a specific EpiUnit should include site visits, clinical exams and necropsy, as well as a review of existing records (e.g. water quality, animal movement, etc.) and history (anamnestic data, earlier veterinary records, diagnostic reports, etc.) received prior to the visit or on site. Samples for disease diagnostics should be collected during necropsy examination and sent to a veterinary diagnostic laboratory for evaluation. It is important that samples are collected and shipped properly by the authorised individual (either a veterinarian or a person directly supervised by a veterinarian) in order to keep the chain of custody in the event that there is a suspicion of a reportable disease or other regulated disease. The choice of disease diagnostic tests is also of importance, since they may need to conform to the regulations – this should be reviewed with a government official prior to sampling (O.I.E. 2017i, O.I.E. 2017g). Veterinary clinical evaluations, diagnostic laboratory results, and farm records therefore need to be included in the biosecurity plan in order to document presence or absence of a selected disease at given time.

Circumstances that determine which diagnostic tests to use, and how the results are interpreted are often complex. Therefore, keeping the complete (or as complete as possible) information about diagnostic tests and their interpretations as part of the biosecurity records on a farm/EpiUnit will help the biosecurity team (and auditors) to establish a baseline for disease presence or absence on the farm through disease surveillance. As part of this process, continuous monitoring of animal morbidity and mortality, and screening of new animals designated to enter the farm or EpiUnit, is required

BIOSECURITY IN AQUACULTURE: PRACTICAL VETERINARY APPROACHES FOR AQUATIC ANIMAL DISEASE PREVENTION, CONTROL, AND POTENTIAL ERADICATION

511

19

in order to maintain a disease status as recorded or awarded by the authorities or third party auditors. The following examples of decisions that a biosecurity programme development team has to make as part of determining needs for disease diagnostics may be helpful in focusing on priorities and help provide the information required in the diagnostic testing record log (Caraguel et al. 2015). As a first decision, producer and veterinarian need to consider what testing is required in the biosecurity plan: i.e. should we rely on official services or use our suppliers' own testing, or do we have to provide third party (external testing) evidence? For example, in many countries, some form of government assistance is offered to fish farmers as part of the broader disease surveillance following national or regional programmes and usually focus on reportable diseases. The decision needs to be made as to whether these programmes comply with the goals laid down in the biosecurity plan, and if additional testing needs to be carried out. In other circumstances, diagnostic laboratory test results provided by the supplier of animals brought into to the EpiUnit/Farm may be considered adequate for monitoring purposes and certifying the disease status, especially if there are no other entry routes for potential disease apart from fish deliveries. However, if an export trade partner or government requires independent testing to confirm the disease status of the EpiUnit, an external testing service, usually involving private veterinary practitioners and accredited laboratories, may need to be engaged to ensure compliance with contractual or other regulatory obligations (O.I.E. 2017c, O.I.E. 2017e).

The decision about which laboratory or laboratories to use for testing is also closely related to the goals laid out in the biosecurity plan, as well as the desired level of certification, contractual obligations or regulatory requirements. If a government agency is involved in the surveillance programme and offers assistance in diagnostic testing, it usually requires diagnostic samples to be sent to government accredited (official) laboratories. However, in other cases, diagnostic assays can be performed by private, university, or even in-house facilities, and the choice may be based on accessibility, cost, and turn-around time for producing diagnostic reports. During the preparation of this section of a biosecurity plan, it is advisable to include contact information of the diagnostic laboratories where samples should be sent. The attending veterinarian would in most cases have the contact information for diagnostic laboratory services, but an aquatic diagnostic laboratory such as www.AquaVetMed.info, can be found online. The OIE also maintains a list of reference laboratories for aquatic animal diseases in case a biosecurity plan is prepared at government or regional level (such as zone or compartment) (O.I.E. 2017i).

When determining which diagnostic assays are suitable and appropriate for achieving the goals of the biosecurity plan, one should also consider: sensitivity and specificity of tests; whether lethal or non-lethal sampling is required for collecting test samples; how easy it is to collect samples; and the costs involved with sampling and the tests required (Caraguel et al. 2015). The OIE Manual provides lists of available and validated tests for specific disease diagnostics (O.I.E. 2017i), but the expert assistance of a veterinary epidemiologist may be needed to select the appropriate test, as well as determine the number of animals to be tested and the sampling frequency. Detailed analyses of sampling approaches such as standard versus risk-based sampling, decision making based on scenario trees, and probability/risk of the introduction of a disease via a supplier need to be considered for deciding on optimal testing procedures for disease status determination and surveillance.

6 Maintaining Biosecurity – Surveillance, Monitoring and Keeping Records

The most essential step in establishing and maintaining a biosecure facility is ongoing disease surveillance and monitoring (O.I.E. 2017b) to determine which diseases are present or absent in a EpiUnit. While there are subtle differences in the initial determination of the presence or absence of disease (usually thought of as surveillance) and monitoring situations on farms to determine if anything has changed, both require periodic sampling for diseases and numerous publications address the appropriate ways to sample and determine the absence or presence of disease in aquaculture and other animal populations (Kenton 2015) that

BIOSECURITY IN AQUACULTURE: PRACTICAL VETERINARY APPROACHES FOR AQUATIC ANIMAL DISEASE PREVENTION, CONTROL, AND POTENTIAL ERADICATION

513

19

can be applied to most EpiUnits. Depending on the goals of the producer, the physical layout of the facility, the process flow for operations and the epidemiology of the pathogen(s) of concern, a surveillance programme should be discussed and determined by a veterinarian, in consultation with the producer and in compliance with regulatory requirements. While initial surveillance is usually carried out on a regular basis (e.g. twice per year, every year, etc.), especially during the initial years of establishing a biosecurity programme, monitoring disease status can either be continued on a regular basis or implemented according to changing circumstances (e.g. new animals of unknown status introduced, or a disease outbreak). In some cases an EpiUnit may be certified free of specific diseases or pathogens and diagnostic sampling may not be deemed necessary, until circumstances change (Kenton 2015). However, if there is a change in biosecurity status, surveillance and monitoring may need to be re-initiated (Oidtmann et al. 2013).

Although it is not necessary to outline a process in order to certify that all biosecurity processes described in this chapter (figure 19.1) are in place and that a farm is free of specific diseases or pathogens, the OIE has processes for recognising other larger EpiUnits (zones, regions or countries) as disease-free (O.I.E. 2017g). However, the IAVBC has considered, but has yet to implement, a process to certify progress towards achieving disease-free status for a farm, as illustrated in figure 19.1.

To ensure that appropriate records are maintained, attention should be given to the following:

1. Records regarding biosecurity procedures discussed in all previous exercises should be maintained.
2. Who is responsible for record keeping and how these records are maintained?
3. How frequently these records need to be updated, reviewed, and how long should they be maintained?
4. What information might be needed for a 'Biosecurity Certificate' that provides assurance that this farm is free of specific diseases or pathogens?

5; Who needs to audit and certify that a farm (or other EpiUnit) is free of specific diseases or pathogens?

Maintaining good farm records for biosecurity activities that contribute to achieving disease-free status is an absolute necessity. On-farm records, supported by periodic farm visits and reviews by attending veterinarians form the basis for auditing and certification. The auditors use on-farm and veterinary records to certify and confirm that adequate biosecurity procedures are being implemented on the farm.

7 Veterinary Auditing and Certification for Freedom from Disease and Achieving Government Recognition

Preventing, controlling and eradicating disease on farms or EpiUnits has obvious advantages for improving production and increasing economic returns (Lafferty et al. 2015). Moreover, it forms the basis for ensuring sustainable aquaculture development in all counties, and possibly sustainable fisheries by reducing the impact of disease on wild fish populations.

However, biosecurity practices that result in freedom from disease or pathogens on a farm or EpiUnit need to be well documented. In order to get full recognition from third parties for disease/pathogen freedom (e.g. other farms or countries to which the animals or animal products are sent), a certification of specific disease or pathogen freedom needs to be obtained. While there has been no formal adoption of a biosecurity certification system that leads to disease-free certification of aquaculture farming operations, a step-by-step system under consideration by IAVBC is outlined in figure 19.1.

BIOSECURITY IN AQUACULTURE: PRACTICAL VETERINARY APPROACHES FOR AQUATIC ANIMAL DISEASE PREVENTION, CONTROL, AND POTENTIAL ERADICATION

515

19

Certifying disease or pathogen freedom (often referred to as 'health certification, 'quarantine,' or 'inspection' procedures) should usually be carried out by one or more individuals (the attending veterinarian, or other knowledgeable and experienced individual) who:

1. have full knowledge of all biosecurity procedures implemented on the farm;
2. are able to audit and verify that these biosecurity processes are in place and, in particular, who examine all documentation and results of diagnostic tests;
3. are given the authority to certify disease/pathogen-freedom by the government regulatory agency (veterinary or competent authority) that has jurisdiction over animal health;
4. are held accountable for the accuracy of their certification.

Some countries or government agencies are unable to employ sufficient numbers of veterinary or other personnel to perform this work and they have drawn up programmes to accredit or approve private practice veterinarians who are allowed to perform animal health audits and certify disease/pathogens freedom on behalf of government agencies. In Europe, these veterinarians are referred to as 'Official Veterinarians'; other countries give them the 'Accredited Veterinarian' designation. However, when animals or animal products are moved between countries, the Certificates of Veterinary Inspection (often called 'health certificates'), require endorsement by a National government official from the agency with responsibility over animal health (veterinary or competent authority)
(Starling et al. 2007).

8 A Way Forward for Aquaculture to Meet International (OIE) and National Biosecurity Requirements

Developing, implementing, auditing and certifying comprehensive biosecurity programmes may be complex and therefore comes at a cost. The benefits and costs, along with developing practical approaches for implementing and applying biosecurity principles, and the need for education, training, credentialing and certification programmes for all involved, will need to be carefully assessed (Oidtmann et al. 2011, Peeler and Otte 2014, Reed and Royales 2014, Lafferty et al. 2015). This will be particularly important for the large number of resource-limited, small-scale producers that are involved and who represent a considerable share of the world's aquaculture production.

Implementing, auditing and certifying biosecurity programmes may be driven by industry and/or government needs, but inevitably the most palatable, feasible and practical will be those implemented voluntarily by the aquaculture industries and individual farms, that involve government-industry partnerships and cost-sharing. Several voluntary, industry-driven biosecurity or certification programmes are emerging that may have some application to animal health and biosecurity (O.I.E. 2017f). Some examples include: U.S. Marine Shrimp Farming SPF Program; World Wildlife Fund-led Aquaculture Dialogues; Global Partnership for Good Agricultural Practice (GLOBALGAP); and Global Aquaculture Alliance's Best Aquaculture Practices (BAP) certification standards. Currently, no voluntary biosecurity certification schemes have fully integrated the veterinary biosecurity principles, approaches and infrastructure required to effectively meet biosecurity objectives. Several national programmes with industry-government involvement are being considered for example in Europe, North America and Australia (E.U. 2006, AQUAPLAN 2014, USDA-APHIS-VS 2017). Mainly in response to disease-free and biosecurity requirements being addressed in legislation and regulations (e.g. 2006/88/EC) and government-endorsed international standards (e.g. OIE Code) for use in live animal trade and commerce (E.U. 2006, O.I.E. 2017a). However, a new industry-government effort involving a voluntarily, non-regulatory 'Commercial Aquaculture Health Program Standards' approach that includes many elements of the IAVBC approach described here (USDA-APHIS-VS 2017), is currently being tested.

Implementation of biosecurity plans or programmes to meet the primary objectives outlined above will require the input, documentation and vigilance of many individuals, including the personnel

BIOSECURITY IN AQUACULTURE: PRACTICAL VETERINARY APPROACHES FOR AQUATIC ANIMAL DISEASE PREVENTION, CONTROL, AND POTENTIAL ERADICATION

517

19

overseeing animal and facility care and maintenance, veterinary and diagnostic service providers, and competent government officials (Palić et al. 2015). Education and training programmes will be needed for producers and private and government sector service providers to ensure that everyone involved has a full understanding of all the biosecurity principles, including: hazard identification and prioritisation; risk assessment/ evaluation, risk management/ mitigation and risk communication; analysis and remediation of critical control points where disease could enter or leave the epidemiological unit; epidemiological principles, diagnostics, surveillance, monitoring and determining the status of, or freedom from diseases; and emergency readiness and contingency protocols for disease control and eradication. Equally important will be record keeping, auditing and the use of certificates that address declarations related to biosecurity procedures which are not typically found in existing model certificates used for documenting animal health or disease freedom. The complexity and time involved in implementing these requirements and achieving and maintaining freedom from disease (SPF) may require a biosecurity certification system that progressively recognises increasing levels of biosecurity. As has been done elsewhere, web-based, train-the-trainer, and on-farm workshops will be effective tools for disseminating this information (Scarfe et al. 2009, Palić et al. 2011, Scarfe et al. 2011b, Scarfe et al. 2011a, Scarfe and Palić 2017)

Auditing biosecurity procedures and records, and certifying disease-freedom for specific pathogen need to be undertaken by a credible, knowledgeable and experienced independent third-party, as these responsibilities are accompanied by legal and professional liability. Traditionally these responsibilities are assigned to veterinarians but, in some countries that have a reduced veterinary workforce, veterinary para-professionals (e.g. fisheries officers) are sometimes brought in. In some countries many regulatory activities involving disease diagnosis, surveillance, monitoring and verification of disease presence and absence, are performed by private practitioners that are approved by the national veterinary authority. Examples include the National Veterinary Accreditation Program (NVAP) in the United States and similar programmes in Australia, Canada, New Zealand and elsewhere, where these responsibilities are delegate to 'Accredited Veterinarians.' Within the European Union similar programmes are being delegated to 'Official Veterinarians' in accordance with the European Directive 97/78/EC (European Council, 1998) and subsequent amendments. Currently only the U.S. and Canada have incorporated training modules dealing with aquatic veterinary procedures into their NVAP requirements. Other countries are expected to follow given the recent OIE recommendation for implementation of a Performance of Veterinary Services (PVS) and Aquatic Animal Health Services tool (O.I.E. 2013).

Validation, verification (auditing) and certification that effective biosecurity plans or programmes have been developed are also the basis for issuing Certificates of Veterinary Inspection, often referred to as 'health certificates'

(Starling et al. 2007). These certificates are a very effective risk communication tools to confirm that the epidemiological unit has been evaluated, that appropriate disease risk mitigating procedures (prevention and control) are in place, and to validate that animals have been examined and tested to verify the absence (or prevalence) of disease. When endorsed by the government agency with regulatory authority over aquatic animal health (competent authority), biosecurity certificates provide the official credibility that the primary biosecurity objectives have been met. Having a sufficiently experienced and credentialed workforce to provide these services to support aquaculture is imperative, particularly if done with government oversight or involvement and if used for international trade purposes (DeHaven and Scarfe 2012). Evaluating this workforce capacity using the OIE PVS Tool may be warranted in some countries, and a system for competent authorities to accredit these workforces as competent officials to perform aquatic regulatory functions (similar to existing national veterinary accreditation systems in many countries) would substantially expand national capacities to support aquaculture industry growth and trade (O.I.E. 2013).

BIOSECURITY IN AQUACULTURE: PRACTICAL VETERINARY APPROACHES FOR AQUATIC ANIMAL DISEASE PREVENTION, CONTROL, AND POTENTIAL ERADICATION

519

19

Acknowledgements

The principles presented here are the result of the collaboration of a very large number of individuals. In particular we thank our IAVBC colleagues who have contributed significantly to the development of the concepts presented here, in particular James A. Roth, Roar Gudding, Atle Lillehaug, Larry Hammell, Edgar Brun, Angus Cameron, Lori Gustafson and Chris Walster. Members of the OIE Aquatic Animal Health Commission (Barry Hill) and FAO Fisheries and Aquaculture (Rohana Subasinghe) provided constructive criticism and suggestions for improvement of the concepts on multiple occasions. Numerous other stakeholders, speakers and attendees of the 2009, 2011, and 2017 International Aquaculture Biosecurity Conferences, workshops and other venues where these concepts have been presented, have been instrumental in helping refine the concepts presented herein, for which we are deeply indebted.

REFERENCES

AQUAPLAN (2014) *AQUAPLAN 2014–2019: Australia's National Strategic Plan for Aquatic Animal Health*, Canberra.

Arthur, J. R., Bondad-Reantaso, M. G., Campbell, M. L., Hewitt, C. L., Phillips, M. J. and Subasinghe, R. P. (2009) 'Understanding and applying risk analysis in aquaculture: a manual for decision makers', *FAO Fisheries and Aquaculture Technical Paper*, (519/1).

Caraguel, C. G. B., Gardner, I. A. and Hammell, L. K. (2015) 'Selection and Interpretation of Diagnostic Tests in Aquaculture Biosecurity', *Journal of Applied Aquaculture*, 27(3), 279-298.

DeHaven, W. R. and Scarfe, A. D. (2012) 'Professional education and aquatic animal health: a focus on aquatic veterinarians and veterinary para-professionals', in *Proceedings of OIE Global Conference on Aquatic Animal Health*, Panama, World Organisation for Animal Health.

E.U. (2006) 'Council Directive 2006/88/EC of 24 October 2006 on animal health requirements for aquaculture animals and products thereof, and on the prevention and control of certain diseases in aquatic animals ', *Official Journal of the European Union*, L(328), 14-58.

Gudding, R., Lillehaug, A. and Tavornpanich, S. (2015) 'Immunoprophylaxis in Biosecurity Programs', *Journal of Applied Aquaculture*, 27(3), 220-227.

Huchzermeyer, K. D. A. and Colly, P. A. (2015) 'Production of Koi Herpesvirus-Free Fish: Implementing Biosecurity Practices on a Working Koi Farm in South Africa', *Journal of Applied Aquaculture*, 27(3), 318-329.

Karreman, G., Klotins, K., Bebak, J., Gustafson, L., Osborn, A., Kebus, M. J., Innes, P. and Tiwari, A. (2015) 'Aquatic Animal Biosecurity: A Case Study of Bioexclusion of Viral Hemorrhagic Septicemia Virus in an Atlantic Salmon Hatchery', *Journal of Applied Aquaculture*, 27(3), 299-317.

Kenton, M. (2015) 'Surveillance to Determine Disease Status and Freedom: A Practical Overview of Methods and Measures', *Journal of Applied Aquaculture*.

Lafferty, K. D., Harvell, C. D., Conrad, J. M., Friedman, C. S., Kent, M. L., Kuris, A. M., Powell, E. N., Rondeau, D. and Saksida, S. M. (2015) 'Infectious Diseases Affect Marine Fisheries and Aquaculture Economics', *Annual Review of Marine Science*, 7(1), 471-496.

Lillehaug, A., Santi, N. and Østvik, A. (2015) 'Practical Biosecurity in Atlantic Salmon Production', *Journal of Applied Aquaculture*, 27(3), 249-262.

Moore, D. A., Leach, D. A., Bickett-Weddle, D., Andersen, K., Castillo, A. R., Collar, C. A., Higginbotham, G., Peterson, N., Reed, B. and Hartman, M. L. (2010) 'Evaluation of a biological risk management tool on large Western United States dairies', *Journal of Dairy Science*, 93(9), 4096-4104.

O.I.E. (2013) *OIE Tool for the Evaluation of Performance of Veterinary Services and/or Aquatic Animal Health Services, First Edition*, Paris: World Organisation for Animal Health.

O.I.E. (2017a) *Aquatic Animal Health Code*, Paris: World Organisation for Animal Health.

O.I.E. (2017b) *Aquatic Animal Health Code Chapter 1.4. Aquatic animal health surveillance*, Paris: World Organisation for Animal Health.

O.I.E. (2017c) *Aquatic Animal Health Code Chapter 2.1. Import Risk Analysis*, Paris: World Organisation for Animal Health.

BIOSECURITY IN AQUACULTURE: PRACTICAL VETERINARY APPROACHES FOR AQUATIC ANIMAL DISEASE PREVENTION, CONTROL, AND POTENTIAL ERADICATION

521

19

O.I.E. (2017d) *Aquatic Animal Health Code Chapter 4.4. Contingency planning*, Paris: World Organisation for Animal Health.

O.I.E. (2017e) *Aquatic Animal Health Code Chapter 4. General recommendations: disease prevention and control*, Paris: World Organisation for Animal Health.

O.I.E. (2017f) *Aquatic Animal Health Code Chapter 5.1. General obligations related to certification*, Paris: World Organisation for Animal Health.

O.I.E. (2017g) *Aquatic Animal Health Code Chapter 5.3. OIE procedures relevant to the Agreement on the Application of Sanitary and Phytosanitary Measures of the World Trade Organization*, Paris: World Organisation for Animal Health.

O.I.E. (2017h) *Aquatic Animal Health Code Glossary*, Paris: World Organisation for Animal Health.

O.I.E. (2017i) *Manual of Diagnostic Tests for Aquatic Animals*, Paris: World Organisation for Animal Health.

Oidtmann, B., Peeler, E., Lyngstad, T., Brun, E., Bang Jensen, B. and Stärk, K. D. C. (2013) 'Risk-based methods for fish and terrestrial animal disease surveillance', *Preventive Veterinary Medicine*, 112(1–2), 13-26.

Oidtmann, B. C., Thrush, M. A., Denham, K. L. and Peeler, E. J. (2011) 'International and national biosecurity strategies in aquatic animal health', *Aquaculture*, 320(1–2), 22-33.

Palić, D., Scarfe, A. D. and Walster, C. I. (2015) 'A Standardized Approach for Meeting National and International Aquaculture Biosecurity Requirements for Preventing, Controlling, and Eradicating Infectious Diseases', *Journal of Applied Aquaculture*, 27(3), 185-219.

Palić, D., Scarfe, A. D., Walster, C. I., Lillehaug, A., Gudding, R., Hammel, K. L. and Gustafson, L. (2011) 'Biosecurity Workshop Workbook', in IAVBC, ed., *International Aquaculture Biosecurity Conference*, Trondheim, Norway, International Aquatic Veterinary Biosecurity Consortium.

Peeler, E. J. and Otte, M. J. (2014) 'Epidemiology and Economics Support Decisions about Freedom from Aquatic Animal Disease', *Transboundary and emerging diseases*, n/a-n/a.

Reed, K. and Royales, S. (2014) 'Shrimp disease in Asia resulting in high U.S. import prices: Beyond the Numbers', *Global Economy – U.S. Bureau of Labor Statistics*, 3(14).

Scarfe, A. D. and Palić, D. (2017) *Aquaculture Biosecurity Workbook and Manual*, Cape Town, South Africa: International Aquatic Veterinary Biosecurity Consortium.

Scarfe, A. D., Palić, D. and Walster, C. I. (2011a) 'Aquatic Veterinary Biosecurity Workshop', at *30th World Veterinary Congress*, Cape Town, South Africa, WVA.

Scarfe, A. D., Palić, D. and Walster, C. I., eds. (2009) 'Proceedings of the International Aquaculture Biosecurity Conference – Practical Approaches for the Prevention, Control & Eradication of Disease', in Scarfe A.D., D. P., and C.I. Walster, ed., *International Aquaculture Biosecurity Conference*, Trondheim, Norway, 17-19 August, 2009, International Aquatic Veterinary Biosecurity Consortium, LMU Munich, Germany. 62 pp.

Scarfe, A. D., Palić , D. and Walster, C. I., eds. (2011b) 'Proceedings of the 2nd International Aquaculture Biosecurity Conference – Practical Approaches for the Prevention, Control and Eradication of Disease', in Scarfe A.D., D. P. a. C. I. W., eds., ed., *2nd International Aquaculture Biosecurity Conference*, Trondheim, Norway, August 14-16, 2011, International Aquatic Veterinary Biosecurity Consortium, LMU Munich, Germany. 42 pp.

Starling, D. E., Palić, D. and Scarfe, A. D. (2007) 'Refinement and Use of Certificates of Veterinary Inspection (Health Certificates) for Optimal Assurance of Disease Freedom in Aquatic Animals', *Developments in biologicals*, 129, 91-102.

USDA-APHIS-VS (2017) *United States Commercial Aquaculture Health Program Standards (CAHPS) Concept Paper*, Riverdale, Maryland, USA.

BIOSECURITY IN AQUACULTURE: PRACTICAL VETERINARY APPROACHES FOR AQUATIC ANIMAL DISEASE PREVENTION, CONTROL, AND POTENTIAL ERADICATION

523

19

CPSIA information can be obtained
at www.ICGtesting.com
Printed in the USA
LVHW071306230519
618874LV00019B/282/P